Compliments of Bayer,
Manufacturer of

TRASYLOL®
(aprotinin injection)

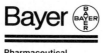

Bayer

**Pharmaceutical
Division**

Biological Products

The
JOHNS HOPKINS
MANUAL
of
Cardiac
Surgical Care

William A. Baumgartner, MD

Cardiac Surgeon-In-Charge
Professor of Surgery
Division of Cardiac Surgery
The Johns Hopkins Hospital
Baltimore, Maryland

Sharon G. Owens, MSN, RN

Nurse Manager CSICU
Division of Cardiac Surgery
The Johns Hopkins Hospital
Baltimore, Maryland

Duke E. Cameron, MD

Associate Professor of Surgery
Division of Cardiac Surgery
The Johns Hopkins Hospital
Baltimore, Maryland

Bruce A. Reitz, MD

Professor and Chairman
Department of Cardiothoracic Surgery
Stanford University School of Medicine
Stanford, California

*with **90** illustrations*

Ⓜ Mosby

St. Louis Baltimore Berlin Boston Carlsbad Chicago London Madrid

Naples New York Philadelphia Sydney Tokyo Toronto

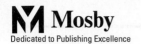
Mosby
Dedicated to Publishing Excellence

Editor: Susie Baxter
Developmental Editor: Anne Gunter
Project Manager: Peggy Fagen
Manufacturing Supervisor: Karen Lewis
Designer: Susan Lane
Cover Designer: Julia Taugner
Production: Graphic World Publishing Services

Copyright © 1994 by Mosby–Year Book, Inc.

Printed in the United States of America
Composition by Graphic World
Printing/binding by R. R. Donnelley

Mosby–Year Book, Inc.
11830 Westline Industrial Drive
St. Louis, Missouri 63146

Library of Congress Cataloging in Publication Data

The Johns Hopkins manual of cardiac surgical care /   William A.
  Baumgartner . . . [et al.].
      p.   cm.
  Includes bibliographical references and index.
  ISBN 0-8016-2248-4
  1. Heart—Surgery—Handbooks, manuals, etc. 2. Therapeutics,
Surgical—Handbooks, manuals, etc. 3. Johns Hopkins Hospital.
Division of Cardiac Surgery—Handbooks, manuals, etc.
  I. Baumgartner, William A.
  [DNLM: 1. Heart Surgery. 2. Intensive Care Units. 3. Monitoring,
Physiologic.   WG 169 J65 1994]
  RD598.J58   1994
  617.4'12059—dc20
  DNLM/DLC
  for Library of Congress   94-9655
                                                                CIP

    95   96   97   98   /   9   8   7   6   5   4   3   2   1

Contributors

Except where noted, the contributors are affiliated with The Johns Hopkins Hospital, Baltimore, Maryland.

Michael A. Acker, MD

Sharon M. Augustine, MS, RN

William A. Baumgartner, MD

Diane M. Burnett, MSN, RN

Duke E. Cameron, MD

Alfred S. Casale, MD

Peter W. Cho, MD

Charles D. Cousar, MD

Cathy Custer, MSN, RN

Patrick DeValeria, MD

R.C. Stewart Finney, Jr., MD

Kirk J. Fleischer, MD

Charles D. Fraser, Jr., MD

Timothy J. Gardner, MD

Vincent L. Gott, MD

Timothy S. Hall, MD

Eugenie S. Heitmiller, MD

David Johnson, MD

Mary Lohmann-Edwards, MS, RN

Pamela Meyer, RN

Karen Michael, RN

Helen O. Michalisko, MSW

Sharon G. Owens, MSN, RN

Bruce A. Reitz, MD
Professor and Chairman
Department of Cardiothoracic Surgery
Stanford University School of Medicine
Stanford, California

Dennis Rivard

R. Scott Stuart, MD

Eric Taylor, MD

Steven Thompson, CCP

Steve Trexler

Susan Ullrich, MSN, RN

Eloise J. Wagner, MSN, RN

Sandra M. Walden, MD
Park Medical Associates, P.A.
Baltimore, Maryland

Janice Wallop, MSN, RN

Jo Marie Walrath, MS, RN

Levi Watkins, Jr., MD

G. Melville Williams, MD

Preface

Care of the cardiac surgical patient has evolved significantly over the half-century history of our surgical specialty. As operative procedures have become more complex and patient age and co-morbidity have increased, so has the challenge of providing comprehensive perioperative care. It has become increasingly important for participating medical and surgical disciplines to coordinate their efforts. The purpose of this manual is to provide a practical guide for coordination of that care and to outline specific management protocols for common clinical situations in the intensive care unit. Although sophisticated technology is an integral part of medical care in the twentieth century, there is an emphasis on bedside clinical care, which remains a key component of the cardiac surgical effort. The later chapters of this text provide the reader with reference information on common cardiac surgical procedures and the corresponding postoperative care issues.

This manual brings together the experience of Hopkins' faculty, residents, nurses, and multiple support services who have cared for our adult patients. We recognize that a variety of other methods and protocols are used at other institutions with excellent results; those presented here have worked well for us and serve as an example of an effective team approach, an approach we believe is of paramount importance to patient survival, safe convalescence, and early hospital discharge.

We wish to acknowledge all of the physicians, nurses, and other personnel who have been and are involved in the care of our cardiac surgical patients. Their dedication and perseverance have resulted in excellent patient care. We also wish to thank Mr. Leon Schlossberg for his many excellent illustrations and Lynn M. DiMarcantonio for her expert secretarial assistance.

William A. Baumgartner
Sharon G. Owens
Duke E. Cameron
Bruce A. Reitz

Contents

The Johns Hopkins Manual
of Cardiac Surgical Care

The Team Approach to the Cardiac Surgical Patient

Sharon G. Owens and William A. Baumgartner

Studies have shown that 84% of cardiac surgical patients realize two to three expected benefits from their surgical procedure.[2] These benefits include prolonged life, improved quality of life, increased exercise and activity, and freedom from pain. The realization of these benefits does not seem to vary according to age or severity of illness preoperatively.[2] These data, in view of the overall decreased hospital stay for most patients undergoing open heart procedures, seem to suggest both an improvement in surgical procedures and a well-coordinated perioperative care plan designed to enhance recovery of the patient. This recovery is not merely physical but also includes the psychosocial adjustments observed in both patients and their families after discharge. Affecting this recovery and adjustment are a variety of factors including patient encouragement to discharging the patient in a fiscally and medically responsible time frame.[1] Increased quality of care despite fiscal restraints has been achieved by a coordinated effort from surgeons, nurses, and an entire team of health care specialists and consultants who treat the patient from a multidisciplinary viewpoint. These specialists, ranging from surgeon to discharge planner, approach problems such as postoperative bleeding, respiratory compromise, and physical rehabilitation in a coordinated and planned manner.

Table 1-1   Multidisciplinary Team Members and Roles

Physicians
  Faculty
  Residents
	Preoperative assessment, evaluation, treatment; surgical interventions; postoperative assessments, treatments, prescription

Nurses
  Primary care
  Associate
	Initial assessment, planning; coordination of care; assessment, revision of plan; coordination of team members and care conferences

Clinical nurse specialist/case manager	Communication, preoperative and postoperative coordination of care, discharge instruction; resource to patient's family for postdischarge questions and concerns
Physician assistant	Preoperative evaluation, intraoperative assistance
Respiratory therapist	Pulmonary assessment and care
Physical/occupational therapist	Rehabilitative assessment and planning
Social worker	Psychosocial assessment and planning; financial counseling
Perfusionist	Intraoperative cardiopulmonary support, postoperative assist device support
Technicians	Assistance to patients, RNs, and physicians in patient care and treatments
Support services	Housekeeping, dietary services, secretarial duties, equipment supply and repair

Many health professionals, out of desire or situational need, have become extremely specialized. Nurses who once chose the medical/surgical area to practice have now specialized into the fields of trauma, cardiology, or transplantation. They have also specialized into specific phases of care such as operating room, inpatient, or intensive care. Social workers and physical therapists have followed the same route in specialization. Not only do the various disciplines have individualized goals for the patient (Table 1-1), but the goals may vary within the group. With all these different perspectives it is essential that these specialists interact as a team; although each specialty has its own focus for the patient, the overall plan needs to be the same. No one person or discipline has the total expertise to diagnose and treat all the varied conditions that confront the cardiac surgical patient.[3,4] Each relies on the skills and background of the others to compliment his or her own skills. For this to work efficiently, each member must realize the multiple needs of the patients. The entire team must be aware of the skills and knowledge each has to offer and the process by which to consult and use these talents in an efficient manner.

Some hospitals have accomplished this through a case management or managed care approach.[5] A critical pathway or plan is developed around a specific diagnosis or surgery or case type and is used by all disciplines in caring for the patient. The critical pathway is a common tool for all the disciplines so that communication is consistent and more efficient. Other models may work as efficiently in various institutions. The key to success is collaboration and coordination to achieve quality and efficiency.

Like spokes of a wheel, the team members work together to produce a successful outcome for the patient and family. It is a complex endeavor requiring all members to participate as a team. At times some team members may be more visible to the patient than others.[3,4] The individual focus of each member may vary, but overall each has the goal to improve the lifestyle of patients and to assist with their adjustment back into the community.

References

1. Bower KA: *Managed care: doing more with less.* Presented at the meeting of the American Organization of Nurse Executives, Philadelphia, Sept 1987.
2. Gortner SR et al: Expected and realized benefits from cardiac surgery: an update, *Cardiovasc Nurs* 25:4, 1990.
3. Guzetta CE, Dossey BM: *Cardiovascular nursing: body-mind tapestry,* St Louis, 1984, Mosby.
4. Stein LI, Watts DT, Howell T: The doctor-nurse game revisited, *N Engl J Med* 322:8, 1990.
5. Zander K: Case management in acute care: making the connections, *Total Case Management* I:39 1991.

2

Preoperative Assessment

Duke E. Cameron, Steve Trexler, and Charles D. Cousar

Patients referred to the cardiac surgeon for a surgical procedure have usually undergone an extensive examination for heart disease and have had concurrent medical problems identified. It remains vitally important, however, for surgeons and their teams to reexamine patients for correct diagnosis and to identify important illness or disorders that could affect the surgical approach or adversely affect surgical outcome. This redundancy of effort is not mandated by lack of trust or faith in those conducting the previous examination, but rather constitutes an important component of the safe practice of surgery to minimize the possibility of human error.

The purpose of the preoperative assessment is threefold:
- Confirmation of the primary cardiac diagnosis
- Identification of relevant medical conditions (e.g., cerebrovascular disease in a patient about to undergo coronary revascularization during cardiopulmonary bypass)
- Determination of the patient's ability to endure the procedure

These goals should be kept in mind by those conducting the preliminary examinations. Indeed, whether the preoperative assessment is conducted by the surgeon, nurse, physician assistant, cardiologist, or house staff is less important than whether that person understands the objectives of preoperative evaluation and has the necessary experience, skills, and judgment to perform the task.

The majority of patients having heart surgery today undergo coronary revascularization to prevent the complications of coronary artery disease. Accordingly, this chapter focuses primarily on those patients, although patients with valvular heart disease, rhythm disturbances, and aortic disease are also considered. The preoperative evaluation of children with congenital heart disease is not discussed.

Standardized History and Physical Examination

The cardiac surgical patient, like any other preoperative surgical patient, should be approached and examined in a comprehensive, systematic, and standardized manner. This is necessary to assure that all necessary precautions are taken and that the diagnosis and planned treatment are appropriate. To this end, a standard history and physical form can be employed to assure a standard of quality and comprehensiveness in preoperative assessment. Many such forms exist; the one used at The Johns Hopkins Hospital for the past several years is included to serve as an example and a template for related efforts (Fig. 2-1). It can be regarded as a checklist to be completed before embarking on a highly technical and complex task, much as the pilot of an aircraft must systematically work through a checklist to determine that the aircraft is safe and prepared for flight.

History

The medical history obtained from the patient is the most important part of the preoperative assessment. Indeed, the correct diagnosis can be achieved more frequently from a careful review of the history than with any other single test. The patient is usually the most reliable source for this history, although occasionally patient denial of symptoms may render a spouse or family member the more accurate source. It is best to let patients recount their own version of the events leading to hospitalization, although this can sometimes be tedious and time consuming. It is important to ascertain the precise nature of the symptoms, their first onset, their frequency, and factors that exacerbate or alleviate, such as activity, position, medications, or time of day.

The symptoms of greatest interest in the evaluation of heart disease are chest pain, dyspnea, syncope, and peripheral edema.

Chest pain may originate from angina, pericarditis, or expansion or tear of the aortic wall. Angina is typically felt as pressure or squeezing in the center of the chest; it may radiate into the arms, neck, or back. Occasionally an "angina equivalent" is felt

Text continued on p. 13

CARDIAC SURGERY
HISTORY AND PHYSICAL
THE JOHNS HOPKINS HOSPITAL

*(Stamp Addressograph
Plate Here)*

PATIENT'S NAME (Last, First, Middle)   Date

JHH History #

Age   Gender M/F   Race   W   B   Other
Attending   Cardiologist   Internist/General Practitioner

I. HISTORY OF PRESENT ILLNESS

_____

_____

_____

_____

_____

CARDIAC RISK FACTORS   Smoking   ALLERGIES
                              Hypertension
                              Obesity
                              Hyperlipidemia
                              Family History
                              Diabetes

MEDICATIONS   1   5
                  2   6
                  3   7
                  4   8

EXERCISE STRESS TEST

ECHOCARDIOGRAM

CARDIAC CATHETERIZATION

    Date, Location

    LV Ejection Fraction   %   Coronary Lesions   L Main
                                                                LAD
    LV Function   Good   Fair   Poor   LADD1
                                                                LADD2
    Cardiac Output   LMD
                                                                CFX
    Valves   Aortic   CM1
           Mitral   CM2
           Pulmonary   CM3
           Tricuspid   RCA
                                                                PD1
                                                                PD2

PREVIOUS ANGIOPLASTY?

Fig. 2-1 History and physical examination form.

Continued.

II. MEDICAL HISTORY (Circle relevant events and explain)

CHILDHOOD DISEASES

		(Addressograph plate)
Polio	Mumps	
Rheumatic Fever	Rubella	
Scarlet Fever	Tuberculosis	

ADULT DISEASES

Arrythmia	Lung Disease
Arthritis	Myocardial Infarction
Bleeding Disorder	Pericarditis
Cancer	Prostatitis/BPH
Diabetes	Peptic Ulcer
Gallstones	Peripheral Vascular Disease
Gout	Stroke/TIA
Kidney Disease	Thromboembolism
Liver Disease	Thyroid Disease

BLOOD TRANSFUSION HISTORY

III. HOSPITALIZATION HISTORY (Illnesses, Operations, Injuries)

1	4
2	5
3	6

IV. SOCIAL HISTORY

Employment/Occupation

Marital status   S   M   D   W   SEP

Smoking History: Cigarette   Pipe   Cigar

   # packs/day
   # years smoked
   # years ago quit
      current practice

ETOH: Rarely   Occasional   Often

Other Substance Abuse History

V. FAMILY MEDICAL HISTORY (Specify serious illnesses or cause of death)

   Siblings
   Mother
   Father
   Maternal Grandmother
   Maternal Grandfather
   Paternal Grandmother
   Paternal Grandfather

   Comments

Fig. 2-1, cont'd. History and physical examination form.

VI. REVIEW OF SYSTEMS (Circle relevant symptoms and specify frequency & intensity)

GENERAL
- fever
- chills
- night sweats

(Addressograph plate)

SKIN
- infections
- rashes

HEAD
- headaches
- colds
- migraines
- trauma

EYES
- diplopia
- blurred vision
- scotoma

EARS
- tinnitus
- vertigo
- balance problems

NOSE
- discharge
- epistaxis

MOUTH & THROAT
- dysphagia
- hoarseness
- sore throat

NECK
- pain
- stiffness

CARDIO-VASCULAR
- angina (exertional, rest)
- claudication
- dyspnea on exertion
- dizziness/syncope
- edema
- fatigue
- palpitations
- paroxysmal nocturnal dyspnea

Patient's NYHA Functional Class *(circle one)*

I No Symptoms
II Symptoms on Heavy Exertion
III Symptoms on Mild Exertion
IV Symptoms at Rest

Symptom *(circle one):* Angina/CHF

THORAX & PULMONARY
- chronic cough
- hemopytsis
- sputum
- wheeze

GASTRO-INTESTINAL
- constipation
- diarrhea
- indigestion
- melena
- nausea/vomiting
- weight change

Fig. 2-1, *cont'd*. History and physical examination form.

Continued.

GENITO-URINARY	discharge dysuria frequency hematuria incontinence nocturia pyuria urgency	*(Addressograph plate)*

GYNECOLOGIC   vaginal changes
               post-menopausal

MUSCULO-   back pain
  SKELETAL   joint pain / tenderness
               muscle weakness

NEUROLOGIC   aphasia
               depression
               memory loss
               paralysis
               seizures
               stroke
               syncope
               transient ishemic at-
                   tacks
               vision changes

VIII. PHYSICAL EXAMINATION
(Circle relevant findings and explain)

GENERAL   NAD Mild distress Distress

VITAL SIGNS   Temp (Oral / Rectal)

               pulse   BP left arm   /
                                                right arm   /
               respirations
               weight (kg / lbs)   height (cm / ft-in)

SKIN   clubbing
               color
               cyanosis
               edema
               pigmentation / moles
               rash
               scars
               temperature
               wounds
               comments

HEAD   tenderness
               scars
               comments

Fig. 2-1, cont'd. History and physical examination form.

EYES	conjunctiva
	fundus
	PERRLA
	sclera	*(Addressograph plate)*
	visual acuity
	visual fields
	comments

EARS	canals
	hearing acuity
	tympanic membranes
	comments

NOSE	nares
	rhinnorhea
	septum
	comments

MOUTH &	dental prostheses
THROAT	exudates
	lips
	mucosa
	teeth/gums
	tongue
	comments

NECK	bruits
	flexibility
	lymph nodes
	masses
	thyroid
	trachea
	scars/incisions
	comments

HEART	inspection
	jugular venous distention
	murmurs
	palpation
	rhythm
	rub/heave/gallop
	S1 S2 S3 S4
	comments

PERIPHERAL VASCULAR

[Pulse strength: 0 = absent, 1 = Doppler, 2 = weak, 3 = strong]

Left   radial brachial carotid femoral popliteal dorsalis ped post tib
Right radial brachial carotid femoral popliteal dorsalis ped post tib

carotid bruits
abdominal bruits
femoral bruits
comments

Fig. 2-1, *cont'd.* History and physical examination form.

Continued.

THORAX	breasts
	breath sounds
	chest wall
	percussion
	comments

(Addressograph plate)

ABDOMINAL	bowel sounds
	hernias
	masses
	organomegaly
	palpation
	scars
	comments

RECTAL	masses
	prostate
	sphincter tone
	stool guiac
	comments

GENITALIA	M/F
	masses
	skin lesions
	comments

MUSCULO-SKELETAL	joint pain/tenderness/swelling
	range of motion
	strength & muscle mass
	comments

NEUROLOGIC	cranial nerves
	gait
	judgement
	orientation
	reflexes
	comments

IX. IMPRESSION

1.
2.
3.
4.
5.

X. PLAN

_____

(signed)

Fig. 2-1, *cont'd.* History and physical examination form.

as left arm heaviness, shortness of breath, or epigastric or throat discomfort. Angina is graded in severity from 1 to 10, with 10 being the most severe. It is further characterized as exertional or rest angina, depending on the level of activity required to produce it. Rest angina is also known as unstable angina if it comes and goes without relation to stress or level of activity; as such, it represents a precarious relationship between myocardial oxygen supply and demand and is usually considered an indication for invasive procedures to improve coronary blood flow: coronary artery bypass grafting (CABG) or percutaneous transluminal coronary angioplasty.

Chest pain may exist in other forms. The pain of pericarditis is constant but may be aggravated by deep inspiration and at times be sharp and stabbing. The pain of aortic expansion, such as from thoracic aortic aneurysm, is usually dull and constant, and can be felt at the base of the neck or in the upper part of the back. Persons caring for cardiac patients must recognize the pain of aortic dissection, because early recognition and intervention are critical to survival. This pain is sudden in onset (the patient can usually describe the precise moment at which it began) and severe ("the worst pain I ever felt"), and is often associated with hypertension. There is some correlation between location of the pain and site of the dissection: ascending dissection usually produces anterior chest or neck pain, whereas descending dissection produces back pain, but this relationship is not reliable enough for diagnosis and preoperative planning of major surgical procedures.

Dyspnea, the sensation of shortness of breath, has multiple causes. It may result from an increase in left atrial pressure as a result of mitral stenosis, mitral regurgitation, aortic stenosis or aortic regurgitation, or left ventricular dysfunction. Alternatively, the inability to raise cardiac output in response to demand, such as in exercise, can limit oxygen delivery to the periphery and produce a sensation of dyspnea and fatigue. **Syncope** also has multiple causes, some cardiac in origin, some not. Among the cardiogenic causes, arrhythmia (either bradycardia or tachycardia) and obstructive lesions of the heart (aortic stenosis) are the most important. Arrhythmia may result in a sudden decrease in cardiac output and blood pressure and a subsequent fall in cerebral perfusion pressure, culminating in syncope. Obstructive heart lesions produce a "ceiling" on cardiac output; during exercise, peripheral vascular resistance falls as muscle vascular beds open. If cardiac output is fixed, blood pressure falls and may lead to syncope. Obstructive lesions can coexist with arrhythmia, such as in the patient with aortic stenosis in whom arrythmia develops during exercise.

The extent to which chest pain or dyspnea limits the patient's activity can be graded according to established scales. The most commonly used scale is the New York Heart Association Functional Class, in which class I is associated with no symptoms, class II with symptoms on heavy exertion, class III with symptoms on mild exertion, and class IV with symptoms at rest.

Peripheral edema is a sign of congestive heart failure, or obstruction of the right side of the heart, such as in tricuspid stenosis. It represents retention of sodium and water to expand intravascular volume. Alternatively, it may be produced by venous insufficiency of the lower extremities.

Other signs and symptoms of relevance to the cardiac history are fever (endocarditis); transient loss of vision, speech, sensation, or movement (carotid artery disease or emboli from within the heart); palpitations (arrhythmia); headache (hypertension); and cough (pulmonary venous congestion).

Other aspects of the remote medical history are important. Childhood experience with rheumatic fever or tuberculosis raises suspicions of valvular disease and pericardial disease, respectively. Important adult diseases are listed in Table 2-1, together with the specific reason for their significance among cardiac surgical patients. In practice, the conditions of greatest significance among cardiac surgical patients are bleeding disorders, history of stroke or recent neurologic events, diabetes, active infection (skin, teeth, lung, urinary tract), and chronic lung disease. Careful recording of the patient's medications is essential, particularly those medications for noncardiac conditions. Unintentional withdrawal of sedatives and anxiolytics can obscure and complicate the postoperative course. With the exception of anticoagulants, most medications can be taken up to the morning of the operation. Aspirin should be withheld for 7 to 10 days before elective operations, to minimize its antiplatelet effect. Whether bleeding time determinations are useful to determine risk for postoperative hemorrhage in patients taking aspirin preoperatively is controversial; in our hospital we use bleeding time in these patients and prefer to postpone *elective* surgery until the bleeding time is less than 6 minutes.

Table 2-1 Important Diseases to Record in Preoperative Examination

Disease	Significance
Bleeding disorders	Perioperative hemorrhage
	Unsuitability for chronic anticoagulation
Cancer	Increased perioperative morbidity
	Appropriateness of surgery?
Diabetes	Increased risk of wound infection
	Increased risk of stroke
Gallstones	Perioperative cholecystitis
Gout	Perioperative gouty attacks
Kidney disease	Aggravation of kidney failure perioperatively
	Sepsis if urinary tract obstructed
Liver disease	Coagulopathy
	Hepatic encephalopathy
	Systemic vasodilation during cardiopulmonary bypass
Lung disease	Ventilatory insufficiency
	Pneumonia
Prostatism/prostatitis	Difficulty passing urinary catheter
	Urosepsis
	Urinary retention postoperatively
Peptic ulcer disease	Postoperative hemorrhage
	Gastritis
Peripheral vascular disease	Stroke
	Poor leg wound healing
	Aggravation of peripheral ischemia from vein harvesting sites
	Mesenteric ischemia
Thyroid disease	Postoperative hypothyroidism or hyperthyroidism

Sodium warfarin (Coumadin) should be withheld at least 5 days before operation, depending on the level of anticoagulation, the presence of liver disease, thrombotic risk from stopping anticoagulation, and the nature and extent of the planned operation. In some patients such as those with mechanical valves, it is advisable to stop warfarin therapy at least 7 to 10 days before surgery and admit the patient when the prothrombin time falls to less than 1.5 times control. Heparin infusion is then begun and continued until the morning of surgery. Established universal guidelines for these practices are lacking, so optimal treatment must be tailored to the patient.

Allergies to medications should be documented. Allergy to penicillin is the most frequently elicited allergy, yet the majority of patients professing such an allergy do not have it. This creates a liability dilemma, which is partly addressed by skin testing. In the absence of a skin reaction, penicillin or a cephalosporin (cefazolin is presently used) can be given safely, but if a reaction is present, vancomycin is substituted as the perioperative prophylactic antibiotic. At some centers vancomycin is substituted whenever the patient relates a penicillin allergy, regardless of skin test results.

Previous exposure to blood transfusion products increases the risk of transfusion reaction in cardiac surgical patients and may make cross-matching of blood difficult. A history of transfusion reaction is of obvious concern.

Previous operations figure prominently in formulation of surgical plans. The records of previous cardiac operations should be reviewed; in the era of facsimile machines, there is rarely an excuse for not having a detailed operative note from the previous surgery. Serious pitfalls can be avoided by making such information available. Previous harvesting of saphenous veins (greater saphenous and lesser saphenous) and use of the internal mammary artery at prior CABG should be noted. Important notations regarding the size of coronary arteries, coronary artery endarterectomy, previous vent sites, or pacemaker wires can aid during dissection of the mediastinum. Previous radical mastectomy and/or chest wall irradiation may affect the decision to use the internal mammary artery graft for coronary revascularization. Similarly, previous abdominal surgery may make use of the inferior epigastric or gastroepiploic arteries inadvisable for myocardial revascularization.

A family history of heart disease is noteworthy, particularly that of early death, familial cardiomyopathy, and connective tissue disorders that can predispose to aortic disease.

Physical Examination

The physical examination begins with recording vital signs (Fig. 2-2). Unexplained fever results in postponement of *elective* surgery; occult sepsis can lead to bacterial contamination of wounds

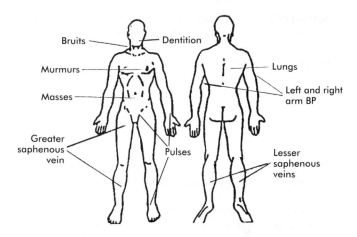

Fig. 2-2 Essential features of physical examination.

and suppurative infection. Pulmonary infection is exacerbated after cardiac surgery, in part because of the effect of inhalation anesthetics, the chest incision with its deleterious effect on functional residual capacity and on the ability to clear secretions, and a diffuse tissue inflammation caused by cardiopulmonary bypass. If the cardiac operation entails placement of a cardiac prosthesis such as a mechanical valve, preoperative infections can be life-threatening if they lead to seeding of the prosthesis perioperatively.

Severe hypertension should be treated medically before the operation to avoid postoperative blood pressure lability and bleeding. Blood pressure should be measured in both arms to detect subclavian or innominate artery stenosis that would preclude use of the pedicled internal mammary artery on the obstructed side.

Examination of the head and neck should focus on detection of dental caries and active gum infection, which might cause postoperative bacteremia. Indeed, all patients scheduled for valve repair or replacement should have a preoperative dental examination to rule out and to treat any oral infection. Carotid bruits are important signs of extracranial vascular occlusive disease. Although not all bruits are associated with significant hemodynamic stenoses and not all patients with severe cerebral vascular disease have bruits, the association between bruit and risk for perioperative neurologic injury is a strong one.[3] In the presence of bruits, especially bilateral bruits, a careful history pertaining to stroke and transient ischemic attacks should be taken and consideration should be given to noninvasive screening examinations of the carotid circulation. If neurologic deficits are present, they should be noted carefully because these deficits may be aggravated after cardiopulmonary bypass.

Auscultation of the lungs may detect rales (a sign of congestive heart failure), ronchi (a sign of consolidation caused by poor clearance of secretions or obstructing bronchial tumor), and wheezes from bronchospastic disease. The cardiac examination should detail heart rate and rhythm, and the presence or absence of murmurs or other sounds. The quality and strength of the pulses (carotid, radial, femoral, dorsalis pedis, and posterior tibial) should be recorded. This is particularly important if the patient requires an intraaortic balloon pump intraoperatively or postoperatively, because the balloon should be placed in the leg with the better circulation. Ischemia of the leg after balloon insertion can be viewed with perspective if the preoperative pulse status is known and recorded accurately.

Abdominal masses suggest malignancy or aortic aneurysm. The presence of an abdominal aortic aneurysm does not preclude proceeding with cardiac surgery but does make placement of an intraaortic balloon pump via the femoral artery inadvisable and mandates avoidance of postoperative hypertension.

Inspection of the legs for saphenous vein (both greater and lesser systems) should be routine, even before valve operations, because coronary grafting is occasionally required unexpectedly. The patient should be asked to stand to engorge the veins; varicosities or gross dilation may be revealed and signal the veins unusable.

Skin lesions such as rashes or pustules on the chest or leg should be treated and cleared whenever possible.

Laboratory Tests

The battery of laboratory tests for cardiac surgical patients is similar to that of general and thoracic surgical patients undergoing major surgical procedures. In general, these include a complete blood cell count, serum electrolyte determination, blood urea nitrogen level, creatinine level, glucose level, and urinalysis. Severe electrolyte abnormalities should be corrected before surgery; transient kidney dysfunction after arteriography usually responds to hydration and the passage of time. Coagulation should be assessed by prothrombin time and activated partial thromboplastin time. Patients with recent aspirin or antiinflammatory ingestion and suspected platelet dysfunction can be assessed by bleeding time. Liver function tests are often obtained but rarely useful; they may occasionally demonstrate elevations of hepatic transaminases, suggesting hepatitis from chronic viral infection or, more likely, drug effect. Routine blood gas sampling is not necessary but may provide valuable baseline data in patients predicted to have difficulty weaning from mechanical ventilation. Accompanying the patient up one flight of stairs and observing ventilatory effort has greater predictive value of postoperative pulmonary dysfunction than pulmonary function tests or arterial blood gas determinations.

For patients undergoing cardiopulmonary bypass, a sample of blood should be taken for typing and cross-matching. Four to six units of blood (packed red blood cells or whole blood) are usually made available for routine operations in average-weight patients. Patients undergoing reoperations and those with established disorders of coagulation require more. Because most operations involving cardiopulmonary bypass involve use of moderate systemic hypothermia (blood temperature 25° to 28° C), identification of cold agglutinins in the patient's blood is of particular value in cardiac surgery. Protocols exist for avoidance of hypothermia in these patients.

When there is a history of hepatitis, the patient's antibody and antigen status should be determined, if only to establish the level of risk to the operative team. A history of thyroid disorder or thyroidectomy should initiate determination of thyroid function; cardiopulmonary bypass itself causes transient depression of circulating thyroid hormone levels, particularly T_3. The significance of this depression is not known, but rarely profound hypothyroidism may occur early postoperatively, manifested as lethargy, obtundation, and inexplicably high inotrope requirements.

Electrocardiography

The 12-lead electrocardiogram (ECG) adds important information about virtually every cardiac surgical patient. A systematic evaluation of the tracing for heart rate, rhythm, axis, evidence of hypertrophy, conduction disturbance (heart block or bundle branch), or previous infarction is conducted. Active ischemia can be an indication for urgent surgical revascularization in some patients but a reason to postpone the operation in others, depending on the status of the patient, the coronary anatomy, and the likelihood of resolution of ischemia by medical means. It is well established that myocardial ischemia within 24 hours of cardiac surgery, particularly active ischemia at the time of the operation, predisposes toward ventricular failure in the intraoperative and early postoperative period (see Chapter 4).

In exercise or stress testing, the ECG is performed before, during, and after a brief period of increased exertion, typically a brief walk on an inclined treadmill. This increases the work and oxygen requirements of the myocardium and may reveal ischemia. Indications for stress testing are (1) to establish or exclude the diagnosis of coronary artery disease, (2) to establish the physiologic severity of coronary artery disease in patients with known disease or history of myocardial infarction, (3) to judge the response to medical or surgical therapy, (4) to detect exercise-induced arrhythmia, and (5) to measure objectively exercise tolerance in patients with cardiac failure. Contraindications include unstable angina, rest angina, acute myocardial infarction, known left main coronary or aortic valve stenosis, obstructive cardiomyopathy, acute myocarditis, or decompensated cardiac failure. Properly selected patients have a 1 in 10,000 risk of death during stress testing and a 1 in 100 risk of myocardial infarction or life-threatening arrhythmia.[4]

Stress testing may be performed in combination with radionuclide imaging to demonstrate regional perfusion abnormalities that might not be evident at rest. These tests are discussed in more detail later.

Twenty-four–hour ambulatory ECG recording (Holter monitoring) enables detection of infrequent dysrhythmias, quantification of frequency of arrhythmic events, and detection of intermittent ischemia.

Imaging Studies

Chest Radiographs

The posteroanterior and lateral chest radiograph is an essential preoperative investigation and should be present in the operating room at the time of surgery. Features to be noted are heart size and contour abnormalities that suggest chamber dilation, lung edema or lobar consolidation, position and size of the aorta, presence of pulmonary masses, prostheses (valves, pacemaker leads, central venous catheters), and calcification of the aorta, cardiac valves, or myocardium. In older patients with diffuse atherosclerotic disease, calcification of the ascending aorta is a marker for increased risk of intraoperative stroke caused by embolization of calcific and atherosclerotic debris from the aorta during cannulation or clamping. Alternate strategies exist for managing this problem, so preoperative awareness of calcification allows for better planning and more accurate preoperative estimation of stroke risk.[1]

In reoperative cardiac surgery the lateral chest radiograph is examined to determine the distance between the back of the sternum and the anterior wall of the heart and aorta. The pericardium is left open after most heart operations to accommodate cardiac edema or saphenous vein grafts; this can lead to adhesion of the heart to the retrosternum, placing the right ventricle, aorta, and innominate vein at risk of laceration during sternal reentry. When a patent internal mammary artery graft is present at reoperative CABG, the metal clips usually placed on branches of the graft mark its course relative to the sternum and lateral border of the heart.

Echocardiography

As a noninvasive study of cardiac structure and function, the echocardiogram is exceedingly useful. Real-time two-dimensional imaging provides data on ventricular size and function (global and regional), valve morphology and function (such as prolapse, perforation, leaflet motion, presence of masses, or vegetations), and septal defects. Although higher-resolution technology may permit precise coronary imaging in the future, this is not possible at present. Most valvular heart disease requiring surgical intervention can be adequately diagnosed and assessed on the basis of history, physical examination, and echocardiogram; in practice, most patients undergoing such surgery are more than 40 years of age and therefore at risk for concurrent coronary disease. For this reason they undergo preoperative cardiac catheterization to define coronary anatomy and to assess ventricular performance, measure chamber pressures, assess transvalvular gradients, and quantify severity of regurgitation.

Although transthoracic echocardiography usually produces good images of the heart, transesophageal echocardiography (TEE) provides complementary and usually superior images because of the proximity of the probe to the heart and the absence of interposed air-filled or bony structures that interfere with ultrasound conduction.[2] TEE is invasive but can be performed with low risk of esophageal perforation (<1:10,000), even in the awake, spontaneously ventilating sedated patient. TEE is particularly useful to evaluate mitral valve disease (especially regurgitant mitral valves being considered for repair), to detect vegetations in the course of investigation for infective endocarditis, and to detect aortic dissection rapidly and accurately. The role of TEE has expanded beyond preoperative assessment into intraoperative and postoperative applications, which are discussed in later chapters.

Cardiac Catheterization

The passage of a catheter into the heart or great vessels to demonstrate anatomy and ventricular function, to record pressures, and to measure oxygen saturations is one of the most commonly performed invasive diagnostic procedures today. Indications for catheterization are lengthy and are not reviewed here but are detailed elsewhere.[4] The approach is usually via the femoral artery (Judkins technique), but the brachial artery (Sones technique) can be used if severe aortoiliac or femoral occlusive disease are present. The risk of catheterization is low: death, stroke, vascular or cardiac perforation, coronary dissection, or severe allergic reaction to the contrast agent occur in approximately 1 in 1000 patients. For the most part, patients seen for catheterization have cardiac problems that pose even greater risks if not diagnosed and treated appropriately. Contraindications to catheterization include previous anaphylactic reaction to the contrast medium, which cannot be prevented by preparatory steroids and antihistamines; patient refusal; and prior agreement that no surgical or medical intervention will be based on the findings.

Ideally, if the patient's condition permits, 1 or 2 days should pass between the catheterization and the surgical procedure, particularly if the procedure requires cardiopulmonary bypass. This allows the patient to ambulate and the kidneys to recover from the nephrotoxic effect of the contrast agents.

Chest Computed Tomography

The imaging modality of chest computed tomography (CT) plays little role in the majority of cardiac surgical patient examinations but is useful when lung masses are discovered incidentally. Other applications of CT include rapid screening for aortic aneurysm and its complications, and detection of aortic dissection and pericardial disease. Refinements in CT scanning may lead to its use for three-dimensional reconstructions in simulated real-time mode, which would demonstrate structural abnormalities within the heart. However, at present, CT scanning is surpassed by magnetic resonance imaging, echocardiography, or angiography in virtually every cardiac imaging application and diagnosis.

Magnetic Resonance Imaging

Magnetic resonance imaging (MRI) scans provide not only two-dimensional imaging of cardiovascular structure but also data pertaining to blood flow. These features make MRI an attractive method to investigate aortic diseases such as aneurysm, coarctation, or dissection. Although the test is noninvasive, its use is hampered by the comparatively long time required to obtain images, the expense and limited availability of scanners, and the high-intensity magnetic fields produced, which make it difficult and sometimes impossible to scan a critically ill patient who requires intensive monitoring. Metallic implanted prostheses also preclude use of MRI. However, the presence of a St. Jude medical prosthesis does not interfere with MRI.

Radionuclide Scanning

Thallium scintigraphy exploits the fact that thallium, like potassium, is taken up by viable myocardium and thus can "light up" healthy muscle under the radionuclide camera. Conversely, areas of infarcted myocardium appear as "cold spots." Thallium scans therefore help distinguish perfused from nonperfused (i.e., infarcted) myocardium; scans are usually repeated 3 to 4 hours after the initial imaging, to detect "redistribution," in which poorly perfused regions of myocardium that appeared cold at first gradually reperfuse with thallium and appear hot later. These are presumably chronically ischemic, or "hibernating," areas of myocardium that may benefit from revascularization.

Thallium scanning can be done in combination with exercise (stress thallium) to demonstrate ischemic zones. Similarly, dipyridamole, a potent vasodilator, can be administered to provoke regional ischemia (Persantine stress thallium).

Gated blood pool imaging uses technetium-labeled autologous blood cells to image blood within the heart. When gated to the ECG, scans allow determination of left and right heart ejection fraction, and detection of regional wall motion abnormalities.

Choice of a Valve Prosthesis

The selection of the appropriate valve prosthesis for a patient is a matter for preoperative discussion; therefore it is included in this chapter on preoperative assessment. Selection of a valve prosthesis depends more on the patient's characteristics than on intraoperative considerations, and because prostheses have major effects on quality of life and the need for reoperation, it is best to involve the patient and family in these planning discussions.

The three categories of valve prostheses are mechanical, bioprosthetic, and human homografts. Each has particular properties, advantages, and disadvantages. Among the commercially available mechanical and bioprosthetic devices, many proprietary models are available, but these various models will not be discussed here.

The mechanical prostheses, of which the St. Jude bileaflet valve is the most popular, consist of metal mechanisms. Their major advantage is durability. Most can be expected to perform for a lifetime without mechanical failure. All, however, require indefinite anticoagulation with sodium warfarin (Coumadin) together with its attendant restrictions on diet and activity, and the need for frequent (monthly) measurements of prothrombin time. In general, mechanical valves are chosen for patients old enough to cooperate safely with anticoagulation (>10 years) yet young enough to avoid the complications of long-term anticoagulation in the elderly (<70 years). Patients in this age range are believed to benefit most from prostheses that minimize the chance that reoperation will be necessary in the patient's lifetime. These prostheses are also preferred in patients who require anticoagulation for other reasons, such as for recurrent pulmonary embolism, atrial fibrillation, intracardiac thrombus, or severe peripheral vascular disease.

Bioprosthetic valves use tissue from animal sources, mounted in polyester and metal housings to facilitate surgical implantation. Of bioprostheses, the porcine aortic valve is most commonly used. These are not vital tissue grafts, because the valve tissue is treated with glutaraldehyde to strengthen it and reduce immunogenicity.

Because they are non-viable, the valves degenerate and require replacement. The rate of degeneration depends on the age of the patient (the older the patient, the better the durability) and the site of implantation (a bioprosthesis lasts longer in the aortic than the mitral position). The principal advantage of these valves is the avoidance of long-term anticoagulation. Because the rate of thromboembolic complications is similar to that of mechanical prostheses *with anticoagulation,* the bioprosthesis is the valve of choice in elderly patients and in those who cannot comply with anticoagulation. The principal disadvantage is limited durability as a result of degeneration. For most patients older than 70 years of age, porcine bioprostheses can be expected to last 10 to 15 years in the aortic position and 7 to 10 years in the mitral position. These valves are not acceptable in children because of accelerated degeneration.

Another subset of bioprosthetic valves are the pericardial valves, which are constructed from tanned animal pericardium. In general, these valves behave much as porcine aortic valves; given current knowledge, their place in the surgical armamentarium is alongside the porcine valves. Long-term anticoagulation is not required, but durability remains their principal limiting feature.

Homografts are human semilunar (pulmonic and aortic) valves, which are taken from organ donors, sterilized, and cryopreserved for later use. Their advantages are superior hemodynamics (smaller gradients for given annular diameter), excellent freedom from endocarditis, and avoidance of anticoagulation. Their disadvantage is durability (which is only moderately better than porcine bioprostheses), availability, and the greater surgical experience and skill required to implant them. Another limitation is that these valves can be used only in the aortic and pulmonary positions. Although homografts retain some viability through the cryopreservation process, much of the graft is replaced in time by nonviable scar, presumably as a result of chronic low-grade rejection. Antirejection medications to improve homograft viability and durability have not been studied carefully, but it is unlikely that gains in durability would significantly offset the risk and cost of decades of immunosuppression.

There is no significant difference in risk of endocarditis between mechanical and bioprosthetic valves, although homografts seem relatively free of this complication. If a prosthesis must be placed in an infected surgical field, homografts are more likely to remain sterile.

It should be evident that choosing a valve prostheses is a complicated decision in which multiple patient and surgical-related factors must be weighed. For most cardiac surgical patients the decision rests mainly on weighing the disadvantages of long-term anticoagulation against the disadvantages of reoperation years later.

References

1. Barzilai B, Marshall WG, Saffitz JE, Kouchoukos N: Avoidance of embolic complications by ultrasonic characterization of the ascending aorta, *Circulation* 80(I):275-9, 1989.
2. Fisher EA, Stahl JA, Budd JH, Goldman ME: Transesophageal echocardiographic procedures and clinical application, *J Am Coll Cardiol* 18(5):1333-48.
3. Gardner TJ, Horneffer PJ, Manolio TA, et al: Stroke following coronary artery bypass grafting: a ten-year study, *Ann Thorac Surg* 40:574-81, 1985.
4. Vlay SC, editor: *Medical care of the cardiac surgical patient*, Boston, 1992, Blackwell Scientific Publications.

3

Preoperative Preparation

Eloise J. Wagner and Steve Trexler

Preoperative preparation is an important part of the cardiac surgical patient's care but one which is becoming more difficult to provide with the need for health care cost reductions. Shorter hospital stays for the patient and the need to stay competitive in the insurance market are making it more complicated to provide a complete introduction and preparation for each patient for their surgery.[30] The surgeon, anesthesiologist, physician's assistant, and nurse each have a role in preoperative instruction that is essential to the patient's successful recovery.

Preoperative preparation and teaching have a positive influence on the postoperative progress of the cardiac surgical patient.[1,2,5,17,20] A multidisciplinary team can provide concise information concerning the patient's surgical care and postoperative recovery in the limited time available. This information can help relieve anxiety and promote collaboration with the patient and family during their recovery. Research has shown that patients with adequate preoperative information and participation have less physical and psychologic problems that may influence their recovery.[5,8,12]

Preoperative patient teaching results in shorter hospitalizations by improving patient compliance and knowledge.[14,26,32,34,35] Cost containment prompted same-day admission for surgery, thereby limiting inpatient preoperative preparation. Because of these time constraints preoperative preparation must be provided in a more organized and collaborative manner.

Managed care[3,4,13,15,16] is a process that defines the achievements and outcomes of care for each patient undergoing coronary artery bypass, transplantation, or valvular surgery at the beginning of care. Shorter hospital stays, many without a preoperative day, have made it impossible to discharge each person with the information he or she needs, without the coordination that managed care provides.[9,22,24,31]

Case Management

Case management is a system developed to maintain quality patient care while efficiently using resources. This system is a part of the managed care organization. Managed care is defined as a unit-based system of care that is organized to provide "specific outcomes" for the patient within a "financially responsible time frame."[3,4,27] This makes use of available resources in a timely and appropriate manner. The patients outcomes are the result of the activities provided by the multidisciplinary team of doctors, nurses, therapists, and other health care providers. Outcome is in measurable terms and includes the patient's health status, satisfaction, and costs.[10,19,22,25,29]

Goals of managed care are as follows:
- To provide a collaboration of practice that promotes coordinated patient care
- To provide continuity of patient care that directs each health care provider in achieving the appropriate patient outcomes throughout the patient's hospital stay
- To provide and promote the appropriate use of resources
- To facilitate an early discharge, by collaborative practice, within an appropriate length of stay for the patient
- To promote professional satisfaction[3,10,28]

The case management team includes the attending physician, primary nurses, respiratory therapists, physical and occupational therapists, social workers, and consultants. Master's prepared registered nurses provide the role of the case manager.[7,33] In cooperation with the physician the case manager is responsible for the coordination and facilitation of patient care throughout the patient's hospitalization. This coordinator evaluates and assesses the patient's daily needs and promotes the continued provision of quality patient care. This care is provided by physicians, nurses, therapists, pharmacists, and other health care providers who take care of the patient on a daily basis and who have an impact on the patient's discharge outcome.

These outcomes can be evaluated by a written "critical pathway"[3,6,7,22,23] that outlines key points in the patient's hospital stay that must occur within a specific time frame for each patient diagnosis. That is, the coronary bypass patient follows a time line that has been developed to include everything the patient should be doing during their entire hospitalization. This includes administration of medications, laboratory work, consultations, treatments, activities, teaching, discharge planning, and physical, occupational, and respiratory therapy. The critical pathway is implemented within 24 hours of the patient's admission by the patient's physician, primary nurse, and the case manager. Any changes that need to be incorporated into the critical pathway standard are done at this point. All deviations from the pathway after this are defined as variances. Actions can then be identified to reestablish the patient on the road to recovery by dealing with these problems (Fig. 3-1).[28,33]

The critical pathway is a guideline that can decrease the redundancies that can occur with each hospitalization. These guidelines are not inflexible and can be individualized for each patient when problems develop. The pathway was developed to provide an outline for fiscally responsible care that still promotes the quality care all patients deserve throughout their hospitalization.

Case management can play a definitive part of the preoperative preparation process by ensuring that adequate information and preparation are completed before surgery. A more simplified version of the critical pathway can be given to the family to show them the basic expectations for a routine hospitalization.

Preoperative Preparation

Preoperative preparation must be started at an earlier stage for the elective cardiac surgical patient. History, physical examination, diagnostic studies, and patient education can be completed 24 to 72 hours before surgery on an outpatient basis. This requires successful collaboration between all hospital departments to provide a rapid and accessible data collection system to prepare the patient for surgery. Studies have shown that outpatient preadmission testing and patient education can be completed cost effectively and still provide patient satisfaction.[5,20,21,23] Outpatient preadmission testing can significantly reduce the average length of stay for the patient and avoid a loss of revenue for the hospital. By identifying problems (e.g., clotting disorders, need for carotid studies, dental evaluation, fever, colds) before the scheduled surgical date, precious hospital days can be saved.

DEPARTMENT OF NURSING
CORONARY ARTERY BYPASS
CRITICAL PATHWAY

MD: _____   Date Discussed with Pt/Family: _____

PN: _____   Date to Begin: _____

Health Parameter	Nursing Diagnosis	INT D-T-D-1	NELSON 6 Pre-OP	OR	ICU Day of Surgery		IMC Day 1
Nutrition			NAS Diet NPO p̄ 2400	OG placed - - -	To Lis - - -	D/C clear liquids D/C	Progress to NAS Diet as Tolerated
Elimination	Fluid Volume Excess			Foley Inserted	I+OQ1* - - - KCL PRN - - - Diuretics PRN - - - -	D/C	Q4* - - - - Colace BID -
Sensory Function	Alteration in Comfort & Pain		Halcion Neurologic Assessment	On call sedatives	Anesthetic agents	Analgesics/ Sedatives Prn - - - - Assess Q2-4* - - -	Analgesics - Prn Assess Q 4-8*
Structural Integrity			Hibiclens scrubs x3 OOB Ad Lib	◄Cautery pad►◄Hypothermia► placed Blanket ◄Padding/ Positioning► Eggcrate - - - - - Bedrest - - - - ┤ - - Turn Q2* - DSD to Chest - - - ┐ DSD to leg c̄ ├- Leg Rewrap ├ ace wrap ┘ Pacing wires -┤- - - - - - Line Placements PA catheter -┤- - - - - - - Central - - ┤- - - - - - - Arterial - ┤- - - - - - - Peripheral - ┤- Hep Lock #2		OOB -►Chair - Ambulate c̄ Suture Assistance Line Care Q Day Pacerwire Care QD D/C D/C D/C	
Respiratory Function	Ineffective Breathing Pattern/ Airway Clearance		Respiratory Assessment CXR O₂ ► NC on call to OR		Intubation - - Pleural Ct - -	Assess Q2-4* - - CXR on Admission ABG Q4-8* - Pulse Oximetry Prn to 20cm suction	Assess Q4-8* CXR QAM FM -► N.C. IS/C+DBQ2* - D/C - - - D/C

***Fig.* 3-1** Coronary artery bypass critical pathway.

for addressograph plate

IMC	NELSON 6					Outcomes	Date Resolved
Day 2	Day 3	Day 4	Day 5	Day 6			
Q8° until fluid restriction D/C D/C when PT at Preop wt t/or no evidence of edema				D/C Meds: Colace	The patient will achieve a decrease or stabilization of fluid volume excess prior to D/C. - V.S. approach normal for age/condition. - Peripheral edema does not increase. - Output is approximately 2/3 of input.	
Assess Q8° x 24° then Q24°				D/C Meds: Tylox	The patient will achieve effective management of pain prior to D/C. - Pain tolerance is sufficient to do ADL's. - PT identifies & demonstrates at least one appropriate relief technique	
D/C DSG if without drainage		◄ Staples D/C ► ◄ Pacing Wires D/C ►				
	D/C					
Assess Q8° x 24° then Q24° D/C	CXR D/C	PRN			The PT will have an effective breathing pattern/airway clearance prior to D/C. - Stabilization of, or improvement in respiratory pattern/mental status. - Demonstrates effective coughing or other mechanism to remove airway secretions.	

Continued.

FORM JHH-PLOT (04-14-92)

JHH 1188 PRINTED BY JHH INFORMATION SERVICES ORGANIZATION

Health Parameter	Nursing Diagnosis	DATE / DAY / UNIT	NELSON 6 Pre-OP	OR Day of Surgery	ICU	IMC Day 1
Circulatory	Decreased Cardiac Output		CV Assess		Assess Q 2-4°	Assess Q 4-8°
			VSQ8°	per Anesthesia Protocol	per ICU protocol 3	Q4°
			12 Lead		12 Lead Q8° x 2	12 Lead/AM
				Cardiac monitor	Rhythm Strip Q shift	
				Pulmonary Artery Pressure Readings/ Cardiac Indicies per Protocol		D/C
				◄Cardioplegia►		
			TNG PRN	Vasoactive Meds: MBP 65-75 CI ► 2.0	Vdemand Pacemaker	D/C
					Antihypertensives Prn	
				Antibiotic x3	q8° x 6	
					ASA QD	
					Auto Transfusion per Protocol	
			Labs: TxC, M7, M12,H8, Pt/Ptt RPR Lipid Profile	Mediastinal Ct	To 20cm suction	D/C
					Admit Labs: Pt/PH,	AM Labs: M7, H8,
					NA/K HcT/ Chem Q4-6° PRN	
Cognitive Response	Knowledge Deficit		Pre-Op Routine Incentive Spirometer or Environment	Family visit by or nurse	Family: Patient Status/Progress ICU Routines	Patient: Orient to ICU Environment	Pt/Family: IMC Routines
			ICU Course & Progression		Concepts of: IS/C+DB Fluid Restriction/ Activity	Concepts of: Medications/ Reinforce Fluid Restriction/ Activity
Consults			Anesthesia		Respiratory Tx	
Daily Evaluation	1. Did the patient's progress correspond to the critical pathway?		Yes No	Yes No		Yes No
	2. Variation? Health parameter?					
	3. Care plan initiated?		Yes No	Yes No		Yes No
	Signature/ Title	D				
		E				
		N				

Critical Pathway

Fig. 3-1 *cont'd* Coronary artery bypass critical pathway.

IMC	NELSON 6					Outcomes	Date Resolved
	Day 2	Day 3	Day 4	Day 5	Day 6		
	Assess Q8° x 24° then Q24° Q4° x 24 then Q8°	12 Lead	---		---	The patient can expect stable cardiac output by discharge. - Pulse, BP, EKG approach normal for age/condition. - Stable or no decrease in baseline mental status. - Baseline or improved peripheral pulses. - Stable or decreased Dyspnea. - The patient will understand how to manage ADL's within tolerance level.	
	D/C D/C						
	D/C						
		---	---	---	D/C Meds: Ecotrin		
	NA/K HcT	AM Labs		AM Labs			
	Patient/ Family: Nelson 6 Routines	Diet Teaching		Discharge Summary		The patient/family will increase knowledge related to the disease process, treatments, and health care practices. - Verbalizes a basic knowledge of disease and related health care practices by discharge. - Demonstrates skills R/T to therapies and health care practices by D/C.	
		Plan date to attend D/C class	◄Discharge Class►				
				Discharge Packet	Discharge Instructions		
	Physical Tx	Nutrition					
	Yes No	Yes No	Yes No	Yes No			
	Yes No	Yes No	Yes No	Yes No			

Same-day surgical patients require the same preoperative care, but the time is considerably limited. Outpatient admission testing can be completed, but the education can be difficult to include. One-on-one teaching can be a problem with the current nursing staff shortages in most institutions today. An organized system of education for the same-day surgical patient can be provided by the following:

- Educational pamphlets or books that explain the hospital process from admission to discharge can include the rehabilitative period for the patient's first few weeks at home.
- Computer programs that are user friendly on a fifth- to sixth-grade reading level can review the hospital course and get the patient involved. (This can be difficult for illiterate, elderly and visually impaired patients. Someone needs to be available to help patients with any questions or computer problems.)
- Use of a video that reviews the postoperative process can be viewed by a group of patients or by a single patient. Hospitals that have their own educational channel can use this medium for the patient to view at preset times.
- Preoperative teaching can be done by the case manager or the primary nurse who has a workable patient load. Providing the patient and family with a booklet or a flip chart on postoperative care can answer many of the basic questions. Follow-up can be done by the case manager preoperatively to answer any remaining questions.[2,11,18]

An organized system of patient education incorporated in the preadmission process can help prepare the patient and the family for the surgical procedure and recovery. The multidisciplinary team that provides this preoperative preparation depends on the collaboration of all involved in the patient's care to expedite the patient's recovery.

Preoperative Visits

Role of the Physician Assistant

The physician assistant (PA) has an important role in providing an accurate history and physical examination and in preparing the patient for surgery. The PA provides the following:

- Preoperative assessment of each patient, including an in-depth history and physical examination concerning prior and current problems

- Ensuring that laboratory work and required diagnostic tests (e.g., chest x-ray film, electrocardiogram, carotid Doppler studies) are completed before surgery
- Preoperative skin preparation (e.g., shaving, and chest and leg scrubs)
- Assistance in the operating room (OR) under the direction of the attending surgeon
- Postoperative follow-up with each patient

The PA reports to the surgeon any problems that warrant a postponement or a cancellation, such as fevers, dental problems, carotid bruits, transient ischemic attacks, or coagulation dysfunctions. The PA is frequently the first person after the primary nurse whom the patient meets. Many of the patients' initial questions about their postoperative care can be answered by the PAs.

Role of the Attending Surgeon

The physician's role in preoperative preparation involves an introduction to the patient and family. After this introduction the surgeon can discuss the upcoming surgical procedure and obtain the informed consent.

Introduction to the patient and family provides a time for the physician to develop a rapport to decrease the anxiety for the entire family, thereby promoting a more rapid recovery. Trust and communication can be the key points of the preoperative process. The patient and family retain more information from the people they trust. An explanation of the operative procedure taking into account the patient's educational level, a basic explanation of the heart's function, the underlying problem and disease process, and how the problem will be repaired are usually part of the conversation between the PA and the patient and family. Informed consent reviews the complications associated with each procedure and operation (i.e., infection, stroke, heart attack, bleeding, arrhythmia, and death).

Role of the Anesthesiologist

The anesthesiologist becomes the important link in preoperative care information. The patient usually is ready to ask questions concerning the immediate postoperative period. The anesthesiologist's knowledge of the intensive care unit (ICU) and their explanations can help relieve the preoperative anxiety. Their responsibilities include the following:

- Assessment of the patient's history and how this relates to their general anesthesia requirements, and review of allergies, transfusions, and current medications that can influence the intraoperative period.
- Discussion of the type of anesthesia, the endotracheal tube, and the invasive procedures required to place central and arterial catheters during and after the anesthetic induction.

Role of the Nurse

The primary nurse

Preoperatively, the primary caregiver is responsible for overall assessment of the patient's physical and psychologic readiness for surgery. The patient needs a stress-free environment that may require limiting visitors and providing extra time to discuss any questions left unanswered. A sedative the night before surgery can assist in an improved night of sleep and help relieve some of the tension.

The primary nurse also reviews the needs for the next day's surgery by doing the following:

- Checking that scrubs are completed appropriately and on time
- Checking to see that the patient is aware of when NPO status begins and what that does and does not include (i.e., necessary medications)
- Discussing where personal belongings can be kept and what should be sent home with the patient's family
- Reminding the patient to remove items such as rings, necklaces, bracelets, watches, dentures, hearing aids, and eyeglasses
- Providing information to the family concerning when they can see the patient before surgery, and the location of the OR and the family waiting lounge

Special care is required to prevent oversaturation of information. The patient sees many people the day or night before surgery with shorter preoperative stays; each of these people has less time to see the patient. An attempt should be made to consolidate some of the visits and coordinate the teaching.

The case manager

The case management process involves the case manager in the role of facilitator and coordinator of patient care. They help the primary care nurse to implement the critical pathway and to define any alterations that require early intervention. Problems such as home care for people that live alone, smoking cessation programs, and family problems can be identified early. Problems that can keep the patient in the hospital, such as no available home care, preexisting disabilities, or financial complications, can be followed up through social services, physical therapy, or financial counseling. If these consulting services are aware of preexisting problems, they can expedite positive results.

The case manager visits the patient and family preoperatively. Because the case managers are familiar with the whole system, they become an important part of the patient's reference guide to the hospital process. They can address unanswered questions and questions the patient may have forgotten to ask.

The role involves assessing the patient, the history and physical examination, and diagnostic tests for anything overlooked before the surgery date. The case manager is the one person who follows the patient from admission to the postdischarge period. In our institution they make rounds twice daily with the resident and intern involved in the patient's care. They provide insights into the patient's recovery process and what needs to be completed in accomplishing discharge goals.

Role of OR and ICU Nurses

The OR nurse

The OR nurse visits the patient preoperatively and discusses the responsibilities of care. This includes greeting patients when they arrive in the induction room. The patient is usually very sleepy as a result of the premedication given about 1 hour before arrival. The nurse provides a quick systematic assessment of the patient's physical status and makes sure they are dressed appropriately for surgery.

The last surgical scrubs and shaving are completed by the PA or technician. After this, the anesthesiologist begins the central lines in the neck and the arterial line in the radial artery. Once these lines are placed, the anesthesiologist induces anesthesia and intubates the patient in preparation for the surgical procedure. The OR nurse assists with the preparation and is available to the patient.

The ICU nurse

The ICU nurse when possible visits the patient the night before surgery and discusses their responsibilities and the ICU environment. This visit includes the following:

- Discussion of the ICU location and the visiting policy for the family
- Explanation of when the family can see the patient postoperatively and for how long
- Review of the ICU environment: The patient has a multitude of tubes that hamper movement at first, but once these are removed, activity is slowly resumed under the direction of their nurse. The rooms can be noisy and brighter than normal, but care is taken to provide privacy and quiet times whenever possible.
- Review of the placement of arterial and central line catheters, and discussion of the placement of chest tubes and urinary catheters and their subsequent removal
- Review of the endotracheal tube, weaning from the ventilator when the patient wakens, removal of the endotracheal tube, and the need for ongoing deep breathing and coughing to prevent atelectasis and pneumonia. Use of the incentive spirometer both preoperatively and postoperatively is necessary for improved lung expansion.
- Explanation of the importance of activity and the necessity of time out of bed in a chair and advancement to short walks
- Explanation of the length of a normal ICU stay, the stepdown unit, and the inpatient unit location
- A critical pathway provided to the patient and the family to review and keep. Use of flip charts, videos, and booklets can assist the patient in gaining the knowledge needed for a successful recovery.

Preoperative Skin Preparation

Preoperative skin preparation to remove surface organisms can be accomplished by the application of a surface bacterial agent and moderate brisk scrubbing of the operative field. We recommend three separate scrubs before the operation and a final intraoperative scrub before the final skin preparation.

Most patients have colonies of gram-positive organisms. Those patients with *Staphylococcus aureus* are at increased risk of postoperative wound infections, and those with coagulase-negative staphylococci are at particular risk of bacterial endocarditis during prosthetic valve surgery. Patients who have been hospitalized for some time before the operation, especially those in the ICU, may have an increased number of organisms.

The efficacy of specific types of antiseptic skin preparation has been well documented in a prospective randomized-observer blind study with chlorhexidine gluconate (Hibiclens), povidone-iodine (Betadine), and a lotion soap (Safe 'n Sure) as preoperative scrubs. This study confirmed that preoperative scrubbing with chlorhexidine gluconate significantly reduced the ability to recover staphylococcal organisms from selected skin sites before surgery. It further showed that the cumulative effect of additional scrubbings would further reduce the ability to recover organisms from the skin. The povidone-iodine was associated with an inconsistent result, and showering with the lotion soap produced a mean increase in staphylococcal colony counts.

We therefore believe that preoperative preparation of the skin is an important step in minimizing postoperative wound infections. We routinely request three scrubs to the chest, abdomen, groin, and leg regions to be performed the evening before the operation for early morning patients. For early afternoon surgery we ask patients to perform two scrubs in the evening before and one on the morning of surgery.

Preoperative Medications

Each patient is assessed by the anesthesiologist before surgery. Any previous adverse reactions to medications is discussed, and any skin testing for penicillin allergics is completed before surgery. If this testing is not feasible, a broad-spectrum staphylococci and gram-positive–sensitive antibiotic is used (e.g., vancomycin).

Currently, preoperative medications include the following:
- Antibiotics: a broad-spectrum cephalosporin (we currently use cefazolin (Ancef) after a 3-year trial evaluating three different cephalosporins (cefazolin, cefamandole, and cefoxitin). Cefazolin was found to be less expensive and as effective as the other antibiotics.)
- Sedatives: Patients are encouraged to use, if needed, a light sleeping pill (e.g., triazolam, diphenhydramine, flurazepam) the night before surgery to help them sleep. Antianxiety drugs (e.g., lorazepam, diazepam-type medications) can also be used to relax the patient preoperatively, especially for patients already using these medications.
- Morning-of-surgery sedatives: Antianxiety medications (e.g., diazepam or lorazepam) are prescribed the morning of surgery in small doses.

- On-call medications: A narcotic analgesic (e.g., morphine sulfate) is prescribed together with scopolamine intramuscularly to prepare for the OR
- Usually the patient's previously prescribed cardiac medications are given at the scheduled times except those which may alter coagulation (e.g., aspirin, ibuprofen, indomethacin)

The future directions of preoperative care must include efficient use of resources while providing the information and education the patient and family need to promote a rapid recovery. This can be accomplished by the close collaboration of all services within the managed care–case management process. The goal is total preparation of the patient and family for the surgical process.

References

1. Barr WJ: Teaching patients with life-threatening illnesses, *Nurs Clin North Am* 24(3):69-644, 1989.
2. Berger MS, Wesley W: Can we educate outpatients effectively? Certainly, *Nurs Management* (17)12:34-37, 1986.
3. Bower KA: Managed care: controlling costs, guaranteeing outcomes, *Definition* 3(3):1-3, 1988.
4. Bryan-Brown CW, Dracup K: Interesting times: managed critical care, *Am J Crit Care* 2(2):108-109, 1993.
5. Christopherson B, Pfeiffer C: Varying the timing of information to alter preoperative anxiety and postoperative recovery in cardiac surgery patients, *Heart Lung* 9(5):855-861, 1980.
6. Coben EL: Nursing case management: does it pay? *J Nurs Administr* 21(4):20-25, 1991.
7. Cronin CJ, Maklebust J: Case-managed care: capitalizing on the CNS, *Nurs Management* 20(3):38-47, 1989.
8. Divine E, Cook R: A meta-analytic analysis of psychoeducational interventions on length of post-surgical hospital stay, *Nurs Res* 32(5):267-274, 1983.
9. Erkel EA: The impact of case management in preventive services, *J Nurs Administr* 23(1):27-32, 1993.
10. Etheridge P, Lamb GS: Professional nursing case management improves quality, access and costs, *Nurs Management* 20(3):30-35, 1989.
11. Goulart DT: Educating the cardiac surgery patient and family, *J Cardiovascular Nurs* 3(3):1-9, 1989.
12. Grady KL, Buckley DJ, Cisar NS, et al: Patient perception of cardiovascular surgical patient education, *Heart Lung* 17(4):349-354, 1988.

13. Gregg SA: How can we achieve more value from our managed care efforts? *Topics In Health Care Financing* 19(2):89-95, 1992.

14. Hathaway D: Effect of preoperative instruction on postoperative outcomes: a meta-analysis, *Nurs Res* 35(5):269-275, 1986.

15. Inglehart JK: The American health care system. Managed care, *N Engl J Med* 327(10):742-747, 1992.

16. Johnsson J: Managed care in the 1990s: providers' new role for innovative health delivery, *Hospitals* 66(6):20-25, 1991.

17. King KB: Measurement of coping strategies, concerns, and emotional response in patients undergoing coronary artery bypass grafting, *Heart Lung* 14(6):579-586, 1985.

18. King I, Tarsitano B: The effect of structured and unstructured preoperative teaching: a replication, *Nurs Res* 31(6):324-329, 1982.

19. Kralovec OJ, Huttner CA, Dixon MD: The application of total quality management concepts in a service-line cardiovascular program, *Nurs Administr Q* 15(2):1-8, 1991.

20. Lepczyk M, Raleigh EH, Rowley C: Timing of preoperative patient teaching, *J Adv Nurs* 15(3):300-306, 1990.

21. Lierman J: Preoperative assessments: can we afford to do without them? *AORN J* 47(2):586-590, 1988.

22. Marr JA, Reid B: Implementing managed care and case management: the neuroscience experience, *J Neurosci Nurs* 24(50):281-285, 1992.

23. Marshall J, Penckofer S, Llewellyn J: Structured postoperative teaching, knowledge and compliance of patients who had coronary artery bypass surgery, *Heart Lung* 15(1):76-82, 1986.

24. McIntosh L: Hospital-based case management, *Nurs Econ* 5(5):232-236, 1987.

25. Merrill J: Defining case management, *Business Health* July/August:5-9, 1985.

26. Miller P, Shada EA: Preoperative information and recovery of openheart surgery patients, *Heart Lung* 7(3):486-493, 1978.

27. O'Connor AC: Quality measurement, management and reimbursement in today's health care environment, *Quality Rev Bull* 19(3):102-103, 1993.

28. Olivas GS, Del Togno-Armanasco V, Erickson JR, Harter S: Case management: a bottom line care delivery model, *J Nurs Administr* 19(11):10-20 [Part I]; 19(12):12-17 [Part II], 1989.

29. Pierog LJ: Case management: a product line, *Nurs Administr Q* 15(2):16-20, 1991.

30. Pointer D, Ross M: DRG cost-per-case management: DRG's kick off a whole new ball game—1984, hospitals need new tactics to win, *Modern Healthcare* 14(3):109-112, 1984.

31. Richardson M: Can managed care control costs without controlling you? *Tex Med* 88(10):36-44, 1992.

32. Steele J, Ruzicki D: An evaluation of the effectiveness of cardiac teaching during hospitalization, *Heart Lung* 16(3):306-311, 1987.

33. Strong AG, Sneed NV: Clinical evaluation of a critical path for coronary artery bypass surgery patients, *Prog Cardiovasc Nurs* 6(1):29-37, 1991.

34. Suter P, Bloch A: Can preoperative care be facilitated by preoperative preparation? In Roskamm H, Schmuziger M, editors: *Coronary Heart Surg* New York, 1979, Springer-Verlag.

35. Worley B: Preadmission testing and teaching: more satisfaction at less cost, *Nurs Management* 17(12):32-33, 1986.

Multidisciplinary Care Involved in Conducting the Operation

4

Eugenie S. Heitmiller, Steven Thompson, Karen Michael, Steve Trexler, and William A. Baumgartner

The purpose of this chapter is to describe the specific and general responsibilities of persons involved in the conduct of a cardiothoracic operation. It provides the reader with a general familiarity with the techniques of anesthesia, an understanding of cardiopulmonary bypass, and an explanation of surgical techniques. Doses, interactions, and side effects of the more commonly used anesthetic and analgesic drugs are described in detail.

Nursing Responsibilities

The operating room (OR) nurse establishes a plan of care and identifies required nursing intervention and actions to provide for a safe, efficient, and comforting environment.[30,42] This is achieved by the use of good observation and interviewing skills, a sound knowledge base, adaptability, and advocacy of patient rights.[44] The OR nurse gathers pertinent information and data through review of the medical record and through patient interviews at time of admission.

The patient is greeted, and warm blankets are provided to reduce and/or prevent shivering, which increases the metabolic rate.[42] Identification is completed by verbal verification and comparison with the medical record and name band.[44] The patient is questioned for confirmation of allergies; NPO (oral intake) status; and the wearing of jewelry, contact lenses, dentures, or any other external or internal prostheses. The presence and location of family members and/or significant others should be verified at this time for dissemination of information regarding the patient's progress during the procedure.

The medical record is reviewed for completion and documentation of informed consent (properly signed and witnessed), laboratory results, diagnostic data, and the medical history and physical.[30,44]

A gross physical assessment is completed and includes the following:

- General appearance
- Skin condition (integrity): Lesions, rashes, contusions, temperature, color, edema, previous incisions
- Level of consciousness: Awake, drowsy, arousable, sedated, obtunded
- Mobility of body parts: Range of motion, joint replacements
- Cardiac condition: Presence of chest pain or pacemaker
- Respiratory condition: Dyspnea, orthopnea, use of accessory muscles
- Gastrointestinal condition: Colostomy, ileostomy
- Genitourinary: Foley catheterization

Patient care in the OR continues as a collaborative approach with other team members as evidenced in the remainder of this chapter.

Anesthesiologist's Responsibilities

Patients undergoing cardiac surgery require preoperative sedation, intraoperative anesthesia, and postoperative analgesia. To care properly for these patients in the postoperative period, it is important to understand the properties and side effects of the various drugs the patient receives in the perioperative period. The number of available anesthetic agents is growing rapidly, and each drug has its own advantages and disadvantages. This section of the chapter reviews the more commonly used anesthetic and analgesic agents for cardiac surgery.

Premedication

The goal in administering a premedication is to reduce the anxiety and stress that accompanies the prospect of cardiac surgery. Much of this normally occurring anxiety can be alleviated by the pre-operative visits of members of the cardiac surgical team who will be caring for the patient. Premedication is then used to relax the patient further before being transported to the OR. Placement of intravascular catheters often occurs before induction of anesthesia. Premedication is therefore designed to facilitate patient comfort during intravascular catheter placement.

The premedication for cardiac surgery is often a combination of a sedative, a narcotic, and a centrally acting anticholinergic, which together deliver analgesia and amnesia during the immediate preoperative period. At The Johns Hopkins Hospital the most commonly used drugs for premedication are diazepam (Valium); 0.1 to 0.2 mg/kg PO or lorazepam (Ativan), 1 to 4 mg PO; morphine, 0.1 mg/kg IM; and scopolamine, 0.2 to 0.4 mg IM.

The premedication is usually given 30 to 60 minutes before the patient's arrival in the operating area. If at that time the patient is not adequately sedated, additional diazepam or midazolam is administered. Oxygen (4 L delivered by face mask) is administered at the time the initial premedication is given.

Induction of Anesthesia

General anesthesia for cardiac surgery is produced by a combination of analgesics, amnesics, and muscle relaxants. The doses vary with the patient's clinical condition and tolerance. The following drugs are most commonly used for anesthetic induction:

- Analgesics: fentanyl, sufentanil, morphine
- Amnesics: diazepam, midazolam, sodium pentothal, etomidate, ketamine
- Muscle relaxants: pancuronium, vecuronium, atracurium, succinylcholine
- Volatile anesthetics: halothane, enflurane, isoflurane

The induction of anesthesia is preceded by delivery of 100% oxygen by mask to denitrogenate the lungs. A working suction must be immediately available. To prevent truncal rigidity caused by narcotic analgesics, a priming dose (usually one tenth of the induction dose) of a nondepolarizing muscle relaxant is given approximately 3 minutes before induction. The narcotic and amnesic or other induction agents of choice are then given in divided doses until the patient is unresponsive. After the ability to ventilate the patient is assured, the remaining dose of muscle relaxant is administered. Additional narcotic and amnesic drugs are given to obtain the desired dose and hemodynamics. After muscle relaxation is achieved, the trachea is intubated and the preparation for surgery proceeds.

Intubation

The most frequently used technique for tracheal intubation in cardiac surgery is direct-vision orotracheal intubation. The head is placed in a sniffing position, the mouth is opened, the laryngoscope is advanced down the right side of the mouth, and the tongue is swept to the left. If a curved (Macintosh) blade is used, the blade is advanced into the vallecula, then raised to draw up the epiglottis and reveal the vocal cords. If a straight (Magill) blade is used, the blade is advanced over the epiglottis, which is then elevated by raising the laryngoscope straight up "toward the ceiling" so that the upper teeth are not used as a fulcrum. As the epiglottis is lifted upward the vocal cords are seen. Once the vocal cords are viewed, the endotracheal tube is advanced through the cords until the cuff of the tube passes into the trachea. The cuff is inflated and the tube is taped into position, noting the tube markings at the mouth. The usual distances are 21 to 23 cm for a man and 19 to 21 cm for a woman. Intubation of the trachea is most often assured by the presence of end-tidal carbon dioxide. Breath sounds should be checked to be sure that both lungs are being adequately ventilated.

Difficult intubations can often be predicted during the preoperative examination. Predictors of difficult intubation include:
- Inability to open the mouth wide enough to see the uvula
- A receding lower jaw
- Protruding upper incisors
- A high, arched palate and narrow, deep mouth
- Inability to extend the neck

If a difficult intubation is suspected, a fiberoptic intubation may be planned before the induction of anesthesia.

Complications can occur any time after intubation and may not be evident until the patient is in the intensive care unit and has been extubated. These complications include:
- Damage to the teeth
- Vocal cord injury
- Dislocation of the arytenoid muscles
- Subglottic swelling
- Contact ulcers

After the induction of anesthesia, hypotension may develop. This is usually managed with fluid administration and small doses of phenylephrine (0.025 to 0.050 mg IV). Bradycardia resulting in hemodynamic compromise is treated with atropine (0.3 to 0.5 mg IV) or ephedrine (5 to 10 mg IV). Tachycardia with hypotension is usually best treated with volume infusion and phenylephrine. Tachycardia with hypertension may be treated with a β-blocker such as esmolol (25 mg bolus or continuous infusion, titrated to effect) or the calcium channel blocker verapamil (2.5 to 10 mg IV).

Antibiotic administration is the responsibility of the anesthesiologist. The standard antibiotic for an adult at The Johns Hopkins Hospital is cefazolin. Each dose of cefazolin for an adult is 1 g and is administered through the central line at the following times during surgery: (1) immediately after central line placement, (2) at the time of incision, and (3) after cardiopulmonary bypass is discontinued. In cases of penicillin allergy vancomycin is administered instead of cefazolin.

Anesthetic Agents

Opioids

The analgesics most often used are morphine, fentanyl, and sufentanil.[6] Morphine is an *opiate,* a drug derived from opium. Fentanyl and sufentanil are *opioids,* drugs with morphinelike actions. The term *opioid agonist* refers to all drugs that bind to opioid receptors and that have agonistic actions. Opioid antagonists such as naloxone (Narcan) bind to opioid receptor sites but do not activate them, so no agonistic action results. The mechanisms of action of opioid agonists are to activate stereospecific receptors in the central nervous system and gastrointestinal tract. Opioids are very effective analgesics but have little amnestic effects. When used for general anesthesia, opioids are often combined with amnestic agents to prevent intraoperative awareness.

Morphine

Morphine is the standard against which new analgesics are measured. It is obtained from opium, which is found in the poppy plant, *Papaver somniferum*. Other clinically used alkaloids derived from opium are codeine and papaverine.

The doses and pharmacokinetics are listed in Tables 4-1 and 4-2, respectively.[21,39,48] Morphine has a short elimination half-life

Table 4-1 Uses and Doses of Commonly Used Opioids

		Dose	
Use	Morphine	Fentanyl	Sufentanil
Premedication (IM)	0.1-0.2 mg/kg		
General anesthesia (IV)			
High-dose	0.5-3 mg/kg	50-150 μg/kg	8-30 μg/kg
Balanced*		2-25 μg/kg	1-8 μg/kg
Analgesia/sedation (IM)	0.1-0.2 mg/kg	0.5-2 μg/kg	0.05-0.10 μg/kg
Intrathecal use	0.1-1 mg		
Epidural use			
Bolus	1-10 mg	25-100 μg	10-60 μg
Infusion	0.1-1.5 mg/hr	25-150 μg/hr (1 g/kg/hr)	5 g/hr (0.1-0.3 μg/kg/hr)

*Refers to its use in conjunction with other anesthetic agents.

Table 4-2 Pharmacokinetics of Commonly Used Opioids

	Morphine	Fentanyl	Sufentanil
Protein binding (%)	30	84	93
Volume of distribution (L/kg)	2-6	3-5	1-3
Clearance (ml/kg/min)	10-23	10-20	9-14
Elimination half-life (hr)	2-3	3-6	2-4
Duration of action (hr)	4-5	1-4	1-4
Metabolism	Glucuronic acid conjugation	90% liver	N-Dealkylation, O-Demethylation
Excretion	~90% conjugated in urine, ~10% in feces	10% excreted unchanged in urine	Liver

but a longer duration of action because of retention in the central nervous system.

Morphine exerts its action on the central nervous system, cardiovascular system, gastrointestinal tract, and other smooth muscle (Table 4-3). Its effects on the *central nervous system* are as follows:

- Analgesia is the primary effect. Continuous dull pain is more effectively relieved than sharp intermittent pain, but with higher doses even severe pain caused by renal or biliary colic can be relieved.
- Drowsiness, changes in mood, and mental clouding may be seen. Some patients experience euphoria, others may sleep.
- Miosis is due to an excitatory action on the autonomic segment of the nucleus of the oculomotor nerve.
- Respiratory depression results from a reduction in responsiveness of the brainstem respiratory centers to increases in carbon dioxide tension, and from depression of the pontine and medullary centers, which regulate respiratory rhythmic-

Table 4-3 Actions and Side Effects of Commonly Used Opioids

System	Effects
Central nervous system	Analgesia
	Drowsiness
	Changes in mood
	Miosis
	Respiratory depression
	Nausea and vomiting
Cardiovascular system	Peripheral vasodilation
	Decreased mean arterial pressure
	Decreased heart rate (fentanyl and sufentanil)
Gastrointestinal system	Decreased stomach motility
	Decreased biliary and pancreatic secretions
	Ileus
	Constipation
	Increased biliary tract pressure
Other smooth muscle systems	Increased ureter tone
	Increased bladder tone

ity. Therapeutic doses depress both *respiratory rate* and *tidal volume*.[2] After a therapeutic analgesic dose, maximal respiratory depression usually occurs in approximately 7 minutes but may be delayed as long as 30 minutes. The respiratory center begins to return to normal function in 2 to 3 hours, but minute volume may be depressed for 4 to 5 hours after a therapeutic dose. Morphine also depresses the *cough reflex* through a direct effect on the cough center in the medulla.

- Nausea and vomiting may be caused by direct stimulation of the chemoreceptor trigger zone in the medulla. Phenothiazines counteract this side effect. Nausea and vomiting are more common in ambulatory patients than in recumbent patients, suggesting involvement of the vestibular system as well. In certain people nausea never develops with morphine, whereas in others vomiting occurs each time a dose is given.

The *cardiovascular effects* of morphine are mainly due to peripheral arterial and venous dilation as a result of histamine release and central suppression of adrenergic tone. Hypotension and increased heart rate can result from the decrease in systemic vascular resistance.[19] There does not appear to be a consistent effect of morphine on cardiac output, but it has been found to decrease oxygen consumption and cardiac work in patients with coronary artery disease.

The effects of morphine on the *gastrointestinal tract* are as follows:[8,13]

- Stomach: Decreased motility is associated with increased tone in the antrum and first part of the duodenum and results in a delay in passage of gastric contents. This delay may decrease the absorption of drugs administered through the stomach.
- Small intestine: Morphine decreases biliary and pancreatic secretions, delaying the digestion of food in the small intestine. Periodic spasms may be present, but propulsive contractions are markedly decreased. Ileus can develop. Chyme viscosity is increased as more water is absorbed from it as a result of delayed passage.
- Large intestine: Colon peristalsis is diminished and may even be abolished by morphine. The delay in passage of colon contents results in desiccation of the feces. Morphine also increases anal sphincter tone. Constipation may result from

morphine. Because of the constipating effects, opiates are very effective in treating diarrhea.
- Biliary tract: Morphine can cause a marked increase in biliary tract pressure and result in epigastric distress or biliary colic. This effect usually occurs about 5 minutes after injection, peaks in approximately 15 minutes, and can persist for 2 hours or more.

Other smooth muscle systems affected by morphine include increased ureter and bladder tone, which may result in urinary retention.

Histamine release is also a well-known side effect of morphine administration. In addition to the decrease in systemic vascular resistance discussed previously, *histamine release* may also be responsible for:
- Dilation of cutaneous vessels
- Pruritus, which is commonly manifested as nasal itching but may be generalized
- Sweating
- Urticaria

Fentanyl

Fentanyl is a synthetic opioid of the 4-anilopiperidine series. It is 50 to 80 times as potent as morphine in producing analgesia. The dose of fentanyl varies with its clinical use, as shown in Table 4-1. The pharmacokinetics of fentanyl are summarized in Table 4-2.[4]

Fentanyl pharmacokinetics differ from morphine in that fentanyl is more lipid soluble and therefore has a shorter onset and duration of action because of its ability to penetrate membranes and dissociate from receptors rapidly.[37]

Fentanyl affects the central nervous system, cardiovascular system, gastrointestinal tract, and other smooth muscle in ways similar to morphine. However, there are some differences:
- Respiratory depression appears to be *biphasic,* with early and delayed respiratory depression. The delayed depression is possibly due to varying degrees of stimulation, release from other tissues (e.g., skeletal muscle), or recirculation from the gastrointestinal tract, which result in secondary peaks during the elimination phase.
- The major hemodynamic effect is a dose-dependent *brady-cardia* caused by vagal stimulation. Fentanyl alone otherwise has little effect on hemodynamics or cardiac function.

- *Chest wall rigidity* can occur within 60 to 90 seconds of fentanyl administration. This rigidity can occur with doses as small as 8 to 9 μg/kg and is abolished by the administration of a muscle relaxant.
- Histamine release resulting from fentanyl is rare.

Sufentanil

Sufentanil is a potent synthetic opioid analgesic that is seven to 10 times more potent than fentanyl.[11,37] Sufentanil is highly lipophilic and therefore is rapidly and extensively distributed to all tissues. Peak tissue levels in the brain are reached in 2 minutes. The uses and doses of sufentanil are listed in Table 4-1. The pharmacokinetics of sufentanil are summarized in Table 4-2.[5]

Sufentanil has a shorter elimination half-life than fentanyl, but its dissociation from narcotic receptors is slower. Sufentanil has the highest (90%) μ receptor specificity of all the opioids. When compared with morphine and fentanyl, sufentanil has a faster time to induction and shorter time until extubation.

The high degree of protein binding by sufentanil is significantly affected by plasma pH. Binding of sufentanil to plasma proteins decreases by 28% when plasma pH rises from 7.4 to 7.8 and increases by 29% when plasma pH decreases from 7.4 to 7.0.

Studies that have compared the effects of sufentanil with other opioids have shown sufentanil to maintain better hemodynamic stability than morphine or fentanyl.[11,15,17] In patients undergoing coronary artery surgery who received sufentanil no significant change was seen in blood pressure after incision, sternotomy, or sternal spread, whereas blood pressure was significantly increased after sternal spread in patients receiving fentanyl.[11]

Nonbarbiturates

In addition to the opioids, intravenous anesthetics that are used as adjuncts include drugs in both the nonbarbiturate and barbiturate classifications. The nonbarbiturates include the benzodiazepines, ketamine, and etomidate.

Benzodiazepines

The doses of the commonly used benzodiazepines are listed in Table 4-4. The actions of the benzodiazepines on the central nervous system result in sedation, hypnosis, decreased anxiety, anterograde amnesia, muscle relaxation, and anticonvulsant activity. Their mechanism of action seems to be related to the metab-

Table 4-4 Doses and Pharmacokinetics of Commonly Used Benzodiazepines

	Diazepam (Valium)	Lorazepam (Ativan)	Midazolam (Versed)
Premedication	0.05-0.2 mg/kg PO	1-4 mg PO	0.05-0.08 mg/kg PO
Sedation (mg/kg IV)	0.05-0.2		0.01-0.05
Anesthesia (balanced) (mg/kg IV)	0.1-0.6		0.1-0.4
Protein binding (%)	96-98	88-92	94-96
Elimination half-life (hr)	20-40	10-14	1-4
Metabolism	Liver	Liver	Liver
Excretion	Kidney	Kidney	Kidney

olism or action of γ-aminobutyric acid. The benzodiazepines are highly protein bound and are metabolized by the liver, and the conjugated metabolites are excreted by the kidneys. Many of the metabolites of benzodiazepines have biologic activity, complicating their pharmacokinetics. A significant amount of biliary secretion of these drugs occurs.

When used alone in lower doses the benzodiazepines have minimal cardiovascular and respiratory side effects. However, in cardiac surgery they are most often used in addition to narcotics and can result in decreased blood pressure, cardiac output, systemic vascular resistance, and respiration. Pain and thrombophlebitis are associated with parenteral administration of diazepam, whereas midazolam, which is water soluble, has a low incidence of injection pain and postinjection phlebitis.

Both diazepam and midazolam are used for anesthesia because of their rapid onset of action when administered intravenously and their excellent anxiolytic, hypnotic, and amnesic properties. Lorazepam is used for premedication but not for induction of anesthesia because of the slow onset of action (20 to 40 minutes) when given intravenously.[46]

Ketamine

Ketamine is a nonbarbiturate intravenous anesthetic that produces a state of dissociative anesthesia.[45] An induction dose of 2 mg/kg has a rapid onset of action (30 to 60 seconds) and a relatively short duration of action (10 to 15 minutes), but complete recovery may be prolonged. The actions of ketamine include dissociative anesthesia, analgesia, nystagmus, and hypertonus.

The cardiorespiratory effects of ketamine include increases in heart rate and blood pressure associated with increased catecholamine levels. The effect on systemic and pulmonary vascular resistance is variable and depends on the patient's clinical state. Patients with ischemic or valvular heart disease and depressed ventricular function may not tolerate the increased heart rate and myocardial oxygen demand associated with ketamine administration.

Ketamine has an elimination half-life of 2.5 to 3.1 hours.[45] It is metabolized by the liver, and the conjugated metabolites are excreted by the kidneys. Postoperative nausea and vomiting have been associated with ketamine administration. In addition, ketamine may produce hallucinations and unpleasant dreams, which may be attenuated by benzodiazepine administration.

Etomidate

Etomidate is a carboxylated imidazole derivative with sedative-hypnotic properties. It is used as an induction agent (0.3 to 0.5 mg/kg) and has a rapid onset and short duration of action because of rapid redistribution. Hemodynamic stability is for the most part maintained with etomidate, and patients with decreased ventricular function or hypovolemia seem to tolerate etomidate better than thiopental for anesthetic induction. However, in patients who are very ill or who have significant valvular heart disease, hypotension with a decrease in systemic vascular resistance may develop. Disadvantages of etomidate include pain on injection, myoclonic activity with anesthetic induction dose, inhibition of adrenal steroidogenesis, and no analgesic activity.

Opiate pretreatment seems to reduce the severity of the myoclonic activity and the occurrence of cough or hiccups.

Barbiturates

Thiopental is a short-acting barbiturate used for induction of anesthesia. Its use in cardiac anesthesia is limited for the most part to patients with normal ventricular function. It may be used in patients who require a rapid-sequence induction in an attempt to avoid aspiration of stomach contents. It may also be used to sedate patients for cardioversion. It has no analgesic properties. Maximum brain concentration is reached in 1 minute and rapidly (5 to 10 minutes) falls as it redistributes to other tissues. The disadvantages of thiopental are myocardial depression and dilation of venous capacitance vessels, which significantly lower preload and cardiac output and subsequently elevates heart rate.

Inhalational anesthetics

The inhalational anesthetics used in the cardiac OR are nitrous oxide, halothane, enflurane, and isoflurane.

Enflurane and isoflurane are the inhalational agents most commonly used in cardiac surgery. The advantages of enflurane include decreased incidence of hepatic toxicity and little effect on systemic vascular resistance. The primary disadvantages of enflurane include myocardial depression, acceleration of heart rate, induction of seizure activity with high concentrations, and renal biodegradation resulting in the liberation of free fluoride ions, which can depress renal function.

When used alone, isoflurane has a minimal effect on cardiac

output. It has vasodilator properties resulting in decreased systemic vascular resistance. The heart is less sensitized to catecholamines with isoflurane use as compared with halothane, and subsequently ventricular arrhythmias occur less frequently. Its disadvantages are related mostly to its vasodilator properties, with tachycardia accompanying vasodilation. This effect may be beneficial for aortic insufficiency but unfavorable for patients with aortic stenosis or coronary artery disease. In addition, it may inhibit hypoxic pulmonary vasoconstriction and has been associated with the phenomenon of "coronary steal."

Neuromuscular blockers

The neuromuscular blockers used most frequently in the care of patients undergoing cardiac surgery are pancuronium (Pavulon), vecuronium (Norcuron), and succinylcholine.

The doses and pharmacokinetics of the neuromuscular blockers are listed in Table 4-5.[38] The pharmacokinetics of pancuronium and vecuronium, which are nondepolarizing (ND) muscle relaxants, and succinylcholine, which is a depolarizing (D) muscle relaxant, may be affected by several factors, which include the following:[47]

- Drug interactions
  — Antibiotics: Increase ND and D neuromuscular blockade
  — Anticholinesterases: Prolong response to succinylcholine
  — Antiarrhythmics: Increase ND neuromuscular blockade
  — Diuretics: Increase ND neuromuscular blockade
  — Local anesthetics: Enhance ND and D neuromuscular blockade
  — Volatile anesthetics: Augment degree and duration of ND neuromuscular blockade
  — Lithium: Prolongs ND and D neuromuscular blockade
  — Chlorpromazine: Prolongs ND neuromuscular blockade
  — Calcium channel blockers: Prolong ND neuromuscular blockade
- Electrolyte disturbances such as hypokalemia, hypocalcemia, and hypermagnesemia increase neuromuscular blockade
- Acid-base imbalance: Acidosis enhances ND neuromuscular blockade
- Hypothermia: Body temperature less than 34° C prolongs neuromuscular blockade
- Renal disease may prolong effect of pancuronium

Table 4-5 Doses and Characteristics of Commonly Used Neuromuscular Blockers

	Pancuronium	Vecuronium	Succinylcholine
Endotracheal intubation (mg/kg IV)	0.1	0.1	1-2
Maintenance relaxation (mg/kg IV)	0.03-0.05	0.025-0.05	
Onset of action (min)	1-3	3	1
Duration of action (min)	30-45	30-70	5-10
Vagolytic effect	Yes	No	Yes
Metabolism (%)	15-40	40%	
Elimination	Renal, 60%-80%; hepatic, 20%	Renal, 10%-20%; hepatic, 80%	Hydrolysis by pseudocholinesterase

- Hepatic disease may prolong effect of ND neuromuscular blockade
- Neuromuscular disease may be associated with an unpredictable response to any neuromuscular blocker

The neuromuscular blockers have the following cardiovascular side effects:

- Pancuronium: Tachycardia, hypertension
- Vecuronium: No undesirable hemodynamic side effects when used alone
- Succinylcholine: Bradycardia, junctional arrhythmias, asystole

In conclusion, this section has reviewed the more commonly used anesthetic and analgesic agents for patients undergoing cardiac surgery. Remember that the patient may have a systemic pathophysiology that can affect the potency, duration of action, and side effects of these agents. Renal and hepatic dysfunction, cerebral vascular disease, pulmonary disease, and endocrine abnormalities can complicate the postoperative care of these patients. Disorders of renal and hepatic systems can prolong the effects of many of the intravenous agents. These factors must be kept in mind when these patients are cared for in the postoperative period.

Operative Procedure

Preparation

Skin preparation consists of:

- Three scrubs with chlorhexidine gluconate
- Shaving of the patient in the OR
- Single application of an alcohol/iodophor solution in a water insoluble polymer base (Dura Prep)

For the majority of open heart procedures the patient is positioned supine on the operating table. Proper positioning of the patient for cardiac surgery is important, to maximize exposure and minimize the risk of skin trauma at pressure areas. The elbows and heels of the patient are appropriately padded. The patient's head is rotated approximately every 20 minutes during the course of the operation to prevent occipital alopecia. The electrocautery grounding pad is placed on the lateral aspect of the patient's thigh. Cautery burns can be reduced if preparation solution is prevented from pooling at dependent skin sites. For routine median sternotomies a double layer of hospital sheets formed into a roll approximately 5 × 24 inches is placed under the patient's shoulders to elevate the chest (Fig. 4-1, *A*).

To reduce brachial plexus injuries, arms are placed at the patient's side and not hyperabducted. Sponge padding is used at the elbows, feet, and head to prevent nerve damage or skin breakdown from pressure at these sites. Previously placed arterial, central venous or Swan-Ganz catheters, and the Foley catheter, are secured and connections are all checked. Lines are brought to the head of the table and carefully positioned to avoid any kinking, obstruction, or pressure on the patient's skin.

A "bat wing" appliance (Fig. 4-1, *A*) is attached to the table to provide protection to the patient's face and endotracheal tube and to support the cardiac drapes. During the course of the operation it also provides a level area for instrument or suction placement (Fig. 4-1, *B*).

We use specially designed cardiac side drapes with adhesive on one side, and a special one-piece cardiac drape with plastic pockets that hold accessory equipment to the table such as cautery, suction tubing, and cold irrigation tubing.

Technique

A standard median sternotomy incision is made. Careful and detailed attention to hemostasis is carried out throughout the operation. Cannulation (Fig. 4-2) is carried out centrally in the majority of patients. The ascending aorta is always palpated before placement of the arterial cannula in an attempt to avoid areas of atherosclerosis. The preferred arterial cannula is a 22F Sarns cannula. Peripheral cannulation with the femoral artery is performed for patients requiring operation on the ascending aorta or certain reoperations, or if diffuse atherosclerosis is present in the ascending aorta.

Venous cannulation is usually performed with a two-stage single cannula. Two venous cannulas are used for operations on the mitral valve because retraction on the left atrium and atrial septum is inhibited by a large single tube and simultaneous obstruction of the superior vena cava can occur. Bicaval cannulation is also used in the majority of congenital heart cases, when the right side of the heart is opened, during tricuspid valve procedures, and during heart and heart-lung transplantations.

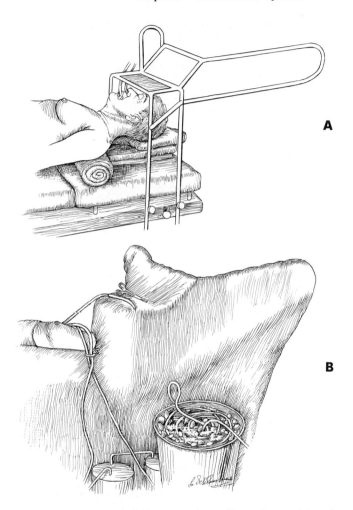

Fig. 4-1 A, Preparation of patient for bypass illustrating shoulder roll and bat-wing appliance for protection of patient's face and for facilitation of draping. **B,** Draping of patient with use of the bat-wing appliance, which provides level area for instrument and suction placement. Coil through which cold saline solution is run for topical cooling of heart during period of ischemic arrest is placed in ice. Automatic suction returns pericardial lavage to multiple containers.

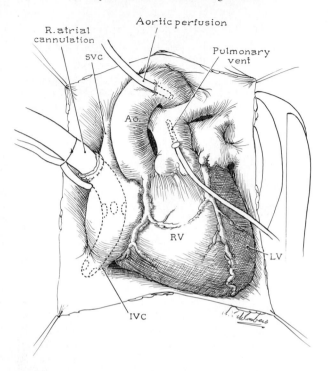

Fig. 4-2 Cannulation of heart with dual-stage venous cannula, a 22-gauge arterial cannula and a 14F vent placed in main pulmonary artery.

A 14F vent (Argyle) is placed in the main pulmonary artery for virtually all operations (Fig. 4-2). Because much effort is expended to maintain the heart temperature at less than 15° C, the pooling of collateral blood (systemic temperature 25° to 30° C) in the left ventricle can warm the subendocardial surface. Because no valves exist in the pulmonary circulation, this simple maneuver reduces noncoronary blood return to the left ventricle and provides a clear field for coronary bypass operations, aortic and mitral valve replacement procedures, and other open heart operations. A left atrial vent placed through the right superior pulmonary vein is used by some surgeons during aortic valvular procedures.

Cardiopulmonary Bypass

Cardiopulmonary bypass is the diversion of venous blood from the right atrium or vena cavae to an extracorporeal pump oxygenator.[20,33-35,41] After gas exchange has taken place, the oxygenated blood is returned to the arterial system of the patient. This technique is so named because the heart and lungs are effectively "removed" from the circulatory system.

Homeostasis

The maintenance of a homeostatic milieu is the primary objective during extracorporeal circulation. Many alterations to normal physiologic principles are caused by this artificial circulatory process. Cardiopulmonary bypass is managed to optimize and correct constantly the changing status of the patient.

Hemodynamic Support

The maintenance of arterial pressure is an important principle of cardiopulmonary bypass.[28,36] The arterial pressure during bypass is critical for homeostasis. Cerebral blood flow is directly determined by pressure. The kidneys and many other organs are highly sensitive to changes in arterial blood pressure. Venous blood pressure is also of critical value during bypass. The gravity drainage of venous blood creates a negative pressure at the cannulation site. This facilitates the drainage of blood and the avoidance of venous hypertension. Increased venous pressure has been associated with edema, and organ and tissue dysfunction, during cardiopulmonary bypass.

The rate of blood flow during bypass is also critical. The flow required to meet metabolic needs must be supplied at all times during extracorporeal circulation.[10,12] Adequate blood flow forestalls anaerobic metabolism. Constant monitoring of blood gases and venous saturation is used as an indicator of the adequacy of perfusion.[18]

Cardiopulmonary bypass must also provide adequate respiratory support in the absence of the patient's pulmonary circulation. Metabolic support is another fundamental requirement of bypass. The perfusate must provide the proper electrolytes and nutritive substrate for cellular function.[23]

Cardiopulmonary Bypass Circuit

The bypass circuit has several components that are chosen and assembled to facilitate optimal performance during a surgical procedure (Fig. 4-3).[43] Components are chosen to minimize the priming volume necessary (Table 4-6). Several components are based on patient size to provide optimal heat and gas exchange.

Table 4-6 Components of a Cardiopulmonary System

Item	Purpose
Oxygenator	Oxygenate and remove CO_2 from blood Cool and warm blood
Cardiotomy reservoir	Collect and filter blood from suction and vent blood
Heat exchanger	Systemically cools and warms patient
Bubble detector	Alarm sounds if bubbles are detected
Arterial filter	Remove gaseous and particulate microemboli from perfusate
Cannulas	Direct blood to and from bypass circuit
Cardioplegia tubing	Holds and administers cardioplegia solution
Monitors	Monitor blood gases, hematocrit, O_2 saturation, arterial line pressure

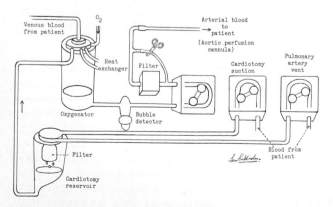

Fig. 4-3 Schematic illustration of heart-lung machine.

Circuit priming

The circuit prime is determined after the patient's requirements are evaluated as previously stated (Table 4-7). The components chosen to accomplish this then dictate the amount of prime necessary. The prime constituents are chosen to facilitate the maintenance of homeostasis.[29,40]

Hemodilution

The addition of an extracorporeal circulatory system in series with the patient will, by definition, greatly increase the circulating blood volume. Hemodilution has both positive and negative effects (Table 4-8). Blood can be added to the prime if the postdilutional hematocrit falls to less than acceptable levels (<20%). The diluted patient's hematocrit (Hct) can be calculated with the following equations:

$$\text{Blood volume} \times \text{Prebypass Hct} = \text{RBC volume} \tag{1}$$

$$\text{RBC volume} \div \text{Blood volume} + \text{Prime volume} = \text{Diluted Hct} \tag{2}$$

Table 4-7   Prime Constituents

Agent	Purpose
Crystalloid agents Ringer's lactate Balanced electrolyte solution	Hemodilution
Mannitol, albumin, hetastarch	Oncotic agents
Heparin	Anticoagulant
Sodium bicarbonate, tromethamine	Buffers
Blood	Increase O_2-carrying capacity

Table 4-8   Hemodilution

Advantages	Limitations	Major determinant
Reduced viscosity Reduced sludging Reduced homologous blood requirement Increased urine output	Decreased O_2 carrying capacity Increased tendency toward edema Dilution of coagulation factors	Patient's preoperative status

Anticoagulation/coagulation

The interaction of blood with the foreign surfaces of the bypass circuit and blood exposure to air necessitates systemic anticoagulation.[9] This is achieved by the administration of the anticoagulant heparin. The anticoagulation effect of heparin is the inhibition of the activated coagulation factors II, IX, X, and XI. The normal loading dose is 200 to 300 U per kilogram of body weight. Coagulation times are monitored frequently to ensure the adequacy of anticoagulation during the procedure.[25]

Protamine sulfate is the pharmacologic agent that reverses the effects of heparin. At the conclusion of the bypass period a protamine dose of 1 to 4 mg/100 U of administered heparin is given (Table 4-9). A return of the coagulation profile to normal is the desired end point.

Conduct of Bypass

Once the operative field has been prepared for bypass, a heparin loading dose is given. Cannulation can then proceed (see Fig. 4-2). Before bypass is started, adequate anticoagulation is confirmed with the activated clotting time. Bypass is initiated by opening the venous gravity drainage line to the oxygenator (see Fig. 4-3). This action rapidly creates a high negative pressure zone in the proximity of the venous cannula(s). Blood preferentially flows to the bypass circuit. The preload to the heart is progressively decreased until the aortic valve no longer opens. This is known as "total bypass." At this time systemic hypothermia may be employed. Cardioplegia is also used at the point when electromechanical cessation of the heart is required. During bypass all the parameters and indicators for adequacy of perfusion are monitored constantly to provide optimal homeostasis.

Table 4-9　Protamine Administration

Protocol: 1-4 mg/100 IU total heparin
Dose-response interpretation: 1-4 mg/100 IU "active" heparin
Protamine titration: 0.3-1.3 mg/100 IU titratable heparin

Protamine dose calculations are determined by any one of the above methods. Each technique differs by the parameter used for evaluating hemostasis (i.e., total heparin, active heparin, or reactive heparin).

Preservation Methods

Systemic hypothermia

Systemic hypothermia is a technique widely employed in conjunction with cardiopulmonary bypass. Hypothermia reduces the metabolic rate of tissues. It provides organ protection and preservation during the altered state of the cardiovascular system during cardiopulmonary bypass. The oxygen requirement for tissue metabolism is reduced 7% per 1° C reduction in core temperature. This translates to 50% reduction at 30° C and a reduction of the basal metabolic rate to 25% of normal value at 26° C. The selective vasodilation and vasoconstriction of central and peripheral vascular beds provides an uneven distribution of blood flow during cardiopulmonary bypass.[16, 22] The decrease in oxygen demand afforded by hypothermia reduces the incidence of anaerobic metabolism and the associated buildup of lactic acid metabolites.[37]

Different levels of hypothermia are employed in different situations. Four levels of hypothermia are summarized in Table 4-10.[31] The complexity of the surgical repair, age and overall medical status of the patient, and the surgeon's preference are all factors that determine the desired level of hypothermia.

Myocardial protection

The majority of open heart operations require a dry and nearly bloodless operative field. This environment is provided by cross-clamping the aorta, which necessitates a method of protecting the heart from ischemic damage. Hypothermia is the cornerstone of all myocardial protection techniques because myocardial oxygen demand diminishes with cooling. Systemic hypothermia to 25 to 30° C is used in virtually all patients.

The present technique of myocardial preservation used by the majority of surgeons at The Johns Hopkins Hospital consists of

Table 4-10   Categories of Systemic Hypothermia

Level of hypothermia	Temperature range (°C)
Mild	32-37
Moderate	28-31
Deep	18-27
Profound	<18

an aortic root infusion of 500 ml of a crystalloid cardioplegia solution (potassium chloride, 25 mEq/L; sodium bicarbonate, 25 mEq/L; mannitol, 12.5 g/L; and D_5W) by hand or pressure bag (150 mm Hg) administration.[1,26,27,32] For patients with aortic regurgitation who are undergoing aortic valve replacement, the aortic root is opened after ventricular fibrillation and cardioplegia is administered directly with cannulas into each of the coronary ostia. Topical cold is simultaneously initiated with cardioplegia administration (Fig. 4-4). Saline solution stored at 4° C is passed through an iced coil, and the topical solution is delivered into the pericardial well at a temperature of 2° to 4° C (Fig. 4-5). An automatic suction removes the solution from the field. This rapid turnover of saline solution prevents warming of the heart and has been documented to maintain temperature at less than 15° C during the course of the operation. For ischemic periods extending beyond 2 hours,

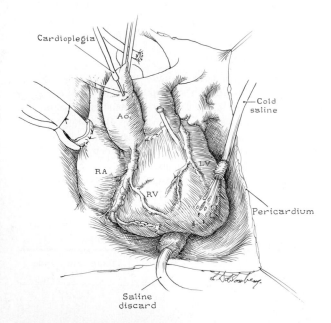

Fig. 4-4 Initial arrest of heart with antegrade crystalloid cardioplegia solution and topical cold saline solution.

low-potassium (5 mEq/L) cardioplegia solution is repeatedly administered to provide additional cooling to the heart.

The route of cardioplegia administration is most often directed in an antegrade fashion.[14] The solution is administered into the aortic root after the aorta is cross-clamped. It is then delivered at a pressure high enough (150 mm Hg) to ensure the complete and constant closure of the aortic valve. This directs the solution into

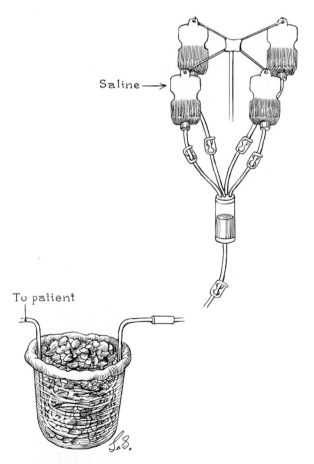

Saline →

To patient

Fig. 4-5 Technique for providing continuous topical cold saline solution to pericardial well.

the coronary ostia and throughout the coronary circulation. This method of administration provides a convenient and rapid achievement of arrest and cooling.

The application of topical cold (4° C) saline solution greatly facilitates cooling of the myocardium, especially with severe atherosclerosis. The combination of aortic root cardioplegia and topical saline solution rapidly (5 minutes) and consistently lowers the myocardial core temperature despite the severity of the coronary artery stenoses. Retrograde administration of cardioplegia through the coronary sinus is a technique receiving increased attention for patients with diffuse disease. It is beneficial in patients undergoing repeated operations for coronary artery disease and in patients with aortic regurgitation in whom the valve is not going to be replaced.

Profound hypothermia with circulatory arrest

For a variety of congenital operations and for those involving the ascending aorta and aortic arch the use of profound hypothermia and circulatory arrest is necessary. Through systemic cooling the patient's temperature is lowered to approximately 13° C. Ice is placed around the head to prevent rewarming.[7] Particular attention is given to protecting the skin from direct contact with the ice by first covering the skin with towels. At this point cardiopulmonary bypass is stopped and blood is drained into the oxygenator. The arterial and venous cannulas can be either clamped or removed to facilitate the operative procedure. While the patient's heart is arrested recirculation of the cardiopulmonary bypass prime continues. This technique has been carried out repeatedly and is relatively safe up to approximately 60 minutes of arrest time.

Important Aspects of the Operative Procedure
Left ventricular dilatation

During the course of the operation, attention should always be directed to the possibility of left ventricular distention. Left ventricular distention, especially in the normothermic heart, can produce severe subendocardial ischemia and result in left ventricular dysfunction. Left ventricular distention results from aortic valve incompetence. This can occur despite a lack of clinical evidence of aortic regurgitation. This is described as "pump aortic insufficiency." The presence of left ventricular distention is checked by direct palpation of the left ventricle. Manual decompression of the left ventricle is sometimes necessary while the heart is fibrillating.

Once the heart is defibrillated it generally remains decompressed. However, if there is any question that left ventricular distension is present, a vent can be placed either through the left ventricular apex or through the right superior pulmonary vein and directed into the left ventricular cavity.

Intracardiac air

We favor pulmonary artery venting for the majority of myocardial revascularization procedures because it prevents the need to open the left side of the heart, thereby minimizing the potential of air accumulation on the left side of the heart. However, during valve replacement, aneurysmectomy, ascending aorta replacement, transplantation, and most congenital defect repair procedures the presence of intracardiac air has necessitated maneuvers to eliminate it. Because air rises, the patient is placed in the Trendelenburg position and a needle stick in the highest point of the ascending aorta usually allows escape of air during left ventricular ejection. Air can also be aspirated from the apex of the left ventricle or from the superior aspect of the left atrium. Generally, however, a simple vent site in the ascending aorta results in the evacuation of the majority of air. The transesophageal echo can be used to assess intracardial air.

Localized dissections and embolization

Friable, diseased, and atherosclerotic aortas are increasingly encountered as the age of the patient undergoing cardiac surgery increases. A local dissection can occur at the aortic cross-clamp site, proximal coronary artery graft anastomosis, aortic cannulation site, or cardioplegia administration site. Once the dissection is recognized, immediate attention and correction are necessary to prevent its extension. Atherosclerotic debris or cholesterol emboli can be dislodged with insertion of the aortic cannula or application of a clamp. Palpation before manipulation is not always successful in detecting aortic plaque.

Blood conservation

Because of the incidence of hepatitis and other blood-borne viruses, recent efforts to decrease blood use have resulted in an increasing number of patients receiving minimal or no blood or blood products. A variety of techniques are used, including:

- Crystalloid priming of the cardiopulmonary bypass circuit
- Autologous blood donation

- Cell saving during the operation
- Preoperative hemodilution
- Postoperative administration of chest tube drainage (auto-transfusion)

Weaning from cardiopulmonary bypass

Systemic rewarming is initiated approximately 30 minutes before the expected time of discontinuation of cardiopulmonary bypass. Although systemic rewarming to a core (nasopharyngeal) temperature of 37° C occurs in the majority of cases, the patient's peripheral (rectal) temperature is often 2° to 5° C cooler, so the core temperature often drifts lower between the completion of cardiopulmonary bypass and chest closure as the temperature equilibrates. This is the primary reason that patients arrive in the intensive care unit with some degree of hypothermia.

During the period of cardiopulmonary bypass the heart is maintained in a flaccid, low-pressure state. Gravity drainage of venous blood and direct cardiac venting ensures this. At the conclusion of the surgical repair the heart is allowed to fill slowly and eject as necessary to support the patient. The cooperative efforts of all members of the OR staff are required for the successful weaning of the patient from cardiopulmonary bypass. Several factors determine the strategy and the manner in which this process is implemented (Table 4-11).

Optimization of the weaning process is accomplished by diligent monitoring of several homeostatic parameters. Acid-base, temperature, and hemoglobin values must be corrected before separation from cardiopulmonary bypass is attempted.

At the direction of the attending surgeon and anesthesiologist the weaning process is initiated. Ventilation of the lungs is initiated in anticipation of the return of pulmonary blood flow. Venous

Table 4-11   Factors Affecting Weaning from Cardiopulmonary Bypass

Preoperative hemodynamics
Preoperative cardiac performance
Adequacy of myocardial protection
Surgical repair
Ischemic time
Postrepair myocardial performance

drainage is then slowly restricted to allow the patient's blood to pass preferentially into the right atrium, through the tricuspid valve, and into the right ventricle. As the wall of the right ventricle is stretched, the pressure surpasses the resistance of the pulmonary circulation, causing pulmonary blood flow. As the flow through the pulmonary circuit increases, a concomitant increase in left heart pressures occurs. The pressure increases until the afterload provided by the aortic valve is surpassed. The blood flow of the cardiopulmonary bypass circuit is decreased as the patient's heart generates a cardiac output. The venous line of the bypass circuit is then clamped, and the patient is "transfused" from the circuit until a satisfactory cardiac output is achieved. When this is accomplished the forward flow of the bypass circuit is discontinued.

A period of stabilization is required because of the transition from artificial circulation. During this time variations in hemodynamic performance may be wide. After a steady state has been reached, the cannulas are removed and hemostasis is achieved by administration of protamine sulfate as described earlier. The remaining contents of the bypass circuit can then be transfused directly to the patient or centrifuged to concentrate the red blood cells.

With present cardiac preservation techniques the majority of patients who have normal left ventricular function preoperatively can be weaned from cardiopulmonary bypass with little to no vasopressor support. The use of the intraaortic balloon pump for postcardiotomy is infrequent. However, in the event that standard vasopressor and inotropic support such as dobutamine, epinephrine, or amrinone are unable to provide effective cardiac output, the intraaortic balloon is placed percutaneously through the right or left femoral artery. The choice of using the right or left femoral artery is based on the preoperative history and physical examination (claudication, pulses), and information (difficulty passing a guide wire), derived from cardiac catheterization. The technique of intraaortic balloon insertion is described in Chapter 7. If the intraaortic balloon pump in combination with vasopressor and inotropic support is inadequate in maintaining cardiac output, left and/or right ventricular assist devices may be inserted if the patient is a candidate for such devices. The details of insertion and maintenance of these assist devices are also described in Chapter 7.

After discontinuation of cardiopulmonary bypass, decannulation takes place and protamine is administered. Protamine is given

74   The Johns Hopkins Manual of Cardiac Surgical Care

slowly because of its potentially harmful effects.[24] It can cause pulmonary hypertension and profound systemic hypotension. Attention to hemostasis is paramount to prevent excessive bleeding and the possible return of the patient to the OR for reexploration.[3] In recent years the takeback rate at The Johns Hopkins Hospital has decreased from 4.5% in 1983 to 2.2% in 1992. Because the internal mammary artery is used as a graft in more than 95% of the patients undergoing bypass operation, two chest tubes are used: one in the mediastinum and one in the left side of the chest. Temporary epicardial atrial and ventricular pacing wires are inserted in the majority of patients. The chest is closed in a standard manner with interrupted wires, and the skin is approximated with either a subcuticular suture technique or staples.

References

1. Addetia AM et al: Study on myocardial contractility after cardiopulmonary bypass versus cardioplegic arrest in an air-ejecting in vivo heart model, *Ann Thorac Surg* 41(3):260-264, 1986.
2. Arunasalam K, Davenport HT, Painter S, Jones JG: Ventilatory response to morphine in young and old subjects, *Anaesthesia* 38:529-533, 1983.
3. Barnette RE, Shupak RC, Pontius J, Rao AK: In vitro effect of fresh frozen plasma on the activated coagulation time in patients undergoing cardiopulmonary bypass, *Anesth Analg* 67:(1):57-60, 1988.
4. Bovill JG, Sebel PS: Pharmacokinetics of high-dose fentanyl: a study in patients undergoing cardiac surgery, *Br J Anaesth* 52:795-802, 1980.
5. Bovill JG et al: The pharmacokinetics of sufentanil in surgical patients, *Anesthesiology* 61:502-506, 1984.
6. Bovill JG, Sebel PS, Stanley TH: Opioid analgesics in anesthesia: with special reference to their use in cardiovascular anesthesia, *Anesthesiology* 61:731-755, 1984.
7. Coselli JS et al: Determination of brain temperatures for safe circulatory arrest during cardiovascular operation, *Ann Thorac Surg* 45(6):638-642, 1988.
8. Daniel EE, Sutherland WH, Bogoch A: Effects of morphine and other drugs on the motility of the terminal ileum, *Gastroenterology* 36:510-523, 1959.
9. Dawids SG, ed: *Physiological and clinical aspects of oxygenator design,* Luxembourg, 1976, Elsevier/North-Holland Biomedical Press.
10. Del Canale S et al: Effects of low flux-low pressure cardiopulmonary bypass on intracellular acid-base and water metabolism, *Scand J Thorac Cardiovasc Surg* 20(2):167-170, 1986.

11. de Large S et al: Comparison of sufentanil-O_2 for coronary artery surgery, *Anesthesiology* 56:112-118, 1982.

12. Dolman J et al: The effect of temperature, mean arterial pressure, and cardiopulmonary bypass flows on somatosensory evoked potential latency in man, *Thorac Cardiovasc Surg* 34(4):217-222, 1986.

13. Economou G, Ward-McQuaid JN: A cross-over comparison of the effect of morphine, pethidine, pentazocine and phenazocine on biliary pressure, *Gut* 12:218-221, 1971.

14. Engelman RM, Levitsky S, eds: *A textbook of clinical cardioplegia,* Mount Kisco, NY, 1982, Futura.

15. Eriksen J, Berthelsen P, Ahn NC, Rasmussen JP: Early response of control hemodyanmics to high doses of sufentanil or morphine in dogs, *Acta Anaesth Scand* 25:33-38, 1981.

16. Feddersen K, Aren C, Nilsson NJ, Radegran K: Cerebral blood flow and metabolism during cardiopulmonary bypass with special reference to effects of hypotension induced by prostacyclin, *Ann Thorac Surg* 41(4):395-400, 1986.

17. Flacke JN, Kripke BK, Bloor BC: Intraoperative effectiveness of sufentanil, fentanyl, meperidine or morphine in balanced anesthesia: a double-blind study, *Anesth Analg* 62:259-263, 1983.

18. Henriksen L: Brain luxury perfusion during cardiopulmonary bypass in humans: a study of the cerebral blood flow response to changes in CO_2, O_2, and blood pressure, *J Cereb Blood Flow Metab* 6(3):366-378, 1986.

19. Hsu HO, Hickey RF, Forbes AR: Morphine decreases peripheral vascular resistance and increases capacitance in man, *Anesthesiology* 50:98-102, 1979.

20. Ionescu MI, ed: *Techniques in extracorporeal circulation,* ed 2, London, 1981, Butterworth.

21. Jaffe JH, Martin WR: Opioid analgesics and antagonists. In Gilman AG, Goodman LS, Gilman A, eds: *The pharmacological basis of therapeutics,* New York: 1985, Macmillan.

22. Johnsson P et al: Cerebral blood flow and autoregulation during hypothermic cardiopulmonary bypass, *Ann Thorac Surg* 43(4):386-390, 1987.

23. Kancir CB, Madsen T, Petersen PH, Stokke D: Calcium, magnesium and phosphate during and after hypothermic cardiopulmonary bypass without temperature correction of acid base status, *Acta Anaesthesiol Scand* 32(8):676-680, 1988.

24. Kesteven PJ et al: Protamine sulphate and heparin rebound following open-heart surgery, *J Cardiovasc Surg (Torino)* 27(5):600-603, 1986.

25. Kesteven PJ, Pasaoglu I, Williams BT, Savidge GF: Significance of the whole blood activated clotting time in cardiopulmonary bypass, *J Cardiovasc Surg (Torino)* 27(1):85-89, 1986.

26. Krukenkamp I et al: Myocardial energetics after thermally graded

hyperkalemic crystalloid cardioplegic arrest, *J Thorac Cardiovasc Surg* 92(1):56-62, 1986.

27. Landymore RW et al: Prevention of myocardial electrical activity during ischemic arrest with verapamil cardioplegia, *Ann Thorac Surg* 43(5):534-538, 1987.

28. Levy JH, Hug CC Jr: Use of cardiopulmonary bypass in studies of the circulation, *Br J Anaesth* 60(suppl 1):35S-37S, 1988 (review article).

29. Lumb PD: A comparison between 25% albumin and 6% hydroxyethyl starch solutions on lung water accumulation during and immediately after cardiopulmonary bypass, *Ann Surg* 206:210-213, 1987.

30. Meeker MH, Rothrock JC: *Alexander's care of the patient in surgery,* ed 9, St Louis, 1991, Mosby.

31. Miyamoto K et al: Optimal perfusion flow rate for the brain during deep hypothermic cardiopulmonary bypass at 20 degrees C: an experimental study, *J Thorac Cardiovasc Surg* 92(6):1065-1070, 1986.

32. Mullen JC et al: Right ventricular function: a comparison between blood and crystalloid cardioplegia, *Ann Thorac Surg* 43(1):17-24, 1987.

33. Pierce EC II: *Extracorporeal circulation for open-heart surgery: pathophysiology, apparatus, and methods including the special techniques of hypothermia and hyperbaric oxygenation,* Springfield, Ill, 1969, Charles C Thomas.

34. Reed CC, Kurusz M, Lawrence AE Jr: *Safety and techniques in perfusion,* Stafford, Tex, 1988, Quali-Med.

35. Reed CC, Clark DK: *Cardiopulmonary perfusion,* Houston, 1975, Texas Medical Press.

36. Rogers AT et al: Response of cerebral blood flow to phenylephrine infusion during hypothermic cardiopulmonary bypass: influence of $PaCO_2$ management, *Anesthesiology* 69:547-551, 1988.

37. Sanford TJ, Smith T, Dec-Silver H, Harrison WK: A comparison of morphine, fentanyl and sufentanil anesthesia for cardiac surgery: induction, emergence and extubation, *Anesth Analg* 65:259-266, 1986.

38. Shanks CA: Pharmacokinetics of the nondepolarizing neuromuscular relaxants applied to calculation of bolus in infusion dosage regimens, *Anesthesiology* 64:72-86, 1986.

39. Stanski DR, Greenblatt DJ, Lowenstein E: Kinetics of intravenous and intramuscular morphine, *Clin Pharmacol Ther* 24:52-59, 1978.

40. Stone JJ et al: Hemodynamic, metabolic, and morphological effects of cardiopulmonary bypass with a fluorocarbon priming solution, *Ann Thorac Surg* 41(4):419-424, 1986.

41. Taylor KM, ed: *Cardiopulmonary bypass: principles and management,* London, 1986, Chapman & Hall.

42. The Association of Operating Room Nurses: *Standards and recommended practices for perioperative nursing,* Denver, 1990, AORN.

43. van Oeveren W, Dankert J, Wildevuur CR: Bubble oxygenation and cardiotomy suction impair the host defense during cardiopulmonary bypass: a study in dogs, *Ann Thorac Surg* 44(5):523-528, 1987.

44. Wells MMP: *Decision making in perioperative nursing,* Philadelphia, 1987, BC Decker.

45. White PF, Way WL, Trevor AJ: Ketamine: its pharmacology and therapeutic uses, *Anesthesiology* 56:119-136, 1982.

46. Wood M: Intravenous anesthetic agents. In Wood M, Wood AJJ, eds: *Drugs and anesthesia,* ed 2, Baltimore, 1990, Williams & Wilkins.

47. Wood M: Neuromuscular blocking agents. In Wood M, Wood AJJ, eds: *Drugs and anesthesia,* ed 2, Baltimore, 1990, Williams & Wilkins.

48. Wood M: Opioid agonists and antagonists. In Wood M, Wood AJJ, eds, *Drugs and anesthesia,* ed 2, Baltimore, 1990, Williams & Wilkins.

General Principles, Organization, and Management of the Intensive Care Unit

5

Jo Marie Walrath, Sharon G. Owens, and William A. Baumgartner

Cardiac surgery is a division of the department of surgical sciences at The Johns Hopkins Hospital (JHH). Patients undergoing cardiac surgery are provided preoperative, intraoperative, and postoperative nursing care within this division. Until 1987 the initial critical care (CC) phase of the postoperative management of cardiac patients occurred in a general surgical intensive care unit (ICU). The disadvantage to this approach was that cardiac nursing was not viewed as a speciality; although nurses brought excellent skills and knowledge to the patient, cardiac care was only one area of their generalized skills. Competition between surgical services for valuable CC bed space was a daily issue. Additionally, patients who could benefit from a slightly prolonged stay were often transferred from the CC area to accommodate patients who required more immediate care. Primarily for these reasons a decision was made to plan an ICU dedicated solely to patients undergoing cardiac surgery.

This chapter focuses on the organization and planning strategies used in expanding an open heart surgical program. Basic principles for planning facility expansion, personnel allocation, supply and equipment procurement, acquisition and inventory, and medical and nursing management are discussed.

Planning

An executive decision was made to allocate space and finances for this project. A cardiac surgical intensive care unit (CSICU) steering committee was established to plan and proceed with determining surgical needs. This committee was interdisciplinary, with representation from medicine, nursing, administration, finance, clinical engineering, pharmacy, and architectural services.

Assessment

The process for designing a new program or expanding an existing ICU for the care of adult or pediatric patients after open heart surgery begins with an assessment (Table 5-1) by the steering committee.

This assessment includes reviewing the internal and external environment. An environmental scan of the community population, health needs, referral base, and required services is done to gain a perspective of the amount of service and beds required and the resources needed to support the defined service level.

Table 5-1   Assessment

External Environmental Scan

Community health needs and resources
Cardiac services provided in local and regional area
Referral base
Labor pool availability

Internal Scan

ICU location
Patient day forecast
Average length of stay by case mix
Cost per patient day
Patient flow (preoperative to discharge)
New program funding
Clinical and support space
Adjacencies to operating suites, inpatient units, labs, etc.
Personnel resources
Ancillary services
Computer information support and interface

The internal assessment consists of identifying the number of patients that will be managed by the institution, the average length of stay, available space for construction, and the facility constraints. Special points to consider in establishing a location are adjacencies to other facilities that are critical to the ICU such as operating suites, cardiovascular diagnostic laboratories, radiologic services, and laboratories.

Plan

Once this assessment is completed, the steering committee uses the data to establish broad goals and objectives, identify subcommittees with specific tasks to accomplish, and define a timetable for task completion (Table 5-2).

The chairs of each subcommittee meet regularly with the steering committee to review progress, discuss problems, and readjust time frames as needed.

The steering committee also meets with other hospital depart-

Table 5-2   Planning Committee Structure

Committee	Prime responsibilities
Steering	Define expected outcomes of planning process
	Establish subcommittees to meet goals and objectives
	Establish and monitor compliance to time-table
Subcommittees	
Patient flow	Identify patient flow from preadmission to discharge
	Define admission and discharge criteria
Personnel	Define staffing requirements
Equipment	Define monitoring system criteria
	Identify major and minor capital needs
	Identify daily par levels of routine stock
Facilities and design	Review floor plans; ensure adequate support and staff space
Finance	Submit operating and capital budgets
Support services	Identify interface with other hospital services

ments to discuss the new program. These departments then become responsible for determining the effect of the new program on their service levels and for requesting appropriate capital and human resources to meet the new demand.

Design and Construction

As the plans are developed, persons who are directly involved in providing care should be involved with reviewing the designs and providing input into the decisions. A mock-up of the floor plan helps to visualize the plans and allows for experimenting with various scenarios before final decisions are made. Developing a strong working relationship among nursing staff, physicians, the architects, and the facility design personnel is critical. The perspective each brings is unique yet extremely interdependent on the other. As plans are implemented, regular on-site visits to the construction site and frequent meetings with the builders and architect are necessary. This expedites problem solving and prevents costly construction errors.

Although the prime goal is to design an environment to provide direct patient care, other considerations critical to the unit design are space allocations that comply with fire and safety regulations and provision of sufficient support space.

During review of the requirements of Joint Commission on Accreditation of Healthcare Organizations (JCAHO),[5] consideration should be given to direct or indirect visualization of patients, central monitors, and the need for a "monitor observer." Design decisions ultimately drive the numbers and types of personnel required; therefore coordination between the personnel task force and the design group is essential.

Categories of support space identified are as follows:

- Supplies and equipment: Capital and daily operating
- Staff: Physician, nursing, secretarial
- Visitors: Family, clergy
- Medication: Preparation, storage, and distribution
- Communication: Rounds, conferences, documentation, computer information, consultations

Equipment

Because of the high technologic needs of the unit, a group was identified to define equipment issues. These included weekly and capital, noncapital, and daily and weekly supply needs. All supplies and equipment requested are reviewed by supply managers and nurses to prevent any oversights and delays. Staging equipment evaluation, ordering supplies, and training becomes critical as the unit approaches opening day.

All equipment should be safety tested through clinical engineering services before installation and operation in the unit. In addition, equipment that requires evaluation before purchase should be procured several months in advance of the unit's opening date to allow time for order, delivery, evaluation, and staff in-services. Staff education should include both a didactic and hands-on experience.

Nursing Organization

Nursing management within the department has responsibility for the development of specific nursing practice standards and policies, daily operations, program planning and implementation, budget and resource allocation, and personnel management. Many of these responsibilities ultimately reside with a nurse manager at the nursing unit level.[2]

The department of surgical nursing at JHH provides nursing services to 23 operating suites (GOH), 14 general surgery intensive care (SICU) beds, 12 cardiac surgery intensive care beds (CSICU), 16 intermediate intensive care (IMC) beds, 180 inpatient beds, outpatient clinics, postanesthesia recovery unit, and a same-day admission/ambulatory care center.

Resources allocated specifically to the care and management of the cardiac patient include 4 cardiac general operating room suites, a 12-bed CSICU, 8 beds within an intermediate care unit, and 30 inpatient beds.

Each of these areas is managed by a nurse manager. Fig. 5-1 depicts JHH's decentralized organizational model as it relates only to the services dedicated to the care of the patient with cardiac disorders.

Personnel

According to the JCAHO, "each special care unit is properly directed and staffed according to the nature of the special patient care needs anticipated and scope of services provided."[5] Staffing patterns can be validated with a reliable and valid patient classi-

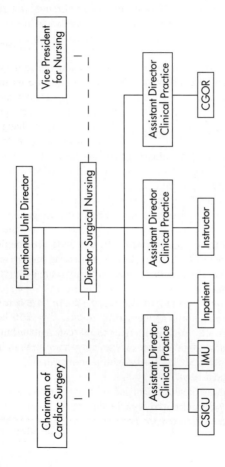

Fig. 5-1 Organizational structure of department of surgery with division of cardiac surgery

fication system. In the absence of a classification system, staffing patterns and standard hours per patient day (HPPD) are determined by the nurse managers' clinical judgment, historical trends, and review of other comparable hospitals' staffing ratios. Although each nursing unit delivers different nursing HPPD, all standards are derived from one staffing method. The following describes the method used to establish the unit personnel budget.

Establish Fixed and Variable Nursing Positions

Fixed staffing is defined as positions that are required irrespective of changes in patient census. Variable positions are those which increase or decrease proportionately with changes in patient census (Table 5-3).[1] A more realistic approach is to have some positions denoted as semivariable; that is, the staffing need changes with volume but not proportionately. It is important to note that if volume consistently dropped or increased, fixed costs would have to be altered accordingly.

Calculate Nonproductive Time

Nonproductive time is defined as time paid but not actually worked[1] (Table 5-4). Historical trends are the basis for the calculation. Time allocated as nonproductive differs among hospitals. Paid hours, 2080 hours per full-time equivalent (FTE) minus nonproductive hours, is the formula for calculating productive or actual worked hours.

Each FTE on an average provides 1824 productive hours (2080 paid hours minus 256 nonproductive hours). The 256 hours of nonproductive time is calculated into the required staffing needs of the unit. Ignoring the replacement of this time results in long-term understaffing.

Table 5-3   Fixed and Variable Personnel Positions

Fixed	Variable
Nurse manager	RN
Charge nurse	
Instructor	
Nursing unit clerk	
Nursing support technician	
Supply clerk	

***Table* 5-4** Nonproductive Paid Hours

Nonproductive time	Paid days	Hours
Sick	7	56
Holiday	8	64
Vacation	15	120
Personal leave	2	16
Total	32	256

Determine Required Staffing at 100% Occupancy

Calculation of required staffing is converted into a staffing standard per patient day. The following formulas give the staffing levels required:

$$\text{Staff per 24 hours} \times \text{Factor for days off} \times \text{Factor for nonproductive time} = \text{Total FTEs required} \tag{1}$$

$$\frac{\text{Required positions per 2080-hour shift/FTE)}}{\text{Forecasted patient days}} = \text{Paid HPPD} \tag{2}$$

Establish Staffing Pattern for Forecasted Annual Patient Days

Staffing patterns are determined once volume is forecasted. Forecasted volume depends on past trends, the potential for expanding market share, or emergence of competition for the same service and patient population. Required staffing is determined as follows:

$$\frac{(\text{Paid hrs/patient day}) \, (\text{Forecasted volume})}{2080 \text{ hrs}} = \text{Required FTEs}$$

Final Staffing Plan

Table 5-5 exemplifies the final staffing plan determined appropriate for the CSICU. Assumptions made by the nurse manager to establish this pattern were as follows:
- 12 beds
- Total capacity 4380 patient days
- Variable staffing
  —Six admissions daily requiring a registered nurse (RN) patient ratio of 1:1
  —Six patients requiring an RN patient ratio of 1:2

Table 5-5 Nonproductive and Productive Hours and FTES for Fiscal Year 1992

	FTE			HPPD		
	NP	P	Paid	NP	P	Paid
Nurse manager	0.13	0.87	1.00	0.07	0.49	0.56
RN	4.80	32.12	36.92	2.69	18.00	20.69
Specialty technician	1.04	6.96	8.00	0.58	3.90	4.48
Nursing unit clerk	0.48	3.23	3.71	0.27	1.81	2.08
Total	6.45	43.18	49.63	3.61	24.20	27.81

Forecasted 1992 patient days for CSICU: 3712.

NP, Nonproductive; *P*, productive.

- Fixed staffing
  - —One nurse manager
  - —Two nursing unit clerks on day shift; one on evening shift
  - —Two nursing specialty technicians per shift

Medical Management

The CSICU is codirected by designated members of the cardiac attending surgical staff. Fig. 5-2 depicts the relationship between the medical structure of the CSICU and the JHH decentralized system. These codirectors are board certified in thoracic and cardiovascular surgery and are qualified to provide care for the critically ill surgical patients and to manage thoracic and cardiovascular emergencies. Other responsibilities include the following:

- Reviewing, revising, and establishing policies, procedures, and protocols in conjunction with nursing and house staff that optimizes patient care.
- Facilitating or limiting the admission and transfer of patients to and from the unit on the basis of preestablished criteria, patient safety, capacity, staffing patterns, and quality care.
- Monitoring and evaluating patient care issues with a quality assurance coordinator. Patient issues and problems are reviewed on a monthly basis with the coordinator and a plan of action is established for the resolution of these issues. Specific issues addressed include the use of infection control, blood products, antibiotics, and invasive lines. Attending physicians, cardiac surgical fellows, and house staff address patient-related problems and issues at a monthly morbidity and mortality conference.[3]

The attending physician of record is responsible for the care and treatment of his or her patients while they are in the CSICU and throughout their hospitalization. Chief residents, first- and second-year cardiac surgical fellows, and second- and third-post graduate-year (PGY 2 and 3) surgical residents (house staff) provide direct care under the supervision of the attending physician and in coordination with the designated plan and critical pathway.

Under direct supervision of the chief resident, PGY 2 and 3 surgical residents are responsible for admission and transfer orders; daily patient orders; documentation of the patient's progress, status, and events; communication of status and events to fellows; chief residents and attending staff; and institution of emergency

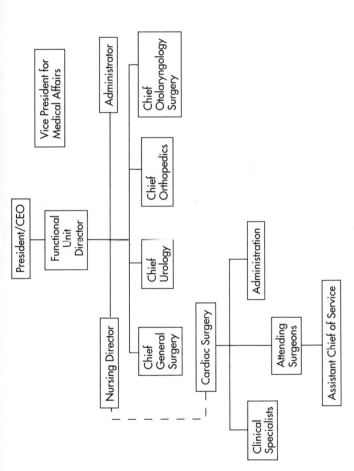

Fig. 5-2 Medical organizational structure of cardiac surgery division.

procedures in the absence of senior cardiac surgical fellows. PGY 2 and 3 residents and first-year cardiac surgical fellows provide in-hospital medical coverage for the CSICU on a 24-hour basis. Chief residents provide 24-hour coverage by telephone or beeper.

Initial orientation and ongoing education of house staff occurs in a variety of forums. A well-established orientation program occurs on the first day of the clinical rotation in the CSICU. The orientation includes but is not limited to the review of location and use of emergency equipment, surgical chain of command for clinical issues and emergencies, written protocols and standards, and general CC management of patients with cardiac disease. Orientation is supplemented with a written manual regarding cardiothoracic patient care.

Ongoing education is provided through monthly in-services by the attending and cardiac surgical fellow staff on topics related to care of patient thoracic and cardiovascular disease, and treatment of complications and interventions in emergency situations. Monthly journal club and morbidity and mortality meetings and daily rounds serve as forums to discuss relevant patient care issues and current trends in cardiothoracic surgery.

Role of the Nurse Manager

The nurse manager of the CSICU plays a critical role in the daily operations of the unit and in long-range planning.

The nurse manager has 24-hour responsibility for the functioning of the unit. This includes assuring adherence to defined standards of care, personnel management and labor allocations, fiscal accountability, supply and equipment standards, quality assurance, and new program planning.[4]

Personnel management includes a wide variety of responsibilities such as:
- Establishing unit staffing needs
- Selecting qualified personnel
- Allocating resources against need
- Providing required specialty education and ongoing in-services
- Evaluating performance
- Terminating personnel if performance is unsatisfactory

The nurse manager is responsible and accountable for the labor budget for the nursing unit.[3] Responsibilities include:
- Defining a staffing pattern based on patient acuity and forecasted volumes

- Determining a standard for paid productive HPPD
- Monitoring labor expense against budget with rationale for all variances
- Managing expenses within a budget level

Procurement of supplies and equipment, establishment of inventory par levels, capital requests, and performance monitoring (use against budget) is a joint responsibility between the nurse manager and the supply and equipment manager. Input by the nurse manager is critical because all supplies and equipment issues are derived from clinical policies, procedures, or protocols.

Each nurse manager defines a unit-based quality assurance program that integrates into the departmental and central hospital programs. The nurse manager oversees three unit committees: monitoring and evaluation, education, and clinical practice.[3]

Nurse managers are key personnel in new program planning. The building of new units, renovations to existing facilities, clinical programs requiring nursing resources, and educational or research protocols that affect the nursing unit or nurse's role require input from the nurse manager.

Clinical Care

The care of patients with cardiac disease occurs in five phases: preoperative, intraoperative, intensive, intermediate, and inpatient care.

The policies and procedures of each of these phases of care meet the standards and requirements of the JCAHO. In addition, operating room personnel are held to standards of the Association of Operating Room Nurses.

Clinical policies and procedures are derived from the knowledge that has been developed around the specialized field of cardiac surgery and by JCAHO standards.

According to the JCAHO, "Written policies and procedures concerning the scope and provision of care in each special care unit are developed by the medical staff and nursing department service."[5] Policies such as admission criteria dictate the type of practice. Protocols (what is to be implemented) and procedures (step-by-step outlines of how to perform a skill) give direction to this practice. Pertinent protocols, policies, and procedures are identified and written by a multidisciplinary task force.

The protocols identify roles and responsibilities, equipment, required documentation, and reportable conditions.[4] Specific protocols for the population undergoing cardiac surgery may include care of the patient with mediastinal tubes, temporary pacing, or cardiac emergency care (Table 5-6).[3]

Although most of the staff are familiar with the existing policies, procedures, and protocols, they serve as a basis for consistent practice and a resource for newer members of the team.

Nurses and physicians must acquire a very specialized body of knowledge to function effectively in the CSICU. Patients require immediate care and intensive invasive monitoring and are often hemodynamically unstable during the CC postoperative phase. Stabilization of the patient requires close monitoring, intricate assessments, and fine manipulations of fluids, medications, temperature, and ventilation.

Care organized within the primary nursing framework results in comprehensive and consistent care of patients and families.

Table 5-6   Care Protocols for Patients with Various Requirements and Conditions*,[3]

Mediastinal tubes
Temporary epicardial pacemaker wires
Temporary pacing
Cardiac monitoring
Hemodynamic monitoring
IV fluid administration via central line
Swan-Ganz catheter
Antidysrhythmic medication (IV)
Intraaortic balloon pump
Ventricular assist device
Blood and blood products
Brevibloc treatment
Alteration in temperature regulation
Inotropic support
Vasoconstricting agents
Medications that alter hemostasis
Pericardiocentesis
Medications for vasodilation
Tracheostomy
Respiratory support
Slow continuous ultrafiltration, continuous arteriovenous hemo-filtration, continuous arteriovenous hemodilation
Foley catheterization

*Not an all-inclusive list.

Nurses work in teams to assure that primary nursing occurs in an environment with variable scheduling needs and fluctuations in the patient's length of stay and acuity of the patient's condition.

In addition to the yearly required cardiopulmonary resuscitation certifications and updates in fire and safety and in infection control, nurses have an 8-week orientation program that involves didactic material and a preceptorship. Advanced classes are provided in intraaortic balloon pump management, care of the transplant recipient, and care of the patient requiring a ventricular assist device.

Emergency procedures such as initiation of the cardiopulmonary support system, sternotomy, or pericardiocentesis are organized around protocols that guide the actions of the health care personnel. It is important that the medical and nursing staff feel comfortable enough with the protocols to integrate them easily into daily practice.

Conclusion

Planning, organizing, and managing care of patients in the CSICU requires close collaboration of medical, nursing, administrative, and support personnel. Although the CC recovery is only one stage in the cardiac surgical patient's hospitalization, it is an integral step in the process toward discharge.

References

1. Finkler SA: *Budgeting concepts for nurse managers,* New York, 1984, Grune & Stratton.
2. Gillies DE: *Nursing management: a systems approach,* Philadelphia, 1982, WB Saunders.
3. *Clinical practice manual,* Baltimore, 1991, Johns Hopkins Department of Surgery.
4. *Personnel policy and procedure manual,* Baltimore, 1990, Johns Hopkins Hospital.
5. *Accreditation manual for hospitals,* Washington, DC, 1990, Joint Commission on Accreditation of Healthcare Organizations.

Monitoring the Cardiac Surgical Patient

6

Eugenie S. Heitmiller

Patients who are to undergo cardiac surgery require basic noninvasive monitoring and more extensive invasive monitoring to manage properly their perioperative care. These include:

- Electrocardiogram
- Monitoring of arterial blood pressure
- Central venous pressure
- Pulmonary artery pressure
- Left atrial pressure
- Transesophageal echocardiography
- Pulse oximetry
- Capnography
- Monitoring of temperature
- Urine output

Electrocardiogram

The *electrocardiogram* (ECG) is indicated for all patients undergoing anesthesia to detect arrhythmias, ischemia, conduction defects, and electrolyte disturbances.[12] Several techniques, both noninvasive and invasive are used to measure the ECG.[10] The noninvasive measurement may be a three- or a five-electrode system. The invasive ECG is used less frequently and includes leads placed in the esophagus, trachea, or pulmonary artery catheter, or monitored epicardial pacing wires.[8,9]

The *three-electrode system* uses electrodes on the right arm,

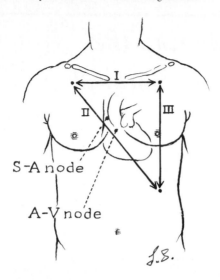

Fig. 6-1 Standard limb leads. Lead I connects two arms; lead II connects right arm with left leg; lead III connects left arm and left leg.

left arm, and left leg to examine leads I, II, and III (Fig. 6-1). These are *bipolar* leads, whereby the potential between two points (a positive and a negative electrode) is measured.[3] Augmented leads (aVR, aVL, aVF) are an expansion of the three-electrode system, with one lead set as an exploring electrode (positive terminal) and the remaining two leads connected and set at zero potential. These are therefore referred to as *unipolar* limb leads, whereby the exploring electrode is placed on one limb and are labeled accordingly:

- aVR, right arm
- aVL, left arm
- aVF, left leg

This unipolar lead system produces larger or "augmented" deflections that are labeled by the prefix *a-*. Thus six frontal plane axes can be obtained from three leads. Leads II, III, and aVF monitor inferior wall ischemia; leads I and aVF monitor the lateral wall.

Modifications of the standard three-electrode system have been used to evaluate arrhythmias and anterior ischemia (Fig. 6-2, Table 6-1.)[3] These modified leads are not often used in the operating room

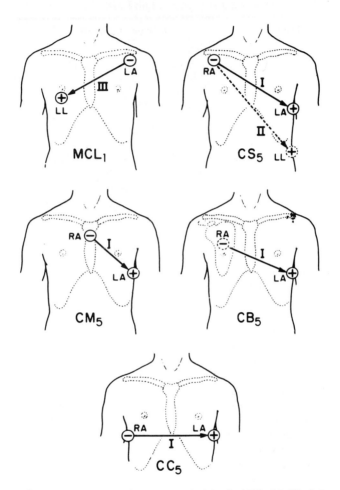

Fig. 6-2 Modified bipolar standard limb leads. *MCL*, Modified chest lead; *CS₅*, central subclavicular; *CM₅*, central manubruim; *CB₅*, central back; *CC₅*, central chest. See Table 6-1 for corresponding areas monitored. (From Griffin RM, Kaplan JA: ECG lead systems. In Thys DM, Kaplan JA, eds: *The ECG in anesthesia and critical care*, New York, 1987, Churchill Livingstone.)

Table 6-1   Standard and Bipolar Limb Leads

Lead	Condition monitored
I	Lateral ischemia
II	Arrhythmias, inferior ischemia
III	Inferior ischemia
aVL	Lateral ischemia
aVF	Inferior ischemia
MCL_1	Arrhythmias
CS_5	Anterior ischemia
CM_5	Anterior ischemia
CB_5	Anterior ischemia, arrhythmias
CC_5	Ischemia

CB_5, Fifth sound on back; CC_5, central chest; CM_5, central manubrium; CS_5, central subclavicular; MCL_1, modified chest lead.

(OR) because they may interfere with the sterile surgical field for median sternotomy or thoracotomy, but they are easily used in the intensive care unit (ICU).

The *five-electrode system* uses one electrode on each extremity and one precordial lead such that all the limb leads act as a common ground for the precordial unipolar lead. The precordial lead is usually placed in the V_5 position. The advantage to having seven leads monitored simultaneously is the enhanced ability to detect ischemic events. It has been reported that 90% of ischemic events are detected by ECG when the five-electrode system is used with simultaneous monitoring.[7]

The ECG recording must follow standard conventions for accurate data interpretation. The ECG output must be calibrated with a 1 mV deflection equaling 10 mm on the strip chart recorder and the paper speed set to 25 mm/sec. The skin where the electrode is placed should be clean and lightly abraded to remove the stratum corneum, which is a source of electrical resistance. ECG artifacts can occur from movement when leads are placed on bony prominences, lead wires are loose or twisted on themselves, or leads are crossed with other monitoring cables.

Arterial Blood Pressure

Both noninvasive and intravascular blood pressure measurements are used in cardiac surgery. A blood pressure cuff is used to take the initial blood pressure on the patient's arrival to the OR or ICU and is left on the patient in case the intraarterial catheter or monitor fails. It is important to use an appropriately sized blood pressure cuff, that is, the width of the cuff is approximately two-thirds the circumference of the arm or limb on which it is used. A cuff that is too large underestimates the blood pressure; a cuff that is too small overestimates it. A cuff that is placed too low on the arm can directly compress the ulnar nerve, resulting in an ulnar neuropathy.[11]

Arterial cannulation for blood pressure measurement is indicated for all patients undergoing cardiac surgery. The *radial artery* is most frequently used because it is easily accessible and has a very low complication rate when the cannula is properly inserted and maintained.[14] It is best to measure collateral blood flow to the hand by an Allen test before inserting a catheter.[1] This is performed by applying pressure over the area of the radial and ulnar arteries at the wrist and having the patient squeeze his or her hand several times until the blood is exsanguinated. The pressure is then released from the ulnar artery, and the time until the nail bed capillaries refill is measured. Collateral flow is considered inadequate if the refill time is greater than 15 seconds. The decision to place the radial artery catheter on the right or left hand most often depends on whether the internal mammary artery is to be used as one of the coronary grafts. The radial artery catheter is placed on the side *opposite* the internal mammary artery to be used, because chest wall retraction and compression of the subclavian artery can dampen or obliterate the radial arterial trace during the dissection of the internal mammary artery of the mammary artery. If the mammary artery is not used, the usual choice is to use the left hand in right-handed persons and vice versa.

The steps for radial artery catheter placement are as follows and are illustrated in Fig. 6-3:

- Dorsiflex the wrist. It is easiest to immobilize the wrist with an arm board and tape.
- Wearing sterile gloves, prepare the skin over the radial artery with an iodine-containing solution and alcohol.
- If the patient is awake, anesthetize the skin with 0.5% to 1% lidocaine with a 25-gauge needle to produce a skin wheal over the radial artery. Inject a small amount of anesthetic below the skin so that the area is anesthetized but the vessel is not disturbed.

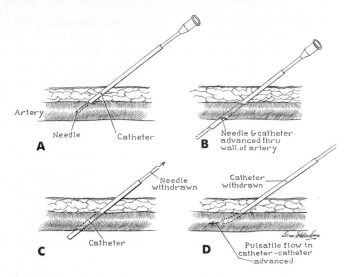

Fig. 6-3 Radial artery cannulation. Catheter-over-needle unit is inserted into artery (**A**). When arterial blood flow is seen in needle hub, catheter may be advanced over needle into artery. Another technique is to advance catheter and needle further until blood flow ceases, thereby transfixing artery (**B**), then remove needle (**C**) and withdraw catheter until blood flow is seen. Catheter is then advanced into artery (**D**).

- Use a 16- or 18-gauge needle to break the skin at the point where the catheter is to be inserted.
- Insert a 20-gauge catheter-over-needle unit over the radial artery. At this point several techniques may be used:
1. Advance the needle and catheter until arterial blood flow is seen. After advancing both the needle and catheter into the artery a small distance, keep the needle stationary and slide the catheter over the needle into the artery.
2. Advance the needle and catheter until arterial blood flow is seen. Continue to advance the needle and catheter until blood flow stops, pull the needle and catheter back until blood flow returns, then advance the catheter over the needle into the artery.
3. Advance the needle and catheter until blood flow stops, remove the needle, then slowly pull the catheter back until

blood flow is seen through the catheter and advance the catheter into the artery.

4. Use the same technique as in method 3 but before pulling back the catheter, attach a syringe with heparinized saline solution. While pulling back the catheter, apply gentle aspiration to the syringe until blood flow returns. Flush the catheter while advancing it into the vessel.

• If it is difficult to advance the catheter despite good arterial blood flow at a particular point, bring the catheter back to the point of good blood flow, advance a flexible wire through the catheter, and pass the catheter over the wire. This technique has a variable success rate but may be worth trying in cases where arterial cannulation is particularly difficult.

Other sites for arterial cannulation include the ulnar, femoral, axillary, brachial, and posterior tibial arteries, and the dorsal artery of the foot. The *ulnar artery* may be used if the radial artery cannot be cannulated, but the Allen test should be repeated to ensure adequate collateral flow from the radial artery. The *femoral artery* is probably the second most frequently used cannulation site at The Johns Hopkins Hospital. It provides central arterial access with reliable blood pressure measurements. However, its use is limited in patients who have had vascular surgery involving the femoral arteries. The *axillary artery* also provides a centrally located catheter, but because of its location close to the aortic arch the risk of cerebral embolus from air or debris is increased when the catheter is flushed. Air embolus can also occur with radial artery cannulation. The femoral and axillary arteries are both most reliably cannulated with the Seldinger technique. The pressure obtained in the femoral artery will be higher than the corresponding pressure measured in the radial artery.

The sites less frequently used are the brachial and posterior tibial arteries and the dorsal artery of the foot. The *brachial artery* is easily accessible but is rarely used because it is a peripheral "end artery" without collateral flow. Thrombosis of this vessel would remove the blood supply to the forearm and hand. The *posterior tibial artery* and the dorsal artery of the foot are not commonly used because they are frequently unreliable after cardiopulmonary bypass and in the immediate postoperative period because of peripheral vasoconstriction and decreased perfusion.

Arterial pressure tracing is a useful monitor in the OR and in the ICU. Electrocautery used in the OR causes interference that interrupts the ECG but not the arterial pressure waveform. Thus the heart continues to be monitored and rhythm disturbances may be seen by changes in the arterial waveform. Changes in the *pulse pressure* (the difference between the systolic and diastolic pressure) can provide very useful information, especially in the ICU setting. *Pericardial tamponade* is associated with a narrow pulse pressure on the arterial waveform. *Aortic insufficiency* is associated with a very low diastolic pressure resulting in a wide pulse pressure. *Hypovolemia* is often accompanied by a respiratory variation in the arterial pressure trace whereby the blood pressure decreases with positive pressure ventilation. This decrease in blood pressure occurs because positive intrathoracic pressure decreases the venous return to the heart. This effect of positive pressure ventilation can be pronounced in the hypovolemic patient.

When central arterial pressures are used (e.g., femoral, axillary), much information can be derived from the pressure waveform (Fig. 6-4). The *upstroke* of the arterial waveform provides information about cardiac contractility. If the rate of rise of the pressure wave is rapid, the contractile state is probably good. A slow upstroke can be a sign of poor contractility but is also associated with aortic stenosis and peripheral vasoconstriction. The position of the *dicrotic notch* is associated with changes in vascular resistance. A dicrotic notch that is high on the downslope of the

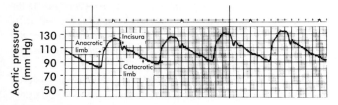

Fig. 6-4 Central arterial pressure trace. Isovolumic contraction is followed by increasing pressure, shown by anacrotic limb, to a peak or systolic pressure. Incisura or dicrotic notch indicates time of closure of semilunar valves. Slower, descending catacrotic notch indicates decreasing pressure after systole. The lowest pressure attained is diastolic pressure. Pulse pressure is difference between systolic and diastolic pressures. (From Abel FL, McCutcheon EP: *Cardiovascular function,* Boston, 1979, Little, Brown.)

arterial pressure trace may occur with increased systemic vascular resistance, whereas low resistance would be indicated by a low-placed dicrotic notch. The *stroke volume* can be correlated with the area under the systolic portion of the pressure curve. These indexes of cardiac contractility cannot be as reliably used with peripheral artery catheters.

Many sources of error exist in intravascular catheter measurements. This applies to systemic arterial and pulmonary arterial catheters. Air within the catheter transducer system is a common cause of monitoring error. Air is very compressible and thus decreases the response of the system, which leads to increased damping. Damping may also be caused by a partial clot or piece of tissue in the catheter. Catheter "whip," which can produce a large pressure swing, is a result of the movement of the catheter in the vessel. This is commonly seen in pulmonary artery catheters. Changes in the electrical zero position of the transducer is a source of measurement error that would not change the waveform but would yield erroneous values. Deviations from the conventional reference level of the transducer at the right atrium produce falsely high or low values that are most significant when low-pressure systems (e.g., central venous pressure) are measured and have less effect on the high-pressure systemic arterial pressures.

The systolic pressure measured by a catheter in the radial or dorsal foot artery is often higher than that measured by blood pressure cuff or even by the pressure measured in the center of the aorta. This is due to the wave-reflection phenomenon. As the pressure wave passes down the arterial tree, it is modified by arterial narrowing, loss of arterial elastic tissue, and the addition of reflected waves until it reaches the distal portion of the catheter (Fig. 6-5).

Complications of arterial cannulation are generally few. These include bleeding, infection, thrombosis, ischemia, and air embolus. Bleeding is usually not a problem in the absence of a bleeding disorder, but a hematoma may result after the catheter is removed or if several attempts were unsuccessful. The risk of infection and ischemia has been reported to be low. (In general, catheters are not placed through areas of infected skin.) The incidence of thrombosis, however, has been found to be high, but studies have shown this not to be clinically significant and recanalization occurs with time.[14]

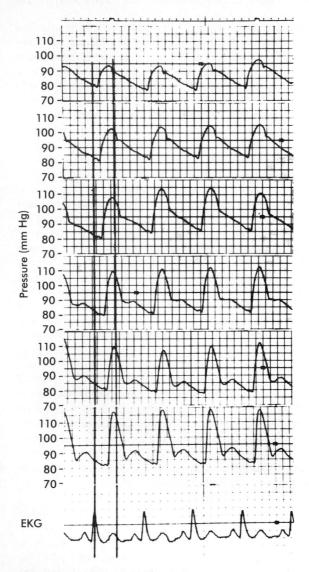

Fig. 6-5 Changes in arterial waveform as it passes down arterial tree. These waveforms are obtained at approximately 10 cm intervals during catheter withdrawal from aorta in a dog. Simultaneous ECG recording is at *bottom*. (From Abel FL, McCutcheon EP: *Cardiovascular function,* Boston, 1979, Little, Brown.)

Central Venous Cannulation

A central venous pressure (CVP) line is indicated for patients who require:

- Cardiopulmonary bypass
- Surgical procedures that entail large blood loss or fluid shifts
- Vasoactive drugs
- Venous access (but who have inadequate peripheral veins)
- Parenteral hyperalimentation

Central venous catheters can be placed through the external or internal jugular, subclavian, or basilic vein.

The internal and external jugular veins are most often used in cardiac surgery because the approach is associated with fewer complications compared with other sites. The subclavian route has the disadvantage of being in the surgical field and cannot be reached by the anesthesiologist during surgery. The subclavian catheter may be kinked when the chest retractor is placed; it carries the highest risk of pneumothorax of any other approach; and other vascular structures such as the subclavian artery and, on the left, the thoracic duct are more frequently injured. The basilic vein has the advantage of having a low rate of complications, but the success rate of central placement is low. Because the arms are tucked at the patient's sides during cardiac surgery, the catheter in a basilic vein is inaccessible to the anesthesiologist.

The complications of internal jugular vein cannulation include infection, local hematoma, air embolism, thrombophlebitis, catheter malposition (resulting in infiltration or extravasation of drugs and fluid into neck tissue, mediastinum, pericardial, or pleural cavities), pneumothorax, hemothorax, trauma to the brachial plexus, and carotid or subclavian artery puncture.

In addition to these risks of cannulation for all patients, some patients have a higher risk of complications because of preexisting clinical conditions, such as patients with obesity, previous neck surgery, contralateral diaphragmatic dysfunction, or recent or repeated internal jugular cannulation.

Before a central venous catheter is placed, the ECG must be monitored because arrhythmias may be induced with the wires or catheters as they enter the heart. The patient is placed in the Trendelenburg position if he or she will tolerate this; otherwise the legs may be raised with the patient flat or in a slightly head-up position. This distends the internal jugular veins and decreases the risk of air embolism. The area is prepared with an iodine-containing solution and draped with sterile towels. If the patient is awake, 1% lidocaine is used to anesthetize the area locally. A "finder" needle (22-gauge) is often used to locate the vein, then the 16-gauge needle is inserted along the same line (Fig. 6-6). When venous blood is freely aspirated a wire is placed through the needle and the needle is removed, leaving the wire in place. If two catheters are to be placed, such as a central venous catheter and a pulmonary artery catheter, the second needle insertion is preformed before the catheter is inserted over the wire, because catheter shearing and embolization can occur if the needle inadvertently cuts into the first catheter. After the catheters are placed over the wires, placement in the vein is confirmed by the lack of pulsatile flow and by measuring the pressure waveforms.

The normal CVP trace has three positive waves; *a, c,* and *v,* and three negative waves, *x, y,* and *z* (Fig. 6-7). The *a* wave,

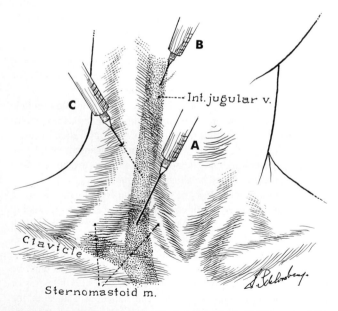

Fig. 6-6 Internal jugular cannulation. Three techniques are demonstrated: *A,* Anterior approach. *B,* Central or paracarotid approach. *C,* Posterior approach.

produced by right atrial contraction, is the largest positive wave in the normal jugular venous pulse and is particularly dominant during inspiration. During atrial relaxation the venous waveform descends and reaches a plateau at the z point. A second positive wave, c, occurs with the bulging of the tricuspid valve into the right atrium during right ventricular isovolumic contraction. The venous pulse wave descends after the c wave because of downward displacement of the tricuspid valve during right ventricular systole and is called the x wave or x descent. When the tricuspid valve closes during ventricular systole, an increase in blood volume in the right atrium and vena cavae results in the positive v wave. The tricuspid valve then opens and blood flows into the right ventricle, resulting in a drop in the venous pressure wave known as the y wave. If diastole is long, a small positive wave, known as the h wave, may appear before the a wave. The normal and abnormal characteristics of the a, c, and v waves of the CVP trace are summarized in Tables 6-2 and 6-3, respectively. The v wave is normally lower in amplitude than the a wave, but in the presence of an atrial septal defect the higher left atrial pressure may be

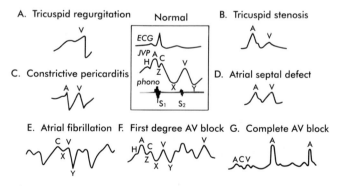

Fig. 6-7 Normal jugular venous pulse and changes seen in structural abnormalities (tricuspid regurgitation and stenosis, constrictive pericarditis, atrial septal defect) and dysrhythmias (atrial fibrillation, first degree atrioventricular block, complete heart block). See text for explanation of a, c, v, x, y, and z waves. (From O'Rourke RA: The measurement of systemic blood pressure: normal and abnormal pulsations of the arteries and veins. In Hurst JW, ed: *The heart*, New York, 1990, McGraw-Hill.)

Table 6-2 Characteristics of the CVP Trace

Wave	Relation to ECG	Physiologic correlation
a	End of P wave	Atrial systole
c	After QRS complex	Bulging of tricuspid valve into right atrium during ventricular systole
v	After T wave	Filling of right atrium

Table 6-3 Abnormal CVP Waveform Patterns

Pattern	Defect
Elevated a waves	Closed or obstructed tricuspid valve
	Tricuspid stenosis
	Right atrial myxoma
	Complete heart block
	Decreased right ventricular compliance
	Pulmonary hypertension
	Pulmonary stenosis
	Right ventricular failure
Absent a waves	Atrial fibrillation
Elevated v waves	Tricuspid regurgitation

transmitted to the right atrium during atrial filling, causing the a and v waves to be equal in amplitude.

The transducer position is particularly important in accurately measuring the CVP. As stated earlier, the transducer position is conventionally at the level of the right atrium. If the patient's position changes, measurements that are erroneously high (if the transducer is too low) or low (if the transducer is too high) result. Because a change in the CVP of just 5 to 10 mm Hg can be a significant finding, one must be vigilant to keep the transducer level in the correct position and accurately zeroed. One must also check the pressure waveform because the catheter may be long enough to pass through the tricuspid valve into the right ventricle in some persons.

Pulmonary Artery Pressure

Pulmonary artery (PA) catheterization is routinely used in patients undergoing operations with cardiopulmonary bypass. The indi-

***Table* 6-4**   Criteria for PA Catheter Insertion in the
Postoperative Cardiac Surgical Patient

Postoperative monitoring
Myocardial infarction
Development of unstable angina
Unstable hemodynamic status as a result of sepsis, massive
trauma, or shock

cations for using a PA catheter are listed in Table 6-4. The PA catheter directly measures: right atrial pressure (CVP), PA pressure, pulmonary capillary wedge pressure, cardiac output (CO), and blood temperature. From these parameters several hemodynamic indices can be derived. They are listed in Table 6-5. With this information the volume status, ventricular function, and presence of pulmonary hypertension can be assessed. The waveforms can give information about valvular disease. The ability to draw blood from separate chambers of the heart can diagnose the presence of shunts. Ischemia can be associated with an increase in PA pressures, reflecting a decrease in ventricular compliance and in the development of a *v* wave (mitral regurgitation), which may represent ischemic papillary muscle dysfunction.

PA catheters are placed through an introducer, which is inserted in the same manner as a central venous catheter. The complications of passing the PA catheter include intracardiac thrombus formation, PA rupture, pulmonary infarction, air embolus, arrhythmias, right bundle branch or complete heart block, catheter knotting or kinking, and valvular damage.

Intracardiac thrombus formation can occur if a thrombus forms from the tip of the catheter. The thrombus can then embolize or lead to thrombocytopenia. PA rupture can occur if the balloon is inflated in a small or diseased PA branch, which may tear. Patients with pulmonary hypertension are at greater risk for this complication. Hemoptysis or blood through the endotracheal tube will immediately develop. Depending on the severity of the bleeding, the therapy ranges from conservative supportive management to use of a double-lumen endotracheal tube to protect the normal lung. In some cases surgery may be required for massive hemorrhaging. Pulmonary infarction can occur if the catheter is allowed to remain in the wedge position for an extended period of time.

Air embolus can be introduced by an attempt to inflate a rup-

Table 6-5 Hemodynamic Indexes Derived from PA Catheter

Derived value	Formula	Normal range
Cardiac index	CO ÷ BSA	2.5-4.2 L/min/m^2
Stroke volume	CO ÷ HR	1 ml/kg
SVI	(CI ÷ HR) × 1000	40-60 ml/beat/m^2
Systemic vascular resistance	[(MAP − CVP) ÷ CO] × 80	700-1600 dynes · sec/cm^5
Pulmonary vascular resistance	[(PAM-PCWP) ÷ CO] × 80	20-130 dynes · sec/cm^5
Left ventricular stroke work index	(MAP-PCWP) × SVI × 0.0136	45-60 g · m/m^2
Right ventricular stroke work index	(PAM-CVP) × SVI × 0.0136	5-10 g · m/m^2

BSA, Body surface area; *HR,* heart rate; *MAP,* mean arterial pressure; *PAM,* mean pulmonary arterial pressure; *PCWP,* pulmonary capillary wedge pressure; *SVI,* stroke volume index.

tured balloon or by the inadvertent introduction of air through one of the ports. This is particularly important in patients with low right atrial pressures or patients who generate large negative inspiratory pressures. If these patients are in the sitting position and the introducer or a catheter port is open to air, a vacuum can develop during inspiration, and cause entrainment of air. In patients with an intracardiac shunt, such as an atrial or ventricular septal defect, this can lead to a left-sided embolus.

Arrhythmias can be precipitated by the catheter's touching the atrium or ventricle. This is more likely to happen if the balloon is not inflated or if the catheter coils in the right ventricle. The administration of lidocaine may help decrease ventricular arrhythmias. The development of a right bundle branch or complete heart block has been reported during passage of the PA catheter through the right ventricle. If a patient has a preexisting left bundle branch block, a PA catheter with pacing capability can be used so that the heart can be paced if complete heart block develops.

Knotting or kinking of the catheter occurs when an excessive length of catheter is passed into the heart in an attempt to enter the PA or to wedge the catheter. The catheter can curl and develop a knot. This is more likely to happen in patients with large atrial or ventricular cavities, and in low-flow states. Damage to tricuspid or pulmonary valves can occur if the catheter is pulled back through a closed valve while the balloon is inflated. For this reason it is important to be vigilant about allowing the balloon to deflate before withdrawing the catheter.

Accurate interpretation of PA catheter data often depends on the location of the catheter tip, the patient's pulmonary status, and the presence of hypovolemia. To obtain accurate PA catheter measurements, the catheter tip must be in an area where the PA blood pressure is greater than the pulmonary venous blood pressure and the pulmonary alveolar pressure (Fig. 6-8). West et al.[15] described the three zones of the lung:

- Zone I; $P_{alv} > P_{art} > P_{ven}$
- Zone II; $P_{art} > P_{alv} > P_{ven}$
- Zone III; $P_{art} > P_{ven} > P_{alv}$

where P_{alv} = pulmonary alveolar pressure, P_{art} = pulmonary artery pressure and P_{ven} = pulmonary venous pressure. If the catheter tip is in zone I, the pulmonary alveolar pressure will be greater than the PA and pulmonary venous pressure, so the PA pressure

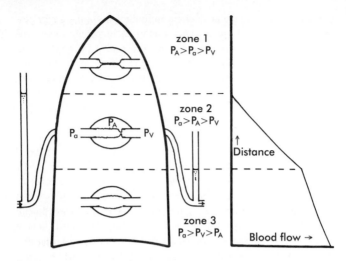

Fig. 6-8 Three zones of lung. Uneven distribution of blood flow in lung is based on pressures affecting the capillaries. (From West JB, Dollery CT, Narmack A: Distribution of blood flow in isolated lung, relation to vascular and alveolar pressures, *J Appl Physiol* 19:723, 1964.)

measurement will be affected by changes in ventilation. If the patient is hypovolemic, and is receiving positive end expiratory pressure, both the PA and pulmonary venous pressures will be low and the alveolar pressure will be high. The alveolar pressures will be transmitted to the PA catheter and erroneously high filling pressures will result.

The PA catheter pressure measurement can be greatly affected by airway pressure transmitted to the pulmonary circulation. If a patient is spontaneously breathing but the breathing is labored or obstructed, a large negative intrapleural pressure can be generated during inspiration and can then be transmitted to the pulmonary circulation. Negative filling pressures will result. If the patient is receiving positive-pressure ventilation, the positive pressure can be transmitted, resulting in falsely high PA pressure measurements. Therefore the PA measurements should be taken at end-expiration.

PA catheters are used to measure CO directly. The CO is measured by the Stewart-Hamilton equation,[4] which relates CO to a change in blood temperature:

$$Q = \frac{V(T_B - T_I)K_1K_2}{T_B(t)dt}$$

where:

Q = Cardiac output
V = Volume injected
T_B = Blood temperature
t_I = Injectate temperature
K_1, K_2 = Computational constants
$T_B(t)dt$ = Change in blood temperature as a function of time

By this equation, the change in blood temperature over time is inversely proportional to the CO.

To obtain accurate CO measurements, several technical factors must be considered. First, the catheter thermistor must be freely floating in the PA. If the thermistor is up against the vessel wall, it will not be in contact with the injectate and the change in blood temperature will not be accurately measured. Second, the injectate volume and temperature must correspond to the settings on the CO computer. If the injectate is too warm or the volume is too small, the CO will be computed to be erroneously high. The speed of the injection should be 10 ml in 4 seconds or less.

In addition to these hemodynamic measurements, mixed venous oxygen saturation ($S\bar{v}O_2$) can be measured by drawing a blood sample from the PA (distal) port of the PA catheter. It is important that the balloon is *deflated* and that the catheter is *not* in a wedged position when the sample is drawn; otherwise, an arterialized pulmonary venous sample will be obtained rather than a mixed venous PA sample. The $S\bar{v}O_2$ reflects the adequacy of perfusion. Under normal circumstances the $S\bar{v}O_2$ is 75% (mixed venous oxygen pressure = 40 mm Hg). The $S\bar{v}O_2$ varies directly with hemoglobin level, CO, and arterial oxygen saturation. The $S\bar{v}O_2$ varies indirectly with metabolic rate. Therefore when $S\bar{v}O_2$ falls, it indicates that the CO, hemoglobin, and arterial oxygen saturation should be directly measured. Stable indices suggest that the metabolic rate may have significantly increased. This can occur, for example, in the postoperative period when a hypothermic patient begins shivering as the muscle paralysis wears off. $S\bar{v}O_2$ is more difficult to interpret under conditions of intracardiac shunts, peripheral shunts, sepsis, cirrhosis, and cyanide poisoning.

Left Atrial Pressure

Direct measurement of left atrial (LA) pressure is indicated when PA catheter monitoring is technically difficult or if the patient's clinical condition does not allow the use of a PA catheter. Such conditions exist with:

- Tricuspid stenosis or atresia
- Pulmonary stenosis or atresia
- Severe pulmonary hypertension
- Right-sided heart failure

The LA pressure waveform has *a, c,* and *v* waves similar to the waveform from the right atrium. The LA pressure measured directly is more accurate than the pulmonary capillary wedge pressure because it does not have the effects of airway pressure and abnormal pulmonary vasculature as does the PA catheter. However, the LA catheter must be placed surgically and has the disadvantage of being a possible site for air entry into the left side of the heart.

Transesophageal Echocardiography

Transesophageal echocardiography (TEE) is a technique whereby echocardiography of the heart is performed with a transducer housed in a gastroscope that is placed in the esophagus just behind the heart. TEE provides high-quality images of the left atrium, mitral valve, atrial septum, thoracic aorta, and left ventricle. TEE is indicated for evaluation of thoracic aortic dissections, native and prosthetic cardiac valve dysfunction, detection of an intracardiac source of embolism, endocarditis, cardiac and paracardiac masses, left ventricular function, and wall motion abnormalities.[13] To date, one Mallory-Weiss tear of the esophagus has been reported as a complication of the TEE probe in a patient undergoing cardiac surgery.[2] It is best to remove an oral or nasal gastric tube before the procedure so that it does not interfere with the study or become misplaced with movement of the probe. In addition, if the patient is intubated, the endotracheal tube should be secured so that the patient is not inadvertently extubated. Because the transducer is housed in a gastroscope, patients in the ICU should be sedated and/or have the throat locally anesthetized before the procedure.

Pulse Oximetry

The pulse oximeter is monitored continuously during all cardiac surgical procedures. It works on the principle of infrared absorbance of blood as it passes through the capillary bed. Pulse oximetry monitors pulsatile delivery of oxygenated blood, which can be measured in the distal part of the extremities, on the earlobes, or over the nose. It has the advantage of being an accurate, continuous, noninvasive monitor of oxygenation that can readily detect reductions in oxygenation caused by pulmonary complications or inadequate perfusion. Situations in which the pulse oximeter reading can be inaccurate or misleading include intravenous use of methylene blue, extraneous or infrared lights, and electrocautery.

The advantages, however, far outweigh the disadvantages, and the pulse oximeter is considered an essential monitor in the operative and postoperative treatment of the patient undergoing cardiac surgery. It is used to wean patients from the ventilator and serves as a signal or marker to check an arterial blood gas.

Capnography

Capnography is indicated in all patients undergoing general anesthesia. It is also becoming increasingly important in monitoring patients in the ICU. It has become essential in providing immediate, accurate evidence of successful (or unsuccessful) endotracheal intubation. It then provides continuous monitoring of expired carbon dioxide. With this information the early diagnosis of hypoventilation or hyperventilation can be made. In addition, if the end-tidal carbon dioxide measurement is different from the partial arterial pressure of carbon dioxide it gives evidence of dead space ventilation, which may be due to hypotension; increased airway pressure with increase in zone I; pulmonary embolus; ventilation characterized by rapid, short inspirations; or anesthesia or ventilator apparatus.

Normally, approximately one third (30%) of each breath takes no part in gas exchange and is therefore termed *dead space ventilation*. The presence of an endotracheal tube increases the total dead space to 46%, and patients with controlled breathing who use a mask have a dead space of 64%.[5] The effects of increased dead space can usually be corrected by increasing the respiratory minute volume. The total dead space normally increases with age.

A hand-held monitor for the presence of carbon dioxide is used to assess the adequacy of tube placement after intubation. If the tube is properly placed in the trachea, carbon dioxide will be detected.

Temperature

Temperature is measured at several sites in patients undergoing cardiac surgery. The most commonly used sites at The Johns Hopkins Hospital are the PA catheter thermistor, nasopharynx, esophagus, rectum, and skin.

In addition, temperature can be measured by a probe placed at the tympanic membrane or through a temperature probe in the bladder catheter. In general, the core temperature represents the temperature of the vital organs. These sites and the corresponding organs they most closely measure are as follows: PA catheter for the temperature of the heart, nasopharynx and tympanic membrane for the brain, bladder for the kidney, and esophagus for the heart.

During cardiopulmonary bypass the temperature of the heat exchanger is measured in the pump arterial line. This represents the lowest temperature during cooling and the highest temperature during rewarming. The pump venous line temperature (blood returning from the patient) represents the general core temperature during cardiopulmonary bypass.

During cardiopulmonary bypass when changes in blood temperature are rapid, a gradient exists between the core temperature (as listed previously) and the peripheral sites (rectum, skin). This occurs because the vessel-rich organs receive a greater proportion of the blood flow so that at the time cardiopulmonary bypass is discontinued the core temperature is 2° to 5° C higher than the rectal or skin temperature. The core heat then dissipates to the cooler periphery so that the final temperature on arrival to the ICU is often closer to what the peripheral temperature had been at the time cardiopulmonary bypass was discontinued.

Urine Output

The urine output is measured for all patients undergoing cardiac surgery. A normal urine output (1 ml/kg/hr) is under most circumstances a reliable indication of adequate blood volume, CO, and peripheral perfusion.

A decrease in urine output (oliguria) can occur in patients during cardiac surgery because of volatile anesthetics, hypothermia, depressed ventricular function or cardiopulmonary bypass.

The volatile anesthetics are known to depress renal function, but the effects are transient and reversible after the volatile agent is discontinued.[6] Intravenous anesthetics have not been shown to alter renal function. Hypothermia and nonpulsatile flow that occur during cardiopulmonary bypass can significantly effect renal function, so that it is not uncommon for little or no urine to be made during that time. Mannitol is routinely given during cardiopulmonary bypass to help maintain normal urine output. When the patient is rewarmed and pulsatile flow restored, urine output returns to normal in most cases.

Hemolysis may occur during cardiopulmonary bypass. This is usually treated with additional diuretics and fluid to avoid damage to renal tubules. If the urine is allowed to become concentrated in the face of hemolysis, hematin precipitation can occur within the renal tubules and the patient is at risk for acute renal failure. If hemolysis develops after a blood transfusion, the possibility of a transfusion reaction must be ruled out.

In summary, this chapter has reviewed the basic noninvasive and invasive monitoring techniques used during cardiac surgery. Knowledge of these basic techniques is essential in treating these patients both intraoperatively and postoperatively. More in-depth information may be found in the suggested readings at the end of this chapter.

References

1. Allen EV: Thromboangitis obliterans: methods of diagnosis of chronic occlusive arterial lesions distal to the wrist with illustrated cases, *Am J Med Sci* 178:237, 1929.
2. Dewhirst WE, Stragand JJ, Fleming BM: Mallory-Weiss tear complicating intraoperative transesophageal echocardiography in a patient undergoing aortic valve replacement, *Anesthesiology* 73:777-778, 1990.
3. Griffin RM, Kaplan JA: ECG lead systems. In Thys DM, Kaplan JA, eds: *The ECG in anesthesia and critical care,* New York, 1987, Churchill Livingstone.
4. Hamilton WF et al: Comparison of the fick and dye injection methods of measuring the cardiac output in man, *Am J Physiol* 153:309, 1948.
5. Kain ML, Panday J, Nunn JF: The effect of intubation on the dead space during halothane anaesthesia, *Br J Anaesth* 41:94, 1969.

6. Kallus FT: Renal function for the anesthesiologist. *Refresher Courses Anesthesiol* 11:143, 1983.

7. Kaplan JA, King SB: The precordial electrocardiographic lead (V₅) in patients who have coronary artery disease, *Anesthesiology* 45:570, 1976.

8. Kates RA, Zardan JR, Kaplan JA: Esophageal lead for intraoperative electrocardiographic monitoring, *Anesth Analg* 61:781, 1982.

9. Lichtenthal PR: Multipurpose pulmonary artery catheter, *Ann Thorac Surg* 36:493, 1983.

10. McCloskey GF, Curling PE: Electrocardiography, *Anesthesiol Clin North Am* 6(4):903, 1988.

11. Miller RG, Camp PE: Postoperative ulnar neuropathy, *JAMA* 24:1636, 1979.

12. Pratila M, Pratilas V: Electrophysiologic effects of anesthetic agents. In Thys DM, Kaplan JA, eds: *The ECG in anesthetic and critical care,* New York: 1987, Churchill Livingstone.

13. Seward JB et al: Transesophageal echocardiography: technique, anatomic correlations, implementation, and clinical applications, *Mayo Clin Proc* 63:649, 1988.

14. Slogoff S, Keats AS, Arlund C: On the safety of radial artery cannulation, *Anesthesiology* 59:42, 1983.

15. West JB, Dollery CT, Naimak A: Distribution of blood flow in isolated lung: relation to vascular and alveolar pressures, *J Appl Physiol* 19:713, 1964.

Suggested Readings

Barash PG, ed: Cardiac monitoring. *Anesthesiol Clin North Am* 6(4):655-929, 1988.

Blitt CD: *Monitoring in anesthesia and critical care medicine,* New York, 1985, Churchill Livingstone.

Hensley FA, Martin DE, eds: *The practice of cardiac anesthesia,* Boston, 1990, Little, Brown.

Kaplan JA, ed: *Cardiac anesthesia,* ed 2, Philadelphia, 1987, WB Saunders.

7

Postoperative Hemodynamics

Kirk J. Fleischer and R. Scott Stuart

As technical and pharmacologic advancements have permitted the safe extension of cardiac surgery to our aging population, expertise in the management of postoperative hemodynamics has assumed an increasingly more important role in the successful care of these patients. Continuous monitoring of the patient's hemodynamic status in addition to a thorough understanding of cardiovascular physiology and the properties of the spectrum of pharmacologic agents currently available are essential for the rational and timely selection of appropriate therapeutic interventions.

Postoperative Evaluation of Cardiopulmonary Status

Admission to Intensive Care Unit

I. Rapid initial assessment
   A. Scan portable monitor for current heart rate (HR) and rhythm, blood pressure (BP), and oxygen saturation. Continue to check monitor periodically.
   B. Auscultate heart and bilateral lung fields while palpating radial artery
   C. Briefly palpate feet for pulses, temperature, and capillary refill
   D. Connect epicardial wires to external pacer; test for capture; set pacer on ventricular demand at rate of 60 beats/min.
II. Attending surgeon, anesthesiologist, and fellows accompany the patient to the intensive care unit (ICU). While they are available, efficient inquiry about the procedure, intraoperative course, and postoperative plan is imperative. Despite its fre-

119

quent brevity, this relay of information is essential for optimal early management in the ICU.

III. Surgical consultation

Address the following issues:

A. In patients who have undergone coronary artery bypass grafting; which vessels were bypassed and which (if any) grafts were believed to be of suboptimal quality by the surgeon? Realize that diagnosis of myocardial ischemia in the early postoperative period can be particularly challenging in the cardiac surgery patient. This information can increase one's index of suspicion when evaluating electrocardiograph (ECG) changes or evolving clinical picture and in turn permit earlier intervention.

B. Target parameters:
   1. BP (particularly important in patients with cerebrovascular or renal disease)
   2. Left ventricular filling pressure (pulmonary capillary wedge pressure, PCWP)

C. General plan for weaning patient from parenteral infusions, fluid therapy, extubation, and other treatment

IV. Anesthesia consultation

Inquire about the following:

A. Intraoperative hemodynamic course

B. Pharmacologic interventions and patient response to each agent

C. Preoperative and postoperative hemodynamic parameters (particularly mean arterial pressure (MAP), cardiac index (CI), systemic vascular resistance (SVR), and PCWP). After treating the patient intraoperatively, the anesthesiologist can fairly accurately assess the patient's response to volume loading and provide some guidelines for optimal filling pressures.

V. Completion of initial cardiopulmonary assessment

A. Admission chest x-ray (CXR) (e.g., endotracheal tube position, baseline size of cardiac silhouette, pneumothorax(?), position of Swan-Ganz catheter), ECG, and arterial blood gas (ABG) determination

B. Assess Swan-Ganz hemodynamic parameters and urine output. Initiate appropriate therapeutic interventions.

C. Document status of pedal pulses (dorsal pedis, posterior tibial) by palpation or Doppler ultrasound. Confirm arterial BP with sphygmomanometer bilaterally.

D. Chest tube: note rate and character of output from chest tube; ensure patency in early postoperative period to prevent pericardial tamponade (if necessary, percuss briskly over developing thrombus in chest tube with clamp)

Basics of Hemodynamic Monitoring in ICU

I. Noninvasive monitoring devices
   A. Continuous telemetry, pulse oximetry, and Foley catheterization are examples of these monitoring methods
   B. Close monitoring of urine output provides a simple but invaluable indicator of adequacy of tissue perfusion. Note: In the early postoperative period urine output may be misleading because mannitol given by the perfusionist often stimulates significant diuresis even in the face of deteriorating hemodynamics.
II. Invasive monitoring devices
   A. Intraarterial catheter (radial artery) is used for continuous arterial pressure monitoring (and serial ABG determinations). Follow MAP.
   B. Swan-Ganz catheter
      1. Although this device can be used to derive a plethora of hemodynamic parameters, three measurements (CI, SVR, and PCWP) together with a careful physical examination are sufficient to identify cardiovascular disturbances and to monitor therapeutic responses in most cases
      2. If a true wedge pressure cannot be achieved because of technical difficulties, pulmonary artery diastolic pressure is a reasonable alternative
III. Mixed venous oxygen saturation (S_vO_2)
   A. Sampled from distal port (pulmonary artery) of Swan-Ganz catheter
   B. Measure of oxygen delivery and adequacy of tissue perfusion
   C. Normal S_vO_2, $\geq 65\%$ to 75%. Low S_vO_2 warrants prompt evaluation to determine its cause; however, normal levels are not necessarily a reflection of adequate perfusion of the microvasculature.
   D. Although a downward treanding S_vO_2 often parallels a falling cardiac output, several other factors (including low arterial oxygen saturation, anemia, intrapulmonary shunting, and increased tissue oxygen consumption) can also

contribute to reduced saturation. Thus S_{vO_2} is best used as an adjunct measurement in combination with cardiac output already measured by the standard thermodilution technique.

IV. For a more detailed discussion, see Chapter 6.

Cardiac Output

Cardiac output (CO) is the cornerstone of cardiopulmonary physiologic assessment. It is measured by the thermodilution technique with a flow-directed pulmonary artery balloon catheter (e.g., Swan-Ganz). To account for differences in patient size, we usually speak in terms of cardiac index (CI), or CO per body surface area in square meters. Average normal CI ranges from 2.5 to 4.0 $L/min/m^2$. The following equations demonstrate the components of CO:

$$CO = HR \times SV$$

where SV is stroke volume and HR is heart rate, and

$$SV = LVEDV - LVESV$$

where LVEDV is left ventricular diastolic volume; and LVESV is left ventricular systolic volume.

The five physiologic determinants of CO are heart rate, preload, compliance, afterload, and contractility. Preload and compliance determine LVEDV, while afterload and contractility determine LVESV. It is important to note that although each variable may be independently defined and evaluated, clinically they are interdependent.

Preload

I. Definition
   A. End-diastolic volume (EDV) of ventricle
   B. Clinically evaluated by pressure correlates of this ventricular filling volume (central venous pressure [CVP] and pulmonary capillary wedge pressure [PCWP])
II. Physiologic determinants
   A. Intravascular volume status
   B. Venovascular tone
III. Frank-Starling curve
      The relationship between resting heart muscle length (determined by EDV or preload) and the tension achieved by the

contracting muscle is defined by the Frank-Starling curve (Fig. 7-1 and 7-2). According to this relationship, increases in preload result in augmented SV and CO. Beyond a certain point, however, the ventricle is placed on the descending limb of the curve and additional increases in EDV result in a reduction in CO and ventricular failure.

IV. CVP and PCWP

CVP and PCWP are the clinical estimates of right and left ventricular preload, respectively. They are a function of both venous return and the ventricle's ability to circulate that volume of blood. Realize that these filling pressures serve only as dynamic guides. Relative changes and trends are considerably more meaningful than absolute values because individual variation may be significant.

CVP is measured through the proximal port of a Swan-Ganz catheter (or other central venous catheter in the right atrium). In most cases it is a poor estimate of circulating blood volume. Furthermore, because of the interposed pulmonary vasculature, CVP cannot be used as a reliable index of left-sided heart pressures. The primary indications for its use are in the diagnosis and management of right-sided heart failure

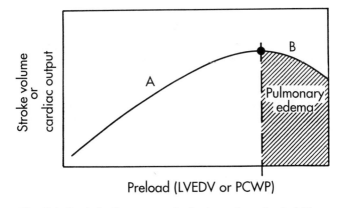

Fig. 7-1 Frank-Starling curve. **A,** Increases in preload yield augmented SV until ventricle-dependent optimal filling volume and pressure are achieved (●). **B,** Beyond this ideal volume and pressure, additional increases in EDV and PCWP result in reduction in CO and evidence of ventricular failure.

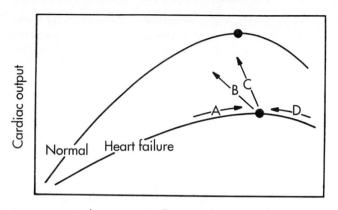

Fig. 7-2 Frank-Starling curve and effects of various therapeutic interventions. *A*, Volume; *B*, inotrope *or* arterial vasodilator; *C*, inotrope *and* arterial vasodilator; *D*, diuretic or venodilator. (Note that only inotropic or arterial vasodilator therapy can shift ventricular function curve toward normal curve.)

and cardiac tamponade. "Normal" CVP values range from 0 to 4 mm Hg.

PCWP is measured via the distal port of the Swan-Ganz catheter. Except for direct measurement via a left atrial catheter, it is the best approximation of LVEDV. Unlike CVP, PCWP is a reliable estimate of volume status. Note that several conditions preclude accurate correlation between PCWP and LVEDV.

Conditions where PCWP *over*estimates LVEDV include the following:
- Increased airway pressures (e.g., positive end-expiratory pressure)
- Mitral valve disease (particularly mitral stenosis)
- Chronic obstructive pulmonary disease
- Pulmonary hypertension
- Hypovolemia

PCWP may *under*estimate LVEDV where there is a noncompliant left ventricle. (In the less compliant heart a greater increase in pressure accompanies the same EDV (preload) compared with a heart of normal compliance.) Optimal PCWP is defined as the highest filling pressure that yields the highest

CO without causing pulmonary edema. "Normal" PCWP values range from 12 to 15 mm Hg in the nondysfunctioning ventricle but may be 20 mm Hg or more in the diseased ventricle.

V. *Note:*
   A. preload is the key determinant of CO in the heart with normal ventricular compliance
   B. arterial BP tracing can frequently be used for rapid diagnosis of inadequate preload. The patient with hypovolemia exhibits a sine wave variation in BP with the respiratory cycle.

Compliance

I. Definition: Tendency of the ventricle to permit distention with blood
II. Physiologic determinants (myocardial)
   A. Acute
      1. Myocardial oxygenation, (e.g., ischemia results in reduced compliance)
   B. Chronic
      1. Fribrotic myocardial scarring (caused by infarction)
      2. Ventricular hypertrophy
III. *Note:*
   A. Ischemia results in reduced compliance
   B. In the early postoperative period higher filling pressures may be required because of the reduced ventricular compliance that accompanies hypothermia and intraoperative ischemia associated with aortic cross-clamping
   C. Severe pericardial scarring may also reduce compliance
   D. PCWP (LVEDP) is a reliable absolute measure of LVEDV only in ventricles with normal compliance

Afterload

I. Definition: Tension in the wall of the ventricle during systole; force opposing ventricular ejection
II. Physiologic determinants
   A. Vascular resistance
   B. Ventricular outflow obstruction (valvular, septal)
III. Vascular resistance
   Vascular resistance accounts for more than 90% of afterload in most patients. Systemic (SVR) and pulmonary (PVR)

vascular resistance are the key determinants of left and right ventricular afterload, respectively. Using the basic physiologic premise, Pressure = Resistance × Flow, one can easily calculate these hemodynamic measures:

$$\text{SVR [resistance]} = \frac{\text{MAP} - \text{CVP [pressure]}}{\text{CO [flow]}} \times 80,$$

where SVR is resistance, MAP − CVP is pressure, and CO is flow.

$$\text{PVR} = \frac{\text{MPAP} - \text{PCWP}}{\text{CO}} \times 80,$$

where MAP is mean arterial pressure and MPAP is mean pulmonary artery pressure.

Normal range for SVR is 900 to 1400 dynes/sec/cm^{-5} and is 150 to 250 dynes/sec/cm^{-5} for PVR.

BP is an insensitive index of myocardial performance because it is a function of both SVR and CO. If CO falls, BP is initially maintained by compensatory sympathetic discharge with resultant arterial vasoconstriction. Hence, monitoring BP alone often does not signal early myocardial failure.

IV. *Note:* Afterload is the key determinant of CO in the diseased heart with reduced ventricular compliance

Contractility

I. Definition: Intrinsic contractile performance independent of the other determinants of CO

II. Physiologic determinants: Microenvironment of the myocyte (oxygen tension, pH, electrolytes, temperature, etc.)

III. Reduced contractility

A. *"Stunned" myocardium* is a term coined to describe the reversible myocardial dysfunction seen in the early postoperative period after cardiac surgery. The cause is uncertain, but reperfusion injury, ischemia, and intramyocardial edema have been implicated.

More than 95% of patients with normal preoperative ventricular function exhibit depressed contractile performance during the first 8 to 24 hours postoperatively. Although some patients require pharmacologic support during this period, the vast majority demonstrate full recovery within 48 hours. In clinical practice myocardial stunning becomes a factor only in patients with preexisting ventricular dysfunction, where this additional insult may significantly complicate early hemodynamic management.

IV. Increased contractility is seen most commonly in patients with ventricular hypertrophy (caused by preexisting systemic hypertension, aortic stenosis, or idiopathic hypertrophic subaortic stenosis). It may exacerbate ischemia by increasing myocardial oxygen consumption.

Low Cardiac Output Syndrome

Low cardiac output syndrome (LCOS) is a multifaceted syndrome of inadequate tissue perfusion and is clinically defined as a CI less than 2.0 L/min/m². As with other hemodynamic parameters, CI is subject to individual variation, but the criterion of CI greater than 2.0 L/min/m² is generally accepted as the minimal requirement for effective perfusion of the microcirculation. Diagnostic sensitivity can be enhanced when mixed venous oxygenation is used as an adjunct measure. It may reveal regional perfusion insufficiency that might go undetected in patients with normal CI.

LCOS is associated with an increased risk of cardiac death and a higher probability of postoperative complications such as respiratory failure, renal insufficiency, and neurologic sequelae. Prompt diagnosis and intervention are essential for this potentially life-threatening condition.

Clinical Features

I. *Rapid bedside assessment* can be performed by merely palpating the patient's feet. In patients without significant peripheral vascular disease, weak or absent pedal pulses (dorsal pedis, posterior tibial) in a cool foot with poor capillary refill indicates inadequate peripheral perfusion. Serial examinations of the foot can provide a reliable and sensitive means of detecting low CO.

II. Sequence of hemodynamic changes associated with evolving ventricular dysfunction is illustrated by the following equation:

$$\uparrow \text{PCWP} \rightarrow \ \downarrow \text{SV and } \uparrow \text{HR} \rightarrow \ \downarrow \text{CO and } \uparrow \text{SVR} \rightarrow \ \downarrow \text{BP}$$

A. Earliest sign is an increase in PCWP

B. Then SV begins to fall while a compensatory tachycardia

Table 7-1 Signs and Symptoms of LCOS

1. Cool, clammy skin
2. Slow capillary refill
3. Oliguria (<0.5 ml/kg/hr)
4. Restlessness, agitation, depressed mental status
5. Tachypnea
6. Reduced mixed Svo_2 (<65%-70%)
7. Metabolic acidosis

maintains the CO. (Remember that CO = HR × SV.) Therefore do not be deceived by an "adequate" CI in the setting of tachycardia. In the normovolemic patient elevated HR often represents this compensatory response.

C. Finally, low CO develops after the elevated HR is no longer able to compensate for diminishing SV. Initially, increased SVR maintains BP, but eventually the increased afterload further exacerbates ventricular dysfunction, and hypotension ensues. Thus the clinician must be vigilant for the signs of the failing myocardium before decompensated state of the LCOS.

III. Signs and symptoms of low CO (Table 7-1)

A. Sympathetic overactivity results in cool, clammy skin and slow capillary refill

B. The best quantitative indicator of inadequate tissue perfusion is oliguria. Minimal acceptable urine output is 0.5 ml/kg/hr (30-40 ml/hr). *Beware:* Diuretics (mannitol) and glucosuria confound this index of CO.

C. Reduced cerebral perfusion results in restlessness, agitation, and depressed mental status

D. Reduced mixed S_Vo_2

E. Metabolic acidosis: It is often difficult to interpret the significance of lactic acidosis in the postoperative cardiac patient because elevated serum lactate levels are very common as constricted vascular beds (with some degree of anaerobic metabolism intraoperatively) dilate during rewarming

Postoperative Causes of Low CO

I. Hypovolemia (caused by third spacing, diuresis, bleeding)*

---

*Most common cause of LCOS.

II. Elevated SVR (caused by hypothermia, circulating catechol-amines, hypovolemia)

III. Myocardial dysfunction (caused by ischemia, acidosis, hypothermia, volume overload, hypercarbia)

IV. Cardiac tamponade

V. Dysrhythmia (bradyarrhythmias/tachyarrhythmias)

VI. Increased intrathoracic pressure (caused by positive pressure ventilation and positive end-expiratory pressure, tension pneumothorax)

Management

General principles

I. Proper management of LCOS is best achieved by a *systematic and physiologic approach to the optimization of the determinants of CO*. Although the following discussion addresses each variable individually, remember that they are interdependent and that in the unstable patient several determinants may require simultaneous manipulation.

II. *Constant reexamination* of these frequently labile patients is crucial for appropriate therapeutic interventions. This is particularly important when pharmacologic agents or dosages are changed. Even if the patient appears stable, recheck hemodynamic parameters 30 to 60 minutes after each intervention.

III. *Follow trends in hemodynamics* instead of absolute numbers

IV. *Consult the attending surgeon or fellow* if patient becomes unstable. Seek early assistance any time one is uncertain about treatment.

Cardiovascular pharmacologic agents

I. Drug appendix
  A. For rapid reference of the pharmacologic agents discussed in this chapter, refer to Appendix A (p. 497).
  B. The detailed discussion of each drug or drug class includes pharmacologic effects, indications, dosage, untoward effects, and other pearls regarding their use

II. Parenteral infusions: Basics
  A. Parenteral cardiovascular drugs must be infused through a central venous catheter with a radiographically confirmed intravascular position
  B. Avoid polypharmacy. Select agents for the patient's specific hemodynamic profile. Critically reassess situation if

more than two continuous infusions are required concurrently.
   C. When several simultaneous infusions are indicated,
      1. manipulate one drug at a time so that observed hemodynamic changes can be attributed to a particular agent
      2. the last drug added is usually the first discontinued
   D. Unless unstable hemodynamics warrant a rapid change of agents, gradually titrate infusion rates. While the patient is weaning, periodically reassess to ensure that adequate parameters are maintained.

Sequence of hemodynamic parameter management

Address hemodynamic parameters in the following order:
1. HR and arrhythmias
2. Preload
3. Afterload
4. Contractility

Heart rate and arrhythmias

 I. Goal: Normal sinus rhythm at a rate of 60 to 90 beats/min. In general, rates greater than 110 to 120 beats/min are not hemodynamically advantageous and increase myocardial oxygen consumption.
II. Bradycardia (and heart block)
   A. Etiologies
      1. Ischemia to sinoatrial (SA) or atrioventricular (AV) node (most frequently seen with inferior myocardial ischemia or infarction)
      2. Excessive hypothermia
      3. Preoperative use of β blockers or calcium channel blockers
   B. Pharmacologic management
      1. *Atropine*
      2. *Isoproterenol (Isuprel)*
   C. Temporary pacemakers
      1. In the early postoperative period, intraoperatively placed atrial and ventricular pacing wires can be used. If the wires are nonfunctional or have been removed, various transvenous catheter pacers can be floated via the internal jugular or subclavian vein approach.

2. Atrial (for bradycardia) or AV sequential (for AV block) pacing are preferable to ventricular pacing, because atrial kick accounts for 15% to 30% of CO. (The more severe the preexisting ventricular dysfunction or hypertrophy, the greater the contribution of the atria.) Nevertheless, if atrial pacing is not possible (malfunctioning wire; atrial fibrillation or flutter), ventricular pacing often significantly improves CO.

III. Sinus tachycardia
  A. Etiologies
    1. Hypovolemia
    2. Pain and/or anxiety
    3. Postoperative hypercatecholamine syndrome
    4. Reduced oxygen delivery (caused by hypoxia or anemia)
    5. Withdrawal (β blockers, alcohol, narcotics, etc.)
  B. Management
    1. Optimize volume status with intravenous (IV) fluids or blood (if hematocrit <30%) (see following section)
    2. Supplemental oxygen to maintain oxygen saturation greater than 92%
    3. Pharmacologic management
      a. Morphine and/or anxiolytic agent
      b. *Esmolol (Brevibloc),* a short-acting β blocker
        Although occasionally seen in the patient with incomplete revascularization, tachycardia-induced ischemia is uncommon in the cardiac surgery patient postoperatively. In the vast majority of cases the risk of precipitating heart failure in patients with marginal ventricular function is greater than the negative chronotropic benefits of β blockers. *Thus the initiation of β-blocker therapy should be approved by the attending surgeon or fellow!*
      c. Other agents (digoxin, calcium channel blockers, and neostygmine [novel therapy that lacks negative inotropic effects])
  C. *Note:* Be aware that in some clinical settings (e.g., cardiac tamponade, ventricular failure) tachycardia may maintain CO until definitive therapy can be instituted. Rule out these causes before inhibiting this potentially life-saving reflex.

IV. Other tachyarrhythmias
   A. Most frequently caused by electrolyte disturbances, myocardial ischemia, or arrhythmogenic inotropic agents
   B. See Chapter 10 for discussion of diagnosis and management

Preload

  I. Goal: Highest filling pressure (PCWP) that yields the highest CO without causing pulmonary edema
 II. Decreased preload
   A. Cause
     1. Intravascular hypovolemia (most common cause)
        a. Total body third spacing of fluids (into the interstitial space) associated with cardiopulmonary bypass (CPB)
        b. Diuresis caused mannitol given intraoperatively
        c. Mediastinal bleeding
     2. Vasodilation associated with rewarming (relative hypovolemia)
     3. Increased intrathoracic pressure
        a. Positive pressure ventilation or positive end-expiratory pressure
        b. Tension pneumothorax
     4. Cardiac tamponade
   B. Straight leg raise or Trendelenburg position immediately but transiently augments preload
   C. Volume therapy
     1. Crystalloid versus colloid versus blood products
     2. Controversy continues regarding choice of replacement fluid. Although proponents of colloid point to reduced third spacing associated with its use, the literature (primarily in sepsis and trauma patients) has been inconclusive. Therefore because of the significant increase in cost of colloid, we recently discontinued its use except in selected patients. An increased incidence in pleural effusions and cases of massive edema (delaying time to extubation and requiring aggressive diuresis) was observed. As a result, a large prospective study is under way at our institution to determine definitively the indications for colloid in post-CPB patients.

3. *Follow electrolytes!* Hypokalemia and hypomagnesemia are frequent causes of arrhythmia in the cardiac surgery patient.
4. Occasionally patients have a dramatic response to the mannitol given intraoperatively, with urine outputs of 500 to 1000 ml/hr. A reasonable regimen is milliliter per milliliter replacement with lactated Ringer's solution every 1 to 2 hours (remember to subtract IV fluid volume given during that period in drips).

D. Control mediastinal bleeding (see Chapter 9)
E. Cardiac tamponade
   1. Precipitates low CO by decreasing atrial filling (preload)
   2. Presentation
      a. Tachycardia, hypotension, pulsus paradox, Kussmaul's sign
      b. Equilibration of right- and left-sided heart filling pressures
   3. Classic scenario: Patient with initially heavy bleeding from chest tube suddenly stops bleeding and becomes hypotensive. CXR reveals widening of the cardiac shadow.

      However, because the blood collecting in the pericardial sac is often loculated, it is important to realize the following:
      a. Less than 100 ml of strategically located blood can cause tamponade (compromise of left atrium)
      b. Freely draining chest tubes and tamponade are *not* mutually exclusive
      c. The frequently encountered posterior loculated collection does not widen the cardiac silhouette

III. Increased preload
   A. Etiologies
      1. Volume overload
      2. Ventricular dysfunction
   B. Management of volume overload
      1. Minimize IV fluids
      2. Diuretic therapy
         a. *Furosemide (Lasix):* first-line agent
         b. *Bumetadine (Bumex)* and *chlorothiazide (Diuril):* second-line agents

    c. *Metolazone (Zaroxolyn)*
3. Dopamine ("renal dose")
C. Management of ventricular dysfunction: Follow strategy for LCOS

Afterload

I. Goal: SVR 900 to 1200 dynes/sec/cm^{-5}

    Generally aim for MAP of 65 to 80 mm Hg. However, target BP must be individualized for elderly and other patients with suspected vascular disease to prevent cerebral and renal ischemia. The best goal for these patients is preoperative BP.

II. Increased SVR
A. Predominant vascular resistance derangement encountered in the cardiac surgery patient postoperatively
B. Etiologies
1. Hypothermia
2. Hypovolemia
3. Low CO (compensatory response)
4. Elevated circulating catecholamines (mechanism uncertain but common postoperatively)
C. Management
1. Warming or hydrating patient may be sufficient to improve CO. *Note:* Until these interventions take effect, some form of pharmacologic afterload reduction is often still necessary.
2. Pharmacologic management: Vasodilator therapy

III. Vasodilator therapy: General principles
A. Vasodilators exert their beneficial effects via reduction of preload and/or afterload with resultant reduction in myocardial oxygen consumption and improved ejection fraction
B. Effect of vasodilator on BP depends on the following:
1. Volume status

    Beware: If intravascular volume status is significantly reduced, rapid life-threatening hypotension may occur with the initiation of vasodilator therapy. *It cannot be overemphasized to optimize preload before administering vasodilators.* Furthermore, while these agents are titrated, volume status must be continually reevaluated and fluids administered to maintain an adequate preload.

    2. Pharmacologic target (artery vs. vein): three basic types of vasodilators
   a. Arteriodilators (reduce afterload)
   b. Venodilators (reduce preload)
   c. Mixed (combined arteriodilator and venodilator)
   As one would expect, arteriodilators provide a more dramatic reduction in systemic BP

  C. Duration of therapy
   Often several hours of therapy are sufficient. Most patients can be weaned off all vasodilators by early morning the first postoperative day. However, occasionally postoperative hypertension persists for more than 24 hours and these patients must be weaned to an oral regimen.

  D. Relative contraindications: Obstructive valvular disease (aortic, pulmonary, mitral); hypovolemia, tachycardia, cardiac tamponade

IV. Vasodilator therapy: Specific agents

  A. Parenteral vasodilators
   1. Rapid onset and short-acting, thus easily titratable
   2. Slow changes in infusion rates minimize degree of reflex tachycardia
   3. *Sodium nitroprusside (SNP; Nipride)* is the parenteral drug of choice for afterload reduction in most cardiac surgery patients
   4. *Nitroglycerin (TNG)* is less efficient than SNP but can significantly reduce SVR when administered in high doses. It has the added benefit of coronary artery and collateral vasodilation; hence it is the drug of choice in setting of ischemia.
   5. *Esmolol (Brevibloc)* is used primarily for its negative chronotropic effects but can also provide some reduction in afterload
   6. *Morphine or furosemide (Lasix)* given as bolus can provide rapid, transient venodilation. Particularly useful in acute congestive heart failure (CHF).

  B. Oral and sublingual vasodilators
   1. *Nifedipine (procardia)* is the oral or sublingual drug of choice. When given sublingually, it acts within several minutes and its afterload-reducing effect can be dramatic. It can be used as a first-line agent before initiation of parenteral therapy.

2. Other agents that can be used to wean patient from continuous vasodilator infusion include *clonidine (Catapres), propranolol (Inderal),* topical *nitroglycerin (Nitropaste),* and *hydralazine (Apresoline)*

V. Increased PVR (see section on right ventricular failure)

Contractility

I. Goal: Difficult to define a specific goal; however, pharmacologic manipulation of contractility should be undertaken only *after* attempts to optimize HR, rhythm, preload, and afterload have been ineffective in improving CO. This is a key concept because the use of inotropic agents can have significant adverse sequelae.

II. Reduced contractility
   A. Causes
      1. Myocardial ischemia (including postoperative stunned myocardium)
      2. Acidosis
      3. Hypothermia
      4. Hypercarbia
      These insults attenuate myocardial responsiveness to catecholamines
   B. Management
      1. Alleviate ischemia (see section on myocardial ischemia)
      2. Correct acidosis, warm patient, and increase ventilation
      3. Pharmacologic management: Inotropic therapy
      4. Mechanical assist devices

III. Inotropic therapy: General principles
   A. Basic strategy: Start with a first-line inotrope. If this is ineffective, add the other first-line inotrope or change to a second-line inotrope. If an adequate CO still cannot be maintained, use of a mechanical assist device is indicated.
   B. Inotropes increase myocardial oxygen demand and often possess arrhythmogenic potential. Use judiciously.

IV. Inotropic therapy: Specific agents
   A. *Dopamine (Intropin)* and *dobutamine (Dobutrex)* are the *first-line* inotropic agents. Their hemodynamic profiles are very similar; however, each has several key distinguishing beneficial effects:

1. Dopamine
   a. Splanchnic and renal vasodilation
   b. Pressor effect (at high doses)
2. Dobutamine
   a. Lower incidence of tachycardia and arrhythmia (at standard doses)
   b. Systemic vasodilation (skeletal muscle bed)
   c. Pulmonary vasodilation; reduction of PCWP
   d. Does not impair coronary artery autoregulation*

B. *Epinephrine* is the most frequently used *second-line* inotropic agent. Tachycardia and arrhythmogenic potential limit use to refractory cases.

C. The following inotropic agents used infrequently because of particularly high incidence of untoward side effects:
   1. *Amrinone (Inocor)* has a hemodynamic profile similar to dobutamine including its systemic and pulmonary afterload-reducing effects. It is indicated in cases refractory to standard therapy or in cases of right-sided heart failure or pulmonary hypertension.
   2. *Isoproterenol (Isuprel)* also possesses systemic and pulmonary vasodilating capabilities and is primarily indicated in right-sided heart failure or pulmonary hypertension
   3. *Norepinephrine (Levophed)*, a potent vasoconstrictor, is almost exclusively reserved for septic shock (low SVR) refractory to phenylephrine. Occasionally it is used to manage severe cardiogenic shock or right ventricular failure.

V. Combination pharmacologic therapy
   A. Combined inotropic therapy
      1. Permits reduction of untoward effects
      2. When dopamine alone is not effective, one may gradually add dobutamine. The patient can then be weaned from dopamine to reduce incidence of tachyarrhythmias.
      3. Although the issue is controversial, many clinicians

---

*It is essential that the coronary arteries respond to the increased demand for oxygen associated with the positive inotropic or chronotropic effects of these drugs. Dopamine (but not dobutamine) disturbs this protective autoregulatory mechanism and thus increases risk of myocardial ischemia.

assert that renal vasodilation may be maintained during infusions of epinephrine or norepinephrine with renal-dose dopamine. Unfortunately, high doses of these inotropes abolishes this beneficial dopaminergic effect.

B. Combined inotropic and vasodilator therapy

  1. This therapy can be life saving in patients with severe myocardial depression by providing a greater augmentation of CO and fewer side effects than inotropes alone. Vasodilators permit improved visceral perfusion and help to minimize myocardial oxygen consumption.

  2. Furthermore, the damaged or diseased myocardium may become resistant to inotropic support alone and rely more on the reduction of afterload to increase stroke volume

  3. Nitroglycerin or nitroprusside are not infrequently combined with inotropes

VI. Mechanical assist devices (see following section)

Mechanical assist devices

I. Devices

  A. Intraaortic balloon pump (IABP) (percutaneous or transthoracic approach)

  B. Ventricular assist devices (VADs) (left, right, biventricular)

  C. Others (ECMO, CPB-portable system)

II. Indications in the postoperative cardiac surgery patient

  A. Cardiogenic shock*

  B. LCOS refractory to pharmacologic therapy

  C. Acute mitral regurgitation

III. Physiology and mechanisms (see Chapter 21)

  IABP only augments existing cardiac function by reducing afterload and increasing diastolic pressure (augmented coronary perfusion). VADs, on the other hand, can completely replace the pumping function of the failing heart.

IV. Basic strategy for use of mechanical assist devices

  In most cases IABP is the first device used. It can be placed percutaneously in the ICU. If IABP counterpulsation in com-

---

Note: Indicated only if cardiogenic shock has a potentially reversible cause or if used as a bridge to heart transplantation.

bination with pharmacologic support (inotropic, afterload reduction) is ineffective in maintaining adequate tissue perfusion, then a left VAD (LVAD) may be indicated. The complete cardiac support afforded by the LVAD may permit the injured myocardium to recover, or, if damage is irreversible, to provide adequate circulation until a heart donor is available.

V. Primary contraindications
   A. IABP:
      1. Aortic valve insufficiency (exacerbates regurgitation)
      2. Dissecting thoracic aortic aneurysm or synthetic thoracic aortic graft
   B. VAD:
      1. Systemic infection
      2. Increased bleeding tendency (e.g., renal failure requiring dialysis, disseminated intravascular coagulation [DIC])

VI. IABP management pearls
   A. IABP support should be considered *early* in the management of myocardial ischemia. Unlike pharmacologic therapy, it exerts its beneficial effects without an increase in myocardial oxygen consumption.
   B. Closely monitor lower extremities for evidence of diminished circulation! IABPs are notorious for causing limb ischemia via emboli from balloon thrombus or from direct occlusion of atherosclerotic iliofemoral vessels.
   C. As the patient improves, the rate of IABP augmentation can be gradually reduced. There is an increased incidence of balloon thrombus formation at low cardiac systole/balloon inflation ratios, and thus it is prudent to wean only to a ratio of 1:4 or more before discontinuing IABP.
   D. Balloon removal (percutaneous)
      1. When balloon is removed from vessel, allow to bleed antegrade, retrograde, and then antegrade again (1–2 seconds each) by alternating compression on artery distal and proximal to puncture site. In addition, during retrograde bleeding, "strip" the artery distal to proximal to milk any thrombus from the vessel.
      2. To prevent hematoma or pseudoaneurysm formation, apply direct pressure for *at least* 30 minutes. During this period check distal pulses with Doppler ultra-

Table 7-2 Review of General Management of Classic Clinical Scenarios

Hemodynamic parameters				Therapy	
MAP	CO	PCWP	SVR	First-line	Possible second-line
↓	↓	↓	↑	Volume	
↓	↓	↑	↑	Volume	Vasodilator
↑↓	↓	↑	↓	Vasodilator	Inotrope/IABP
↓	↓	↑	NL/↓	Inotrope	
NL	NL/↑	NL	↑↓	Vasopressor	
NL	NL	↑	↓	Diuretic	

NL, normal.

sound—one should still hear a minimal flow signal. *Beware:* The arterial cannulation site is actually 1–2 cm *proximal* to the cutaneous puncture site.

Review of general management of classic clinical scenarios (Table 7-2)

Right Ventricular Failure

Etiology

I. Inferior myocardial infarction (most common cause of *primary* right ventricular failure)

II. Increased right ventricular afterload
   A. Pulmonary hypertension (usually a result of long-standing mitral valve disease)
   B. Pulmonary embolism
   C. Left ventricular failure (the most common cause of right ventricular failure is *left* ventricular failure. The key to appropriate management is the ability to recognize the primary dysfunctional ventricle.)

Presentation and Diagnosis

I. Physical findings
   A. Jugular venous distention (JVD)
   B. Kussmaul's sign (augmentation of JVD with inspiration)
   C. *Absence of* evidence of pulmonary edema (rales): Although not always present, this is the most important finding to help distinguish right ventricular failure from left
   D. Cyanosis (infrequently seen; suggests pulmonary embolus or patent foramen ovale permitting a significant right-to-left shunt)

II. Diagnostic studies
   A. CVP
      1. Elevated (generally >10 mm Hg; may mimic cardiac tamponade because right and left atrial pressures approximate)
      2. Prominent y-descent in pressure tracing
   B. ECG may demonstrate ischemic changes in leads II, III, and AVF (inferior territory)
   C. Echocardiography reveals dilated right ventricle and global or regional akinesis in inferior myocardial infarction

Complications

I. Bradyarrhythmia or AV block
II. LCOS
III. Tricuspid regurgitation
IV. Rupture of ventricular free wall or interventricular septum

Management

I. Volume expansion
   A. Foundation of treatment of right ventricle failure
   B. Most beneficial in patients with normal PVR and normal right ventricular contractility. In this group volume loading often is the only intervention required.
   C. In patients with myocardial infarction, fluids are rarely sufficient. Initiate inotropic support early.
   D. *Beware:* Aggressive volume loading can further compromise CO because the dilating right ventricle limits left ventricular filling. If PCWP is greater than 15 to 18 mm Hg, addition of inotrope is usually indicated.
   E. Volume expansion can be used as a crude diagnostic test to distinguish right-sided versus left-sided heart failure. If CVP increases more than PCWP with fluid bolus, right ventricle failure is more likely.

II. Inotropic therapy
   A. Agents used for inotropic support in right ventricle failure include *dobutamine (Dobutrex), amrinone (Inocor),* and *isoproterenol (Isuprel).* Avoid dopamine because it can cause an increase in pulmonary artery pressures.
   B. Indicated in myocardial infarction after appropriate volume loading
   C. These agents are also pulmonary (and systemic) vasodilators

III. Afterload reduction
   A. Agents that reduce pulmonary afterload include *SNP (Nipride), nitroglycerin,* and *prostaglandin E_1 (PGE_1)* in addition to the three inotropic agents listed previously
   B. Indicated in patients with elevated PVR
   C. May be added to pharmacologic regimen if low CO persists despite volume expansion and inotropic support
   D. PGE_1 is also a potent systemic vasodilator. Concurrent infusions of PGE_1 through a pulmonary artery catheter and norepinephrine through a left atrial line maintain systemic BP

IV. Dobutamine is the overall agent of choice and should be the first pharmacologic intervention instituted

V. Maintenance of adequate cardiac rhythm

    A. Bradyarrhythmias and AV block complicate inferior myocardial ischemia

    B. Pharmacologic therapy: *Atropine* or *isoproterenol*

    C. *Beware:* Must have rapid access to pacing capabilities either via intraoperatively placed pacing wires or a transvenous pacing catheter for cases resistant to pharmacologic interventions. Even with this mechanical backup in place, AV block in the setting of large right ventricle infarction can frequently prove fatal because the necrotic tissue is refractory to pacing.

VI. Mechanical assist devices (IABP or right VAD) are indicated for cardiogenic shock if the aforementioned interventions cannot maintain an adequate CO

Postoperative Myocardial Ischemia

Improvements in intraoperative myocardial preservation, anesthetic techniques, and monitoring in addition to advancements in pharmacologic and mechanical support have resulted in a decrease in the prevalence and severity of perioperative myocardial ischemia. However, despite this progress, ischemic events still represent a significant threat to cardiac surgery patients. As the severity of preoperative myocardial dysfunction continues to increase with our aging patient population, even small amounts of injury to the myocardium have proven to be detrimental for those with significant preexisting disease. It is therefore imperative that early supportive management and/or surgical intervention be initiated to minimize permanent myocardial damage.

Incidence

The incidence of myocardial infarction varies dramatically (3% to 15%) depending on diagnostic criteria, patient population, and the experience of the operating room team. Not surprisingly, an increased risk is associated with emergent cases in unstable patients, with patients undergoing coronary artery bypass grafting (as opposed to isolated valve procedure), and with redo procedures. The highest incidence of perioperative myocardial ischemia occurs in the first 6 hours after bypass.

Prognosis

Conflicting evidence exists regarding the morbidity and mortality associated with postoperative myocardial ischemia in cardiac surgery. Its prognostic significance depends primarily on the criteria used for its diagnosis. Exclusive reliance on sensitive diagnostic studies (e.g., scintigraphy) results in detection of injury of little clinical significance. On the other hand, the application of stricter criteria (e.g., combination of ECG, biochemical, and clinical findings) selects for patients with myocardial damage significant enough to influence long-term survival. The majority of the literature supports our experience that only hemodynamically significant ischemic events associated with hypotension, low CO, and/or ventricular arrhythmia adversely affect survival.

Etiology

  I. Mechanical*
     A. Graft occlusion (thrombosis, stenosis)
     B. Distal coronary occlusion (atheromatous debris, air embolus)
     C. Incomplete revascularization
 II. Myocardial hypoperfusion (caused by perioperative hypotensive episode)
III. Increased myocardial oxygen demand (caused by hemodynamic stress)
     A. Tachycardia
     B. Elevated left or right ventricular afterload (SVR or PVR)
 IV. Vasospasm (of native coronary artery, internal mammary graft, or saphenous vein graft)
  V. Inadequate intraoperative myocardial protection

Presentation

  I. Symptoms
     A. More than 85% are silent
     B. Classic symptoms associated with angina include chest pain and tightness, diaphoresis, tachycardia, dyspnea, and nausea
 II. Hemodynamics
     A. Hypotension
     B. Low CO

---

*Technical factors are the most common cause of early graft failure.

    C. Elevated filling pressures (usually PCWP; but if right ven-
tricular infarction is present, CVP is elevated)

III. Malignant ventricular arrhythmias (with or without evidence
of ischemic ECG changes)

    A. Recurrent or refractory ventricular tachycardia or fibril-
lation

Diagnosis

ECG

The ECG is the most relied on diagnostic study for acute myocardial ischemia. It is imperative that the intensive care unit team
be aware of which vessels were bypassed and which (if any) grafts
were believed to be of suboptimal quality by the surgeon. This
information is helpful in the evaluation of postoperative ECG
changes by raising one's index of suspicion in those coronary artery
territories (Table 7-3).

ECG findings suggestive of ischemia or infarction (particularly
if they persist >24 to 48 hours) include the following:

  I. ST segment changes: Significant deviation from baseline (>2
mm) may represent ischemia (ST depression) or infarction
(ST elevation)

  II. T wave changes: Acutely, T waves are peaked; however, they
rapidly flatten and then invert

  III. Q waves

    A. The appearance of new significant Q waves (lasting ≥0.04
seconds) is the diagnostic standard for transmural myocardial necrosis. Q waves are a late finding and signal
irreversible damage.

    B. Be aware that up to 20% of Q waves are falsely positive
and represent transiently altered ventricular depolarization
without associated detectable infarction

Table 7-3   ECG Coronary Artery Territories

Territory	ECG leads	Coronary artery
Lateral	I, aVL, V_5, V_6	Circumflex (marginal) or LAD (diagonal)
Inferior	II, III, aVF	Right
Anteroseptal	V_1-V_4	LAD
Posterior	V_1, V_2*	Right

LAD, Left anterior descending.
*Reciprocal changes: Large R wave, ST depression.

C. Also, many postoperative infarctions in cardiac surgery patients are non-Q wave

IV. New bundle branch block (BBB), particularly a left BBB: Once a left BBB has been established, one is no longer able to evaluate accurately the ECG for further evidence of ischemia

V. *Note:*

A. ECG findings (particularly ST segment and T wave changes) alone are very nonspecific findings. However, acutely in the ICU, they are the best diagnostic tool available and must *not* be taken lightly.

B. Ventricular pacing, like BBB, precludes ability to evaluate for ischemia

Biochemical markers

Kinetics of serum levels after myocardial infarction:

I. Creatine kinase, MB isoenzyme (CK-MB):
Onset 4 to 8 hours; peak 24 hours

II. Lactate dehydrogenase (LDH):
Onset 16 to 24 hours; peak 3 to 6 days

CK-MB and LDH have traditionally been used to detect the presence and severity of myocardial injury. However, in the postoperative cardiac surgery patient, they lack sensitivity and specificity. Elevated CK-MB levels are found in essentially all patients and reflect myocardial mechanical trauma incurred intraoperatively because of the nature of the procedure (from simple manipulation of the heart to the atriotomy or ventriculotomy for cannulas or vents). Furthermore, even in the setting of infarction, there is no correlation between the size of the infarction and the peak CK-MB.

Despite these shortcomings, serial analysis may be useful. If levels rise after the acute postoperative period, it is likely that an ischemic event has occurred and further studies (scintigraphy, echocardiography) may be indicated to determine the extent of injury.

Echocardiography

Echocardiography is used to identify regional or segmental wall motion abnormalities. Higher quality views are achieved with transesophageal echocardiography.

Radiopharmaceutical myocardial imaging

Two types of radiopharmaceutical myocardial imaging are available: Infarct avid (technetium) and myocardial perfusion (thallium) scans. They are the most sensitive and specific tests for evidence of ischemia; however, if only scintigraphy is positive, the injury is rarely associated with early or late myocardial dysfunction.

In summary, no single test can make the diagnosis of significant postoperative myocardial ischemia with absolute certainty in the cardiac surgery patient.

Sequelae

    I. Acute myocardial infarction
   II. LCOS (in most severe form, cardiogenic shock)
  III. Malignant ventricular arrhythmias or cardiac arrest
  IV. Acute mitral regurgitation
   V. Acute ventricular septal defect
  VI. Right ventricular failure
 VII. Ventricular free wall or aneurysm rupture (with associated pericardial tamponade)

Management

Therapeutic goals

    I. Alleviate myocardial ischemia (maximize myocardial oxygen delivery, minimize myocardial oxygen demand)
   II. Treat ventricular dysfunction
  III. Prevent arrhythmias

Basics

    I. Myocardial ischemia must be managed in a *monitored* environment. If patient is on the wards, transfer him or her to the ICU without delay. Place patient on continuous telemetry and pulse oximetry.
   II. Do not forget to perform the standard ABC's of resuscitation (*a*irway, *b*reathing, *c*irculation) while initiating the following outlined regimen for myocardial ischemia. Be vigilant with frequent reassessments as interventions are underway on these potentially labile patients.
  III. *Notify attending surgeon or fellow immediately if a question of ischemia arises!*

Immediate management

I. Oxygen: 100% nonrebreather face mask versus intubation (if patient in severe respiratory distress or in shock). If uncertain, be conservative and intubate. These patients poorly tolerate the increased sympathetic activity (and resultant increased myocardial oxygen demand) associated with respiratory distress.

II. *Nitroglycerin,* 0.4 mg sublingually (SL) STAT (then q 5 minutes) for coronary vasodilation and preload (and afterload) reduction. If systolic BP is greater than 90 mm Hg administer topical nitroglycerin (Nitropaste), 1- to 2-inch.

III. Establish IV access (large-bore [14- or 16-gauge] peripheral line if patient is hypotensive) Maintain adequate BP with fluid boluses as needed.

IV. *Morphine,* 1 to 2 mg IV STAT (prompt pain control is also important to minimize sympathetic activity). May repeat, but beware of hypotension.

Short-term management

I. Perform follow-up 12-lead ECG every 5 to 10 minutes until ischemic changes have resolved or definitive therapy initiated

II. Consider nifedipine, 10 mg sublingually if vasospasm suspected (particularly if internal mammary artery is used as conduit). Beware of hypotension and reflex tachycardia.

III. If ischemia persists and BP is adequate, initiate nitroglycerin infusion (start at 10 μg/min and titrate to 100 μg/min if BP tolerates). *Note:* As rate increased, additional fluid may be required to accommodate increasing venous capacitance.

IV. If patient is hemodynamically unstable, initiate invasive monitoring with intraarterial and Swan-Ganz catheters

V. If hematocrit is less than 30%, transfuse 2 units of packed red blood cells (maximize oxygen-carrying capacity). *Note:* If patient in CHF, diuretic therapy is indicated *before* blood products.

VI. Serum CK-MB should be drawn now and q 8 hours

VII. Indications for heparin and β blockers are patient dependent. Decisions for their use must be made by the attending surgeon or fellow.

Optimize determinants of CO

Tachycardia and increased preload or afterload may exacerbate myocardial ischemia by increasing oxygen debt. On the other hand, the ischemic heart may require an elevated HR or filling pressure to maintain an adequate CO, because of impaired ventricular function. Hemodynamic management must be individualized to patient requirements. See section on low CO for detailed therapeutic algorithms.

Ventricular arrhythmias

Myocardial ischemia is associated with increased risk of arrhythmias as a result of increased myocyte automaticity or irritability. Of most concern are life-threatening ventricular tachycardia or fibrillation, which occur in 5% to 25% of patients with infarction.

I. Correct serum electrolytes ($K^+ > 4.5$ mEq/L, $Mg^{++} > 1.8$ mEq/L).

II. If myocardial infarction is suspected or ventricular ectopy (premature ventricular complexes [PVCs], especially if frequent or multifocal) noted in the setting of ischemia, ventricular arrhythmia prophylaxis is indicated. *Lidocaine* is the first drug of choice. If ectopy is refractory to lidocaine and correction of serum electrolytes, consider *procainamide (Procan)*. Because of its negative inotropic effects, *bretylium (Bretylol)* is infrequently used. (The experimental drug amiodarone can be used for unrelenting ventricular arrhythmias, although acquisition of this agent requires formidable effort.)

III. For a more detailed discussion, see Chapter 10

Mechanical assist devices

I. Indicated in patients unresponsive to pharmacologic treatment. Mechanical assist devices should be initiated *early* in these hemodynamically unstable patients to minimize injury to salvageable myocardium!

II. Percutaneous IABP is the most frequently used device. It decreases afterload on left ventricle and increases diastolic coronary perfusion.

III. For details concerning management, see section on LCOS and Chapter 21

Surgery

I. Indicated in patients hemodynamically or electrically unstable, presumably because of significant myocardial ischemia (resulting from bypass graft failure or insufficient revascularization)

II. Decide whether the risk associated with emergent coronary catheterization is warranted

  A. If patient's condition is stabilized with pharmacologic or mechanical support and the surgeon feels confident about all the grafts, catheterization is a reasonable option. One must avoid the scenario of negative reexploration with documented ongoing ischemia.

  B. Conversely, if the patient is unstable and there is some suspicion concerning a particular graft, emergent surgical intervention must be immediately undertaken

III. After surgery, patient returns to ICU for continued medical therapy (dependent on operative findings and degree of successful revascularization)

Management of cardiac complications associated with myocardial ischemia or infarction

I. Bradycardia or AV block

  A. Caused by ischemia to sinoatrial or AV node. Most frequently seen with inferior infarction (right coronary artery territory)

  B. See section on LCOS and Chapter 10 for discussion of management (atropine, isoproterenol, pacers)

II. Acute Mitral Regurgitation

  A. Resulting from papillary muscle dysfunction or rupture

  B. Diagnosis

    1. Evidence of CHF (rales, JVD, S_3 gallop, etc.)

    2. New holosystolic murmur, radiating to axilla

    3. Large v wave on PCWP tracing (reflective of left atrial pressure tracing)

  C. Management

    1. Pharmacologic

      a. Goal: Afterload reduction (minimize regurgitant flow by maximizing forward flow from left ventricle)

      b. Systolic BP > 90 mm Hg: Nitroprusside (titrate to reduce CHF, while maintaining systolic BP > 90 mm Hg)

      c. Systolic BP < 90 mm Hg: Dobutamine (temporizing measure to maintain BP until mechanical support initiated or surgical intervention)

    2. Use IABP if patient hypotensive

    3. Surgery

III. Acute ventricular septal defect
   A. Usually occurs 5 to 7 days after transmural infarction
   B. Diagnosis
      1. Evidence of CHF (rales, JVD, S_3 gallop, etc.)
      2. New harsh pansystolic murmur and thrill left sternal border
      3. Step-up of O_2 saturation (>10%) between left atrium (proximal Swan port) and pulmonary artery (distal port)
   C. Management
      1. Pharmacologic (analogous to that for acute mitral regurgitation)
         a. Goal: Afterload reduction (minimize left-to-right shunting by maximizing forward flow from left ventricle)
         b. Systolic BP > 90 mm Hg: Nitroprusside
         c. Systolic BP < 90 mm Hg: Dobutamine
      2. Use IABP if patient hypotensive
      3. Surgery
IV. Right ventricular failure (see section on LCOS section for diagnosis and management)

Postoperative Hypertension

Postoperative hypertension occurs in 30% to 60% of cardiac surgery patients. An increased incidence is associated with the following:

- History of preoperative hypertension and/or β-blocker use
- CABG (incidence 30% to 50%) compared with isolated valve procedure (5%)
- Surgery for aortic stenosis (at increased risk for postoperative hyperdynamic myocardium syndrome)

The MAP provides the most reliable parameter of BP (MAP = Diastolic BP + ⅓ [Systolic BP − Diastolic BP]). Systolic BP measured at the radial artery, on the other hand, demonstrates a variable relationship with the central aortic pressure, because of the numerous determinants of systolic amplification (e.g., severity of atherosclerotic disease). Iatrogenic hypotension may result in patients with significant systolic amplification if systolic BP is monitored instead of MAP during vasodilator therapy.

Various criteria exist for hypertension. Some identify an absolute upper level of normal (e.g., MAP > 105 mm Hg), whereas others define a hypertensive state as a specified increase from baseline (e.g., 20 mm Hg greater than baseline).

Etiology

BP is product of SVR and CO. Thus hypertension may be due to (1) elevated SVR and/or (2) hyperdynamic myocardium syndrome (CI $\geq$ 3.0 L/min/m^2 and HR $\geq$ 100 beats/min) (see discussion in LCOS section). Specific etiologies include:

- Pain/anxiety
- Hypothermia
- Hypoxia
- Hypercarbia
- LCOS (with reflex vasoconstriction)
- Hyperdynamic myocardium syndrome
- Other causes include visceral distention (bladder or stomach), fever, drug withdrawal (e.g., β blocker, narcotics, etc.)

Sequelae

I. Myocardial ischemia or infarction*
II. LCOS
III. Cerebrovascular accident
IV. Increased postoperative bleeding
V. Aortic dissection

Management

(See Appendix B on p. 516 for therapeutic summary)

Basics

I. Goal
   A. Reduction of BP to decrease afterload, improve CO, and minimize myocardial oxygen consumption while still maintaining adequate coronary, cerebral, and renal perfusion
   B. MAP approximately 60 to 85 mm Hg (SVR 900 to 1200 dynes/sec/cm^{-5})
   C. *Note:* Target BP must be individualized for elderly and other patients with suspected vascular disease to prevent

---

*Because of increased myocardial oxygen consumption and reduced subendocardial coronary perfusion associated with increased afterload and ventricular wall tension.

cerebral and/or renal ischemia. The best goal for these
patients is preoperative BP, but confirm target parameters
with the attending surgeon or fellow.

II. All patients receiving parenteral vasodilator or β-blocking
agents must have continuous invasive arterial pressure monitoring to permit optimal titration of agent and to avoid iatrogenic hypotension

III. Periodically confirm arterial line readings by manually checking BP in both upper extremities with sphyngomanometer

IV. While treating the hypertension, continue to search for primary
etiology so that definitive therapy may be undertaken

Management

I. Pain and anxiety

A. Sedation: Midazolam (Versed), 1 to 5 mg IV every 1 hour
as needed while the patient is intubated

B. Analgesia: Morphine, 1 to 5 mg IV every 1 hour as needed.
Beware: Narcotics blunt respiratory drive (particularly
dangerous in the early extubation period).

C. Verbal reassurance, especially in the early postoperative
period when patient is still intubated and unable to communicate

D. Extubate as soon as possible

II. Vasoconstriction caused by hypothermia: Use warming lights
and blanket

III. Oxygenation and ventilation: Serial ABG should be monitored
to assure optimal respiratory status (arterial pressure of O_2 and
CO_2)

IV. Determine cardiac hemodynamics (CI and SVR)

A. If CI is adequate but SVR is elevated, use vasodilator
therapy (see following subsection)

B. If CI is supraphysiologic and SVR is normal or elevated,
consider β-blocker therapy (see section on hyperdynamic
myocardium syndrome)

C. If CI is less then 2.0 L/min/m², follow algorithm for
treatment of LCOS. Patient may actually need inotropes
in the setting of hypertension to resolve the compensatory
vasoconstriction of decreased CO.

Note: Do not initiate cardioactive pharmacologic interventions
(i.e., step IV) until steps I. through III. have been addressed or
initiated.

V. Other
   A. Use foley catheter or nasogastric tube if visceral distention is suspected
   B. Antipyretic agent (acetaminophen, 650 mg orally or rectally every 4 hours) if patient is febrile
   C. Administer paralytic agent (pavulon) if intubated patient is shivering.

Vasodilator therapy

   I. Vasodilators exert their beneficial effects via reduction of preload and/or afterload with resultant reduction in myocardial oxygen consumption and improved ejection fraction
   II. Effect of vasodilator on BP depends on the following:
      A. Volume status
         Beware: If intravascular volume status significantly reduced, rapid life-threatening hypotension may occur with the initiation of vasodilator therapy. It cannot be overemphasized to *optimize preload before administering vasodilators*. Furthermore, while these agents are being titrated, volume status must be continually reevaluated and fluids administered to maintain an adequate preload.
      B. Pharmacologic target (artery vs vein)
         1. Three basic types of vasodilators
            a. Arteriodilators (reduce afterload)
            b. Venodilators (reduce preload)
            c. Mixed (combined arteriodilator and venodilator)
         2. As one would expect, arteriodilators provide a more dramatic reduction in systemic BP
   III. Duration of therapy
      Often several hours of therapy are sufficient. Most patients can be weaned off all vasodilators by early morning on the first postoperative day. However, occasionally postoperative hypertension persists longer than 24 hours and these patients must be weaned to an oral regimen.
   IV. Relative contraindications include obstructive valvular disease (aortic, pulmonary, mitral), hypovolemia, tachycardia, cardiac tamponade
   V. Specific vasodilators (refer to Appendix A on p. 497 for complete discussion of each agent)
      A. *Sodium nitroprusside*
      B. *Nitroglycerin*

    C. *Nifedipine (Procardia)*
    D. β-Blocking agents
       1. *Esmolol (Brevibloc)*
       2. *Propanolol (Inderal)*
       3. *Atenolol (Tenormin)*
       4. *Labetalol (Normodyne)*
    E. Other antihypertensive agents (less frequently used at our institution)
       a. *Clonidine (Catapres)*
       b. *Prazosin (Minipress)*
       c. *Hydralazine (Apresoline)*
       d. *Prostaglandin E$_1$*

VI. "Rebound hypertension"
    A. Abrupt discontinuation may result in hypertensive crisis
    B. Classically seen with clonidine and β-blockers
    C. Taper withdrawal of these agents

Standard Johns Hopkins cardiac surgery postoperative antihypertensive regimen

  I. Admission to ICU
    A. Nitroprusside drip: Titrate to MAP of 60 to 85 mm Hg
    B. Midazolam, 1 to 5 mg q 1 hour prn; morphine, 1 to 5 mg every 1 hour as needed; pavulon, 1 to 5 mg q 1 hour prn
 II. Six hours postoperatively
    A. Nifedipine, 10 to 30 mg SL or PO q 1-2 hours to wean from nitroprusside
    B. Nitropaste, 1 to 2 inches, q 1-2 hours prn for additional vasodilation
III. Postoperative day 1: Start preoperative PO antihypertensive regimen in patients with history of hypertensive or new PO agent in those who have not successfully weaned from routine antihypertensive regimen

Postoperative Hypotension

The principal feature defining shock is inadequate perfusion pressures for preservation of visceral function, not hypotension per se. However, although often not the first clinical sign of shock, hypotension is the most readily detectable and requires immediate attention.

A MAP of 60 mm Hg is generally accepted as the lower limit

of normal. Realize that like its counterpart, hypertension, the criteria for defining a hypotensive state are patient dependent (i.e., significant cerebrovascular and renal disease mandate higher pressures).

Rapid assessment of BP can be achieved by palpation of pulses. Detectable pulse in the femoral artery indicates a systolic BP of at least 60 mm Hg; in the carotid artery, 70 mm Hg; and radial artery, 80 mm Hg.

Etiology

I. Hypovolemia (including relative hypovolemia associated with postoperative vasodilation that occurs with rewarming)
II. Myocardial ischemia or infarction (and other causes of cardiogenic shock, as discussed later)
III. Cardiac tamponade
IV. Arrhythmias
V. Decreased SVR
   A. Sepsis
   B. Inflammatory-mediated vasodilation associated with CPB (uncommon)
   C. Transfusion or drug reaction
VI. Pneumothorax
VII. Pulmonary embolus

Cardiogenic shock

I. Defined as a shock state caused by cardiac dysfunction, signaled by CI less than 2.0 L/min/m^2 and elevated PCWP
II. Differential diagnosis includes large myocardial infarction (>30% to 40% of left ventricle), acute mitral regurgitation, acute ventricular septal defect, and right ventricular failure
III. Poor prognosis (mortality rate >75%)

Management

Immediate management of acute hypotension: Address ABC's of resuscitation (airway, breathing, circulation)

I. Place patient in Trendelenberg position
II. Oxygen (100% O_2 via face mask or intubation if indicated)
III. IV fluid bolus (through cordis port or large peripheral IV line)
IV. Calcium chloride 1 amp IV bolus (may repeat)
V. If in early postoperative period, dopamine is often already

infusing at renal dose (0-3 μg/kg/min). Increase dopamine rate to achieve pressor effect (15–20 μg/kg/min).

VI. *Notify fellow or attending surgeon*

Acute management

I. Assessment to determine cause of hypotension
  A. Physical examination (e.g., tachycardia, irregular rhythm, rales, absent breath sounds, wheezes, JVD, new murmur)
  B. ECG or telemetry (ischemia, arrhythmia)
  C. ABG (hypoxia, large alveolar-arterial gradient)
  D. CXR (enlarged heart shadow, pneumothorax)
II. Intraarterial and Swan-Ganz catheters
  A. In the ICU most patients still have these catheters in place. However, if they have been discontinued and initial assessment suggests cardiac etiology or if cause is uncertain, they should be replaced without delay.
  B. Remember also to analyze right-sided pressures for evidence of right ventricular failure or cardiac tamponade

Management of specific etiologies

I. Hypovolemia: Volume expansion (see subsection on preload management in LCOS section)
II. Myocardial ischemia or infarction (see section on postoperative myocardial ischemia for management of ischemia and its potential cardiac sequelae [acute mitral regurgitation or ventricular septal defect])
III. Pericardial tamponade: Acutely volume loading is the temporizing treatment of choice (see subsection on preload management in LCOS section and Chapter 9)
IV. Arrhythmias (see subsection on heart rate management in LCOS section and Chapter 10)
V. Decreased SVR
  A. Volume expansion
  B. Vasopressor therapy
    1. *Phenylephrine (Neo-Synephrine)*
    2. *Norepinephrine (Levophed)* for refractory hypotension
  C. Antimicrobial therapy if caused by sepsis
  D. *Note:* Frequently associated with concurrent high CO
VI. Pneumothorax
  A. If patient is unstable, 14-gauge needle in midclavicular

    line of intercostal space 2 is the temporizing intervention
    of choice
  B. Chest tube
VII. Pulmonary embolus: Heparin infusion and supportive therapy

Hyperdynamic Myocardium Syndrome

Hyperdynamic myocardium syndrome is loosely defined as a condition with elevated CO (CI > 3.0 L/min/m²; often supraphysiologic) with or without tachycardia (HR > 100 beats/min). It is
most commonly encountered in patients with compensatory ventricular hypertrophy caused by preoperative systemic hypertension,
aortic stenosis, or idiopathic hypertrophic subaortic stenosis. However, it may be encountered in the setting of routine coronary artery
bypass grafting presenting as an overall hyperdynamic cardiovascular state with an associated sinus tachycardia. Although the
mechanism is uncertain, evidence points to elevated circulating
catecholamines.

Management involves the following:
- Increased contractility *without* tachycardia rarely requires
  therapeutic intervention
- *Esmolol (Brevibloc)* is occasionally indicated. Because of the
  potential for significant negative inotropic effects, *the initiation of β-blocker therapy should be approved by the attending surgeon or fellow.*

Heart Transplantation: Basics of Unique Postoperative Hemodynamics

The Denervated Donor Heart

The intact heart is innervated by antagonistic sympathetic and
parasympathetic fibers of the autonomic nervous system. Transplantation necessitates transection of these fibers, yielding a denervated heart with altered physiology.
  I. Resting HR
     Normally, the negative chronotropic and dromotropic effects
     of the parasympathetic vagal fibers are dominant over the
     opposing sympathetic signals. Devoid of autonomic input, the
     SA node of the transplanted heart fires at an increased intrinsic
     resting rate of 90 to 100 beats/min.

II. Reflex tachycardia
   A. The transplanted heart relies on distant noncardiac sites as its source for catecholamines. Its response to stresses (e.g., hypovolemia, hypoxia, anemia) is delayed until the circulating catecholamines can exert their positive chronotropic effect on the heart. This also accounts for the frequency of orthostatic hypotension in transplant patients.
   B. Because part of the recipient's atria (including the SA node) is preserved, careful evaluation of the ECG often reveals the simultaneous presence of two different P waves. Although the signal from the innervated remnant SA node is not conducted to the ventricle, an increased rate can be used as an early indication of stress.
III. Response to therapeutic interventions
   Interventions that act directly through the cardiac autonomic nervous system are *ineffective*
   A. Carotid sinus massage and Valsalva maneuver
   B. Atropine and digoxin
IV. Angina
   The denervated heart lacks afferent sensory fibers; thus these patients do not have the characteristic chest discomfort associated with myocardial ischemia (at least in the early postoperative period; some evidence exists that reinnervation may occur later)

Management of Selected Postoperative Complications

I. Low CO
   A. The newly transplanted heart is stiff and noncompliant because of the insult associated with harvesting, cooling, and ischemic time. Therefore a low CO state frequently exists in the early postoperative period.
      1. The denervated heart relies heavily on the Frank-Starling relationship for augmentation of CO. Maintain an adequate preload, particularly in the setting of vasodilation (from rewarming or pharmacologic agent).
      2. The most effective way to initially increase CO is to increase HR (CO = HR × SV). This can be achieved with *isoproterenol (Isuprel)* and/or AV sequential pacing. Maintain HR between 100 and 125 beats/min.
      3. Additional inotropic support may be achieved with *dobutamine (Dobutrex)*.

Note: Isoproterenol is the first-line agent in transplant patients compared with dobutamine (or dopamine) in the general cardiac surgery patient.

B. There is an increased incidence of right ventricular failure in transplant patients. The cause is multifactorial and includes direct injury to the right ventricle (e.g., ischemia) and the elevated pulmonary afterload (PVR) frequently encountered in patients with long-standing left ventricular failure.

    1. Monitor right-sided heart filling pressure (CVP) in all patients for early detection of right ventricle failure

    2. Isoproterenol is the agent of choice because of its pulmonary vasodilatory effect (in addition to its positive chronotropic and inotropic effects).

II. Conduction disturbances

A. Bradycardia or junctional rhythms are common postoperatively

B. Management

    1. Isoproterenol (*Note:* Do not use atropine)

    2. AV sequential pacer

Suggested readings

Baumgartner WA, Reitz BA, Achuff SC, eds: *Heart and heart-lung transplantation,* Philadelphia, 1990, WB Saunders.

Daily EK, Schroeder JS: *Techniques in bedside monitoring,* St Louis, 1989, Mosby.

DiSesa VJ: Pharmacologic support for postoperative low cardiac output, *Semin Thorac Cardiovasc Surg* 3:13-23, 1991.

Gray RJ, Matloff JM, eds: *Medical management of the cardiac surgery patient,* Baltimore, 1990, Williams & Wilkins.

Kotler MN, Alfieri AD, eds: *Cardiac and noncardiac complications of open heart surgery: Prevention, diagnosis, and treatment,* Mount Kisco, NY, 1992, Futura.

Opie LH, ed: *Drugs for the heart,* ed 3, Philadelphia, 1991, WB Saunders.

Sabiston DC, Spencer FC, eds: *Gibbon's surgery of the chest,* Philadelphia, 1990, WB Saunders.

Wilmore DW, ed: *Care of the surgical patient: Perioperative management and techniques,* New York, 1992, Scientific American.

Zaloga GP: *The critical care drug handbook,* St Louis, 1991, Mosby.

Pulmonary Management

8

Sandra M. Walden *and* Pamela Meyer

Management of the patient's respiratory status is an extremely important aspect of the postoperative care of the cardiac surgical patient. A patient with underlying pulmonary problems may have an excellent surgical result only to have difficulty weaning later in the postoperative course. The preoperative medical condition, intraoperative events, and postoperative management all contribute to outcome. Goals for postoperative pulmonary management include the following:

- Successful weaning from ventilatory support as quickly as possible
- Maintenance of adequate oxygenation and ventilation after extubation
- Prevention and treatment of postoperative nosocomial pulmonary-related complications

This chapter focuses on the multiple considerations involved in successful respiratory system management after cardiac surgery. Topics include preoperative evaluation, initial postoperative evaluation and management, strategies for weaning from mechanical ventilation in both routine and complicated cases, and identification and management of ventilator-related and other respiratory complications.

Preoperative Evaluation

A careful preoperative evaluation assists in predicting the patient's response to cardiac surgery, cardiopulmonary bypass, and postoperative weaning. It allows the caregiver to anticipate potential problems, initiate treatment preoperatively where appropriate and possible, and develop guidelines for ventilatory management, from induction of anesthesia to extubation. A thorough pulmonary evaluation should include the following:

- Smoking history and any occupational or travel exposures
- History of frequent upper respiratory or sinus infections, bronchitis, pneumonia, tuberculosis, chronic productive cough
- History of asthma or airway obstruction
- History of previous hospital admissions, surgical operations, response to previous anesthesia, and previous episodes of mechanical ventilation
- Assessment of acute illness, including pneumonia, bronchitis, asthma, congestive failure, sepsis
- Current medications
- Baseline preoperative pulmonary function testing, when indicated
- Review of chest radiograph for infiltrates, masses, atelectasis

In general, preexisting pulmonary conditions such as chronic obstructive lung disease (particularly if the forced expiratory volume in 1 second is <1.0 L), active asthma (particularly steroid-dependent asthma), pulmonary fibrosis, and pulmonary hypertension may result in prolonged mechanical ventilation for more than 72 hours.

It is important to remember that the general medical condition of the patient contributes to the pulmonary response to cardiac surgery and mechanical ventilation. Poor nutritional status may result in weak, ineffective respiratory muscles, poor wound healing, and higher morbidity from postoperative infections. Volume overload or congestive heart failure may result in impaired gas exchange, leading to hypoxemic respiratory failure. Changes in mental status; neuromuscular function; gastrointestinal problems such as reflux, ulcers, or intraabdominal pain; and active multisystemic diseases all affect respiratory system competency and present possible weaning difficulties.

Multidisciplinary patient education is an important aspect of preoperative management. This should include information regarding what the patient should expect postoperatively with respect to nutrition, intubation, ventilator management, and pain control strategies to be used. Patient involvement in the use of the incentive spirometer, cough and deep breathing techniques, and general rehabilitative motivation should be emphasized.

Initial Ventilator Management

In addition to the patient's preoperative medical status, intraoperative events also contribute to the course of early postoperative management. Cardiothoracic surgery reduces functional residual capacity and may cause hypoventilation, early airway closure with microatelectasis, and poor secretion clearance initially. Prolonged cardiopulmonary bypass (CPB) and the intraoperative requirement of a significant volume replacement further contribute to shunting, vascular congestion, and pulmonary vascular endothelial damage that may result in prolonged ventilatory support. In the immediate postoperative period patients continue to receive ventilatory support and are observed for potential problems from anesthesia, CPB, rewarming, sedation, and excessive bleeding. Hypothermia may contribute to respiratory alkalosis and hypomagnesemia. Shivering with warming may lead to respiratory acidosis, if excessive, but can usually be controlled with sedation and paralysis (see Chapter 4). Hypercapnia can usually be controlled by changes in respiratory rate. Another major concern in the early postoperative period is the amount of oxygen consumed with the work of breathing in circumstances of shivering, anxiety, and underlying pulmonary disease. The muscles of respiration may require up to 50% utilization of the oxygen delivered (normal requirement, 2% to 5%). Even with a high fraction of inspired oxygen (Fio_2), other organs and tissues may develop a relative tissue hypoxia and lactic acidosis.

Therefore almost all patients arrive in the cardiac surgical intensive care unit while receiving artificial ventilation. Initial evaluation should include an in-depth review of the intraoperative course and physical examination, arterial blood gas (ABG), and chest x-ray film (CXR). The CXR should determine the presence and position of the following:

- Endotracheal tube
- Central venous catheter
- Pulmonary artery catheter
- Gastric tube
- Internal pacing device and wires
- Intraaortic balloon catheter
- Extracorporeal assist devices

It is important to assess the CXR for the following early complications:

- Atelectasis

- Widened mediastinum
- Hemothorax and pneumothorax
- Pulmonary infiltrates and pneumonia
- Congestive heart failure
- Air trapping and hyperinflation

Postoperative pulmonary care is initiated by protocol and subsequently individualized to fit each patient. Oxygen concentration is set at 90% to 100% and ABG obtained. FIO_2 is then titrated to maintain oxygen pressure between 70 and 100 mm Hg. Whenever possible, the FIO_2 should be maintained at 0.6 or less to avoid complications of oxygen toxicity. The endotracheal tube tip should be 2 cm above the carina. A full discussion of the mode or type of ventilation is included later in this chapter. The synchronized intermittent mandatory ventilation (SIMV) mode is most commonly used. Minute ventilation is set at 120 ml/kg/min with tidal volumes of 10 to 15 ml/kg ideal body weight and the rate at 8 to 15 breaths/min. The rate and tidal volume are then adjusted to keep pH at 7.35 to 7.40 and carbon dioxide pressure at 40 mm Hg. To help restore the functional residual capacity of the lungs to normal and reduce microatelectasis, positive end-expiratory pressure (PEEP) of 5 cm H_2O is added.

Most patients tolerate this level of PEEP well. Air trapping in a patient with obstructive lung disease may result in the development of endogenous PEEP (auto-PEEP), which would be a contraindication to the external application of PEEP. High levels of PEEP may impede venous return and depress cardiac output by reducing ventricular filling. However, levels of PEEP as high as 20 mm Hg may be required to reduce intravascular shunting in such situations as adult respiratory distress syndrome (ARDS). There is controversial evidence that high levels of PEEP may assist in tamponading small blood vessels in the chest wall and mediastinum, which may help control postoperative bleeding (see Chapter 9).

The majority of patients are able to be weaned from the ventilator within the first 6 to 48 hours postoperatively, guided by oxygen saturations and/or ABG measurements and rate of spontaneous respirations. If the patient's acid-base status is stable, oxygen saturation determination is a reasonable substitute for ABG determinants (3,24) (see the box). Generally, the Fio_2 is weaned first, to 0.40 to 0.50. The SIMV rate is then successively reduced by decrements of 2 breaths/min until the patient is receiving continuous positive airway pressure (CPAP). Frequent suctioning, the

Policies, Procedures, and Protocols*

Ventilator weaning: Management of patient requiring the following—

1. *Indications for Use*

Patients who are intubated and patients 1 hour postoperatively who demonstrate the following criteria:
- 1.1 Hemodynamically stable
- 1.2 No physiologic contraindications
- 1.3 ABG within normal parameters on admission to unit
- 1.4 Patient receiving routine postoperative ventilator settings according to standard MD orders

2. *Responsibility*
- 2.1 MD writes order to initiate weaning protocol
- 2.2 RN and RT initiate protocol and monitor progress.

3. *Assessment*

Before implementing the protocol, RN:
- 3.1 Reviews initial ABG results completed on admission to unit
- 3.2 Reviews patient history for contraindications to weaning
- 3.3 Reviews postoperative ventilator settings
- 3.4 Monitors patient condition every hour while weaning
- 3.5 Compares CO_2 from ABG with capnometer reading simultaneously
- 3.6 Assesses ability to maintain total minute ventilation as SIMV rate is decreased

4. *Interventions*
- 4.1 Initiate pulse oximetry
- 4.2 Coordinate with RT initiation of end tidal CO_2 monitoring
- 4.3 Begin weaning FIO_2 after initial ABG is $PaO_2 \geq$ 100-110 mm Hg
- 4.4 Decrease FIO_2 by increments of 20%-40% every 30 min, maintaining O_2 saturation $\geq 92\%$
- 4.5 Begin weaning from SIMV when patient is normotensive, normothermic, and arousable or initiating spontaneous respirations

Continued.

Policies, Procedures and Protocols* — cont'd

4.6   Decrease SIMV by intervals of 2 every 30 min, maintaining end tidal CO_2 ± 10 points from baseline (as previously correlated with ABG). *If MD order is present,* stop at predetermined SIMV rate and go to CPAP.

4.7   Within 2 hours after initiation of weaning, draw ABG

4.8   Monitor and record end tidal CO_2 and O_2 saturation every hour during weaning

4.9   Draw ABG and record end tidal volume when patient receiving CPAP or at anytime patient's respiratory status deteriorates

4.10 RT checks forced vital capacity and negative inspiratory force readings while patient's receiving CPAP

4.11 RT extubates per MD's order

5. *Reportable Conditions*

5.1   Inability to wean per protocol

5.2   Failure to maintain minute ventilation when SIMV rate decreased

5.3 O_2 saturation, end tidal CO_2, ABG, or respiratory rate outside normal ranges

5.4   Change in patient condition

5.5   Clinical condition necessitating increase or change in type of ventilator settings

6. *Documentation*

6.1   RN/RT to sign order on MD order sheet

6.2   RN to document ventilator changes, end tidal CO_2, O_2 saturation on high-frequency observation record

6.3   RN to document respiratory assessment every 4 hr per protocol on high-frequency observation record

Reference: Nursing practice and organization manual: surgical sciences: Volume 2 Clinical Practice.

See Also: Management of Patient Requiring Mechanical Ventilation Protocol.

RN, Registered nurse; *RT,* respiratory therapist.
*From The Johns Hopkins Hospital
Department of Surgical Sciences
Nursing Clinical Practice Manual, May 1992.

use of PEEP, sighs, and hand bagging help reverse atelectasis. Before extubation the patient should be assessed for airway stability, ability to handle airway secretions, adequate level of consciousness and spontaneous breathing, hemodynamic stability, and absence of unstable arrhythmias, excessive bleeding, or other complications that might require return to the operating room. It is important to establish that there is complete recovery from anesthesia, sedation, and paralytic medications used (see Chapter 4). The effect of pain medications on ventilation must also be considered before extubation.[19]

The physiologic criteria for extubation are listed below.[21] The patient should be able to meet several of these criteria before being extubated. It is important to remember that from a pulmonary point of view the patient may no longer be receiving ventilation and may be ready to be extubated, but may possibly require continued intubation for some period of time for the reasons previously described.

Failure to Wean

Approximately 10% of patients fail weaning from the ventilator during the 72 to 96 hours after cardiac surgery.[16,19] Formulation of

---

Criteria for Extubation

1. Arterial O_2 pressure >80 mm Hg with Fio_2 ≤ 0.5
2. pH 7.35-7.45
3. Spontaneous tidal volume >10 ml/kg and/or able to double minute ventilation on request without fatigue
4. Negative inspiratory force >20 cm H_2O
5. Satisfactory ventilation demonstrated with CPAP with respiratory rate <30 breaths/min
6. Patient alert and awake (for most patients without neurologic damage)
7. Ability to maintain airway and clear secretions
8. Patient hemodynamically stable, no unstable arrhythmias (intraaortic balloon pump is not a contraindication if hemodynamics are completely stable)
9. No excessive bleeding or impending reason to return to operating room

a rational weaning strategy should be based on an understanding of the physiologic reasons for respiratory failure. Potential forces contributing to prolonged ventilatory dependence are outlined below. Frequently the medical issues leading to weaning failure are multifactorial. Hepatic and renal dysfunction, poor nutritional status, medications, cerebrovascular accidents, and cardiovascular complications may play significant contributing roles in the development of respiratory failure, particularly with respect to respiratory muscle fatigue. Before initiating a weaning protocol, it is imperative to identify intercurrent problems and to initiate treatment of all which are potentially reversible. As previously described, these may be due to preoperative conditions, intraoperative events, or postoperative complications. Evaluation of the patient may include the following:

- Complete physical examination
- Serum chemistry determination and serial ABG

Conditions Associated with Prolonged Mechanical Ventilation

Gas Exchange Failure with Hypoxemia

Atelectasis of large subsegments of lung parenchyma
Impaired cardiac output with congestive heart failure
Excessive volume replacement with pulmonary vascular congestion
Adult respiratory distress syndrome and/or sepsis
Underlying lung disease causing loss of effective alveolar-capillary gas exchange capacity

Respiratory Muscle Pump Failure Manifested by Hypercapnia and Hypoxemia

Respiratory neuromuscular weakness and/or fatigue
Requirement for extracorporeal devices necessitating sedation and paralysis
Central nervous system depression of respiratory drive
Phrenic nerve injury with diaphragmatic dysfunction
Underlying obstructive lung disease that increases work of breathing
Excessive CO_2 production
Increased dead-space ventilation

- Sputum analysis and culture
- CXR to look for pleural effusions, atelectasis, infiltrates
- Fluoroscopy to assess diaphragm function
- Bronchoscopy to remove mucous plugs and retained secretions; washings for culture (if appropriate)
- Assessment of cardiovascular status with pulmonary artery catheter
- Echocardiogram

In particular, multiple factors may contribute to respiratory muscle weakness and fatigue (see below). High priority must be given on a daily basis to optimizing the patient's nutrition[22,27]; hemoglobin, fluid, and electrolyte status; acid-base status[32]; neuropsychological level of functioning; and cardiorespiratory status. Any infections should be aggressively treated. Maintenance of as normal a sleep-wake pattern as possible allows the patient to gain strength and enthusiasm to participate actively in the weaning process.

Inadequate respiratory drive may be due to nutritional deficiency, sedative medications, central nervous system impairment, or sleep deprivation.[1,13]

Excessive breathing work may occur for many reasons. First, underlying diseases such as pneumonia, sepsis, and pulmonary edema may interfere with gas exchange and the effectiveness of

---

Causes of Respiratory Muscle Weakness and/or Fatigue After Cardiac Surgery

Fever
Sepsis
Anemia
Phrenic nerve impairment
Excessive work of breathing
Poor cardiac performance
Hypoxemia
Hypercarbia
Protein-calorie malnutrition
Hypomagnesemia
Hypokalemia
Hypocalcemia
Hypophosphatemia

respiratory muscles that are relatively hypoxemic. The release of various chemical mediators may interfere with respiratory muscle function. Second, mechanical ventilation itself may increase the work of breathing before the patient is sufficiently ready to do so.[12] The development of auto-PEEP in patients with obstructive lung disease may disrupt length-tension relationships and require excessive work for patients to overcome their own PEEPs to generate a breath. Intermittent mandatory ventilation may increase the work required with spontaneous breathing by increasing airway resistance through the ventilator tubing, thus requiring considerable work to breathe spontaneously when a low rate of assisted breaths is provided. Assist control systems may be set to require excessive work to trigger the assisted breath, or the tidal volume or rate adjustment may be inadequate for the patient's needs.[18]

Choice of Ventilator Mode for Weaning

To plan a strategy for weaning a patient from mechanical ventilatory support, it is important to understand the methods of ventilation available and what work of breathing is required from the patient. Generally, after cardiac surgery patients are weaned from the ventilator with positive pressure ventilation. A superatmospheric pressure is generated at the upper airway, creating a pressure gradient between the upper airway and the lungs such that air flows into the lungs to deliver breaths at a set rate. For most patients this is introduced translaryngeally through an endotracheal tube placed after induction of anesthesia. Patients requiring prolonged mechanical ventilatory support (more than 14 to 21 days) may have a tracheostomy tube placed to manage their airways and deliver air. Tracheostomy tube placement is discussed in more depth later in this chapter.

With positive pressure ventilators inspiratory airflow is determined by limits set on either the total pressure or volume created during inspiration within the lung-airways-ventilator circuit. In pressure-limited ventilators a maximum pressure is established such that when inspiratory airflow occurs, the ventilator delivers gas until this pressure is reached in the lung-airways-ventilator system, at which time inspiratory airflow ceases and passive expiration begins.[12] Thus pressure is preset, and volume is allowed to vary with the compliance of the lung and airway resistance. With asthma the lung has decreased compliance and increased resistance to airflow, and inspiratory volume may be decreased while airway pressure is held constant (Fig. 8-1). In patients with obstructive lung disease, this may prevent hyperinflation and the development of auto-PEEP.

Volume-limited ventilators deliver a preset volume to the lungs with each breath, allowing the pressure generated to vary with the respiratory mechanics of the lung. In the setting of asthma, with decreased compliance and increased resistance to airflow, peak

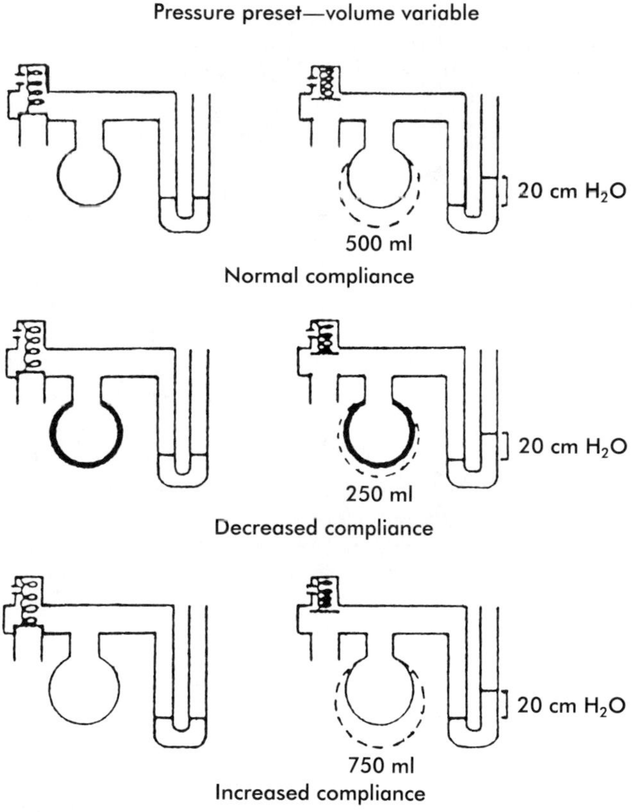

Pressure preset—volume variable

500 ml
20 cm H$_2$O
Normal compliance

250 ml
20 cm H$_2$O
Decreased compliance

750 ml
20 cm H$_2$O
Increased compliance

Fig. 8-1 Principle of operation of pressure-limited ventilator. (From Irwin RS: Mechanical ventilation, Part I. In Irwin RS, Alpert JS, Fink MP, editors: *Intensive care medicine,* ed 2, Boston, 1991, Little, Brown.)

Volume preset—pressure variable

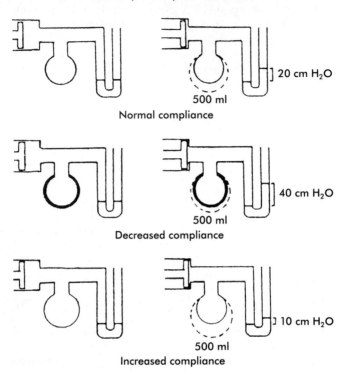

Fig. 8-2 Principle of operation of volume-limited ventilator. (From Irwin RS: Mechanical ventilation, Part I. In Irwin RS, Alpert JS, Fink MP, editors: *Intensive care medicine,* ed 2, Boston, 1991, Little, Brown.)

airway pressure would increase (Fig. 8-2). Limits can be set on the peak pressures allowed to develop, with the remaining volume in that breath discarded. Volume preset ventilators are generally thought to deliver more consistent tidal volumes and are most commonly used in weaning.

The most common modes of delivering cyclic, or intermittent, positive pressure volume-limited ventilation are controlled, assist-control, intermittent mandatory ventilation, synchronized inter-mittent mandatory ventilation, and pressure support. With the exception of pressure support, these are used with volume preset ventilation. With *controlled ventilation* the ventilator is set to deliver breaths at a fixed rate irrespective of the patient's efforts (Fig. 8-3). This is especially useful in the patient with no respiratory drive who has been sedated and/or paralyzed electively, has barbiturate or narcotic overdose, or has impaired central nervous system drive. It is not a mode used for weaning, and prolonged use of this mode may result in atrophy of the muscles of respiration.

Assist-control ventilation (ACV) allows the patient to initiate a breath spontaneously by generating a negative inspiratory pressure (Fig. 8-3). This triggers a positive-pressure, or "assisted," breath, delivered at whatever rate the patient is breathing. If the patient fails to initiate a breath within a set period of time, the ventilator cycles at a preset minimum rate. The amount of negative inspiratory pressure necessary to trigger an assisted breath can be set such that the patient is relatively rested or worked, depending on what is appropriate. Patients with diaphragmatic fatigue can be rested without disuse atrophy of the respiratory muscles. For patients with bronchospasm and increased airway resistance, or ARDS and decreased compliance, the work of spontaneous breathing may be too great, and ACV permits them to breathe spontaneously without complete respiratory muscle fatigue. One potential disadvantage is that the patient may overbreathe and respiratory alkalosis may develop.

Intermittent mandatory ventilation (IMV) is a modification of control ventilation that permits the patient to breathe spontaneously (Fig. 8-3). The patient still receives a set rate of mandatory positive pressure breaths irrespective of the rate of spontaneous breathing. The spontaneous breaths are unassisted. There is some increased work of breathing due to the resistance present in the endotracheal tube–ventilator circuit.[13,18] This mode is good for patients who are ready to be weaned from the ventilator and who have good respiratory muscle strength, are not having to generate excessive work to breathe, and can breathe spontaneously. Most postsurgical cardiac patients without underlying problems can be weaned from the ventilator with this mode by successively reducing the fixed rate of controlled breaths. One concern is that the mandatory breath is delivered irrespective of where a patient is in the cycle of a spontaneous breath, which can be uncomfortable for the patient and create anxiety.[8]

Synchronized intermittent mandatory ventilation (SIMV) was conceived in an effort to avoid the patient receiving IMV having

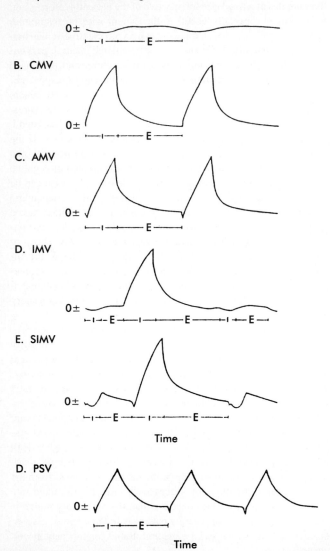

Fig. 8-3 Airway pressure tracings during spontaneous breathing and mechanical ventilation. (From Sassoon CSH, Mahutte CK, Light RW: Ventilator modes: old and new, *Critical Care Clinics* 6(3):605, 1990.)

mandatory breath in the middle of a spontaneous breath, by delivering a positive-pressure assisted breath triggered by the patient's spontaneous respiratory efforts (Fig. 8-3) at a set frequency. In between, the patient is allowed to breathe spontaneously without assistance. However, if the patient fails to trigger the ventilator during the interval between assisted breaths, a controlled breath is delivered. This mode is theoretically believed to be more comfortable for the patient and is a common mode used for weaning. However, SIMV may actually increase the work of breathing required by the patient if the ventilator uses a demand-flow system rather than a flow-by system of delivering fresh gas during an assisted breath.[25] Some of the newer generation of ventilators, such as the Puritan-Bennett 7200 and 7200a and the Siemens 900C, have been able to minimize the extra demands on respiratory work.[15,25] This issue has been nicely summarized by Sassoon and coworkers.[26] IMV and SIMV have become popular modes of ventilator support and weaning.

Pressure support ventilation (PSV) is a newer mode of ventilation that is gaining popularity. PSV is a form of pressure-limited intermittent positive-pressure ventilation in which a preset positive pressure is applied and the patient determines his or her own inspiratory flow rate, inspiratory time, and respiratory frequency.[17] Tidal volume is determined by the patient's effort, the preset pressure, and respiratory system impedance, and may vary with each breath. The degree of machine support depends on the level of preset pressure. The work of breathing is lower, and diaphragm fatigue can be avoided. Higher tidal volumes are achievable at lower peak airway pressures, particularly in patients with obstructive lung disease. PSV can be used as the sole ventilatory support, although all breaths must be triggered by the patient. It is more commonly used in combination with IMV or SIMV, and may decrease the work of breathing and increase patient comfort.[14,17]

Weaning Strategies

Weaning a patient from the ventilator entails allowing the patient to gradually assume the full work of breathing while ventilatory support is withdrawn. The "T piece" method consists of removing the patient from the ventilator for spontaneous breathing sessions with or without CPAP, with oxygen-enriched humidified air. Between sessions the patient is maintained with the ventilator with enough support to prevent respiratory muscle fatigue. Initial trials may last from 5 to 30 minutes, every 30 to 180 minutes. At the end of each trial the patient's clinical status is evaluated for evidence of respiratory muscle fatigue, increases in respiratory rate of more than 10 breaths/min or total rate of more than 40 breaths/min, decrease in pH to less than 7.3, carbon dioxide pressure to increase greater than 5 mm Hg, oxygen desaturation less than 90%, change in blood pressure or heart rate, and use of accessory muscles. The duration of the trials is increased as tolerated until the patient is able to spontaneously breathe for several hours. The patient then rests overnight. Generally IMV is the mode of mechanical ventilation used between T-piece trials.

When a patient is ventilated with the SIMV/IMV mode, with or without pressure support, the patient is weaned by gradually reducing the IMV rate. This can be accomplished in a few hours or gradually during several days, depending on the patient's clinical status. For patients who are slow to wean, the respiratory muscle strength should be assessed on a daily basis, with the criteria for weaning discussed earlier (p. 167). The IMV rate is generally reduced in small increments of 1 or 2 breaths/min. Clinical parameters as discussed previously are measured 30 minutes after each change. As reviewed by Sassoon and colleagues,[26] the type of ventilator used with IMV or SIMV can greatly affect the work of breathing required by the patient to trigger an assisted breath. Some investigators have found that IMV or SIMV was associated with a lower mean airway pressure, increased mean arterial pressure, and improved cardiac output and oxygen delivery compared with ACV. However, the use of one weaning method over another remains highly controversial and is often a matter of personal style and experience of the physician, and the type of ventilator available.

The concomitant use of PSV (usually beginning with ≤20 cm H_2O) is helpful, particularly in patients with obstructive lung disease or asthma. Patients with these disorders may have increased airway resistance to airflow and reduced lung compliance. The ability to determine inspiratory flow, rate (and thus inspiratory/expiratory ratio), and tidal volume may add greatly to patient comfort and help reduce hyperventilation and auto-PEEP. Once the patient is stable and ready to be weaned, the level of pressure support is weaned gradually along with the IMV or SIMV rate.

Often the patient is weaned to an SIMV rate of 1 or 2 per minute, then the PSV is weaned.

Some potential weaning problems are more likely to be seen in cardiac patients after surgery than in other critical care populations.[19,20,33]

Diaphragmatic Dysfunction

The use of cold topical pericardial lavage has been associated with postoperative diaphragmatic dysfunction.[31] This may lead to respiratory muscle fatigue and predispose to atelectasis. Patients can generally tolerate unilateral impairment as long as there are no other significant problems. However, bilateral diaphragmatic dysfunction may take months to resolve and and necessitate a long period of mechanical ventilation. The patient should continue to have daily gentle weaning trials to prevent respiratory muscle atrophy and to assess progress.

Noncardiogenic Pulmonary Edema

Rarely fulminant postoperative noncardiogenic pulmonary edema may develop. It can occur as a result of prolonged CPB or as a reaction to the administration of blood products. The primary clinical feature is the accumulation of interstitial fluid and pulmonary edema, with an ARDS picture. Alveolar epithelial cell damage occurs with concurrent dysfunction and production abnormalities of surfactant. These factors cause changes in lung compliance and resultant hypoxemic respiratory failure with a propensity for shunting caused by alveolar collapse. In addition to the pulmonary edema, severe bronchospasm, anasarca, and myocardial edema may occur. The morbidity rate has been quoted at approximately 50%, without failure of other systems.[4,11]

Ventilatory management with ARDS includes maintaining a Po_2 of approximately 60 to 70 mm Hg with as low an Fio_2 as possible. PEEP is almost always required and must be titrated to optimize Fio_2 without compromising cardiac output. For a more complete discussion of optimization of PEEP, please refer to the discussion by Sassoon and associates[12,26] or by Humphrey and colleagues.[11] The work of breathing may be so great that the patient requires controlled ventilation or very sensitive ACV to prevent respiratory muscle fatigue until ARDS has substantially resolved. Invasive hemodynamic monitoring is likely required to help differentiate cardiac and noncardiac factors and to assist in the optimization of PEEP and pulmonary capillary wedge pressure.[11] Other organ systems must be rigorously monitored as well.

Surgical Incisions

The surgical incision made in cardiac surgery greatly affects post-operative chest wall function and therefore total lung compliance. Several studies have reported the frequent occurrence of left lower lobe atelectasis, which may be in part due to decreased lung excursion, supine position, and poor gas exchange.[19,31] Although atelectasis is not completely preventable, it can be minimized with aggressive management techniques, including cough, deep breathing, and incentive spirometry every few hours while the patient is awake, and by positioning the patient such that the posterior lower lobes are not always dependent. The posterior-basal segment of the left lower lobe is particularly vulnerable.

Tracheotomy

Although controversial, we believe that a cricothyroidotomy in cardiac surgical patients increases the distance from the median sternotomy wound and the tracheotomy and may reduce the incidence of mediastinitis.

A recent consensus conference on artificial airways concluded that translaryngeal intubation is preferred in patients requiring an artificial airway for 10 days or less, whereas tracheotomy is recommended if the need for an artificial airway can definitely be anticipated to be greater than 21 days[23] (see the box below). Tracheotomy has several benefits for the patient requiring ventilatory support for more than 21 days. These include the following[7,9,16]:

Tracheostomy Guidelines

1. Continue oropharyngeal or nasopharyngeal intubation when anticipated need for artificial airway is ≥10 days
2. Between 10 and 21 days, reassess daily whether to convert to tracheostomy
3. Tracheostomy is indicated when anticipated need for artificial airway >21 days

- Provision of a more secure airway
- Sparing of further injury to upper airways, sinuses, oro-pharynx, and larynx
- Lower risk of purulent sinusitis
- Facilitation of weaning by reducing airway resistance, dead space, and work of breathing
- Better management of airway secretions
- Increased patient mobility and independence
- Speech possible
- Oral intake possible without a nasogastric tube
- Psychologic benefit to patient

Potential complications of a tracheotomy include the following[2,10,16]:

- Mediastinitis caused by infection of sternotomy wound
- Tracheomalacia, tracheal stenosis
- Stomal erosion
- Mucosal bleeding
- Innominate artery erosion and bleeding
- Subcutaneous emphysema
- Tracheoesophageal fistula
- Chronic trachcobronchitis
- Aspiration

Controversy still exists regarding the best management of the airway in patients requiring intubation between 10 and 21 days.[16,28] Translaryngeal intubation is well tolerated by most patients for 2 to 3 weeks, provides a reliable airway, and does not require surgical intervention. Disadvantages, which are substantial and increase with time, include bacterial airway colonization, ulcerative glottic inflammation, chronic laryngeal dysfunction after extubation, chronic aspiration, purulent sinusitis, and inadvertent premature extubation.[10] Tracheomalacia or stenosis at the cuff site has been reduced in recent years by the use of low-pressure endotracheal tube cuffs. Laryngeal stenosis remains a significant problem in 10% to 12% of patients after prolonged endotracheal intubation.[5,10,30] If a tracheotomy is delayed, problems that arise may be attributed to the tracheotomy but may really derive from the period of excessive translaryngeal intubation. The importance of timing in tracheostomy placement has recently been reviewed by Heffner.[10]

In the controversial 14- to 21-day period, Heffner[10] advocates an anticipatory approach. In patients for whom the issue is not clear, daily reevaluation of clinical status and weaning progress should be used to determine the optimal timing of tracheostomy.[10] Risks should be compared with benefits. However, at 10 to 14 days after surgery, if it becomes increasingly apparent that the patient is not likely to be extubated during the next week, it may be prudent to place the tracheostomy early.

Postextubation Pulmonary Management

Immediately after extubation the patient should be observed for an adequate breathing pattern without the presence of laryngeal stridor. If the intubation was complicated or traumatic, the patient can be extubated with a fiber-optic bronchoscope to allow observation of the vocal cords and upper airway tissues. If excessive edema is noted, the patient can be reintubated with the bronchoscope and treated with dexamethasone for 24 to 48 hours. During this time the patient may be able to be treated with oxygen supplementation and/or CPAP without returning to mechanical ventilation.

Initially the patient is given an FIo_2 of 0.60 by a humidified face mask. He or she is observed for the presence of adequate oxygenation and respiratory muscle fatigue. Bronchospasm should be treated aggressively with inhaled bronchodilators, including anticholinergics and β_{3-2}-specific β agonists. Incentive spirometry and cough and deep breathing techniques should be instituted immediately. Even with thick secretions, mucolytic agents are no longer recommended, because they can provoke airway irritation and bronchospasm. Secretions can be managed with adequate hydration, guaifenesin, regular suctioning and coughing, bronchodilators, and antibiotics (if appropriate).

After extubation it is common for cardiac surgical patients to have mild relative hypoxemia[19,29] requiring oxygen supplementation by nasal cannula. Contributing factors include persistent microatelectasis, incisional pain, impaired cough, and clearance of secretions, bronchospasm, increased lung water, and pleural effusions. Persistently decreased lung volumes may be due to sluggish or impaired diaphragmatic function caused by phrenic nerve injury during surgery. These factors usually resolve in 5 to 7 days. Patients who fail to improve steadily should be examined (by ABG, complete blood cell count, and CXR) for evidence of pneumonia, atelectasis, effusions, and congestive failure, and treated accordingly. Rarely patients require discharge home with oxygen supplementation until they can maintain oxygen saturation by pulse oximetry greater than 90% in room air.

References

1. Askanazi J, Weissman C, Rosenbaum SH, et al: Nutrition and the respiratory system, *Crit Care Med* 10:163-172, 1982.
2. Astrachan DI, Kirchner JC, Goodwin WJ: Prolonged intubation versus tracheostomy: complications, practical and psychological considerations, *Laryngoscope* 98:1165-1169, 1988.
3. Bolgiano C, Saah ML: Measurement of bedside ventilatory parameters, *Crit Care Nurse* 10(1):60-66, 1990.
4. Culliford AT, Thomas S, Spencer FC: Fulminating noncardiogenic pulmonary edema: a newly recognized hazard during cardiac operations, *J Thorac Cardiovasc Surg* 80:868, 1980.
5. Elliott CG, Rasmusson BY, Crapo RO: Upper airway obstruction following ARDS: an analysis of 30 survivors, *Chest* 94:526, 1988.
6. Gibney RTN, Wilson RS, Pontoppidan H: Comparison of work of breathing on high gas flow and demand valve continuous positive pressure airway systems, *Chest* 82:692, 1982.
7. Grover ER, Bihari DJ: The role of tracheostomy in the adult ICU, *Postgrad Med J* 68:313-317, 1992.
8. Hasten RW, Downs JB, Heenan TJ: A comparison of synchronized and nonsynchronized intermittent mandatory ventilation, *Respir Care* 25:554, 1980.
9. Heffner JE: Timing of tracheotomy in ventilator-dependent patients, *Clin Chest Med* 12(3):611-625, 1991.
10. Heffner JE: Timing of tracheotomy in mechanically ventilated patients, *Am Rev Respir Dis* 147:768-771, 1993.
11. Humphrey H, et al: Improved survival in ARDS patients associated with a reduction in pulmonary capillary wedge pressure, *U Chicago Hosp Clin* 11176-79, 1989.
12. Irwin RS: Mechanical ventilation: part 1—initiation. In Rippe JM, Irwin RS, Alpert JS, Fink MP, eds: *Intensive care medicine,* Boston, 1991, Little, Brown.
13. Irwin RS: Mechanical ventilation: part II—weaning. In Rippe JM, Irwin RS, Alpert JS, Fink MP, eds: *Intensive care medicine,* Boston, 1991, Little, Brown.
14. Kacmarek RM: The role of pressure support ventilation in reducing the work of breathing, *Respir Care* 33:99-120, 1988.
15. Katz JA, Kraemer RW, Gjerde G: Inspiratory work and airway pressure with continuous positive airway pressure delivery systems, *Chest* 88:519-526, 1985.

16. LoCicero J III, McCann B, Massad M, Joob AW: Prolonged ventilatory support after open-heart surgery, *Crit Care Med* 20:990-992, 1992.

17. MacIntyre NR: Respiratory function during pressure support ventilation, *Chest* 89:677-683, 1986.

18. Marini JJ, Smith TC, Lamb VJ: External work output and force generation during synchronized intermittent mechanical ventilation, *Am Rev Resp Dis* 138:1169, 1988.

19. Matthay MA, Weiner-Kronish JP: Respiratory management after cardiac surgery, *Chest* 95:398-405, 1989.

20. Moreno-Cabral CE, Mitchell RS, Miller DC: *Manual of postoperative management in adult cardiac surgery,* Baltimore, 1988, Williams & Wilkins.

21. Morganroth ML, Morganroth JL, Nett LM, Petty TL: Criteria for weaning from prolonged mechanical ventilation, *Arch Intern Med* 144:1012-1016, 1984.

22. Pingleton SK: Nutritional support in the mechanically ventilated patient, *Clin Chest Med* 9(1):101-112, 1988.

23. Plummer AJ, Gracey DR, co-chairs: Consensus Conference on Artificial Airways in Patients Receiving Mechanical Ventilation, *Chest* 96:178-180, 1989.

24. Rotello LC, Warren J, Jastremski MS, Milewski A: A nurse-directed protocol using pulse oximetry to wean mechanically ventilated patients from toxic oxygen concentrations, *Chest* 102(2):1833-35, 1992.

25. Sassoon CSH, Giron AE, Eli EA, et al: Inspiratory work of breathing on flow-by and demand-flow continuous positive airway pressure, *Crit Care Med* 17:1108-1114, 1989.

26. Sassoon CSH, Mahutte CK, Light RW. Ventilator modes: old and new, *Crit Care Clin* 6(3):605-634, 1990.

27. Schlichtig R, Sargent SC: Nutritional support of the mechanically ventilated patient, *Crit Care Clin* 6(3):767-784, 1990.

28. Stauffer JL: Medical management of the airway, *Clin Chest Med* 12(3):449-482, 1991.

29. Vander Salm TJ, Visner MS: Management of the postoperative cardiac surgical patient. In Rippe JM, Irwin RS, Alpert JS, Fink MP, editors: *Intensive care medicine,* 1991, Little Brown.

30. Whited RE: A prospective study of laryngotracheal sequaelae in long-term intubation, *Laryngoscope* 94:367, 1984.

31. Wilcox P: Phrenic nerve function and its relationship to atelectasis after coronary artery bypass surgery, *Chest* 93:693-698, 1988.

32. Yanos J, Wood LDH, Davis K, Mitchell K III: The effect of respiratory and lactic acidosis on diaphragm function, *Am Rev Respir Dis* 147:616-619, 1993.

33. Zin W, et al: Expiratory mechanics before and after uncomplicated heart surgery, *Chest* 95:21-28, 1988.

Hemorrhage and Tamponade

9

William A. Baumgartner and Sharon G. Owens

Although the incidence of returning to the operating room (OR) for bleeding has been reported between 1% and 5%,[1,9,13] the occurrence of postoperative hemorrhage remains one of the more frequent complications associated with open heart surgery. The use of cardiopulmonary bypass and systemic heparinization renders each patient vulnerable to bleeding in varying degrees.[1,9,13,31,33] Meticulous care and surgical technique result in good hemostatic control in the majority of patients.

However, in certain groups of patients with uremia, primary liver disease, other coexisting illnesses, and previous thoracic procedures generalized bleeding can develop. Appropriate treatment requires knowledge of the coagulation system, diagnostic tests, and specific interventional therapeutic modalities. The care of the patient with postoperative bleeding requires close coordination between the physician and nurse and on occasion the hematologist. Management requires control of systemic blood pressure, maintenance of acid-base balance, alertness to the possibility of pericardial tamponade, and occasionally a rapid response to acute hypotension. This chapter describes the preoperative assessment of patients, reviews the contributory factors to postoperative bleeding, details the postoperative management, and summarizes the complications associated with hemorrhage and the administration of blood products.

Preoperative Evaluation

History and Physical Examination

The most important step in determining whether a patient has a bleeding disorder is a careful and accurate assessment of the *pa-*

tient's history. Routine screening tests are often normal in patients with mild defects in the coagulation system. The majority of bleeding disorders are acquired and are usually associated with an underlying disease process such as primary liver disease, uremia, or the ingestion of medications that interfere with hemostasis. Congenital hemostatic disorders, although less common, may also be present.

Specific preoperative questions about bleeding should be asked. These include the following:
- Any unusual bleeding tendencies or bruising
- Whether the process is generalized or local
- Whether it occurs spontaneously
- Whether it resulted from injury
- Degree of injury required to produce bleeding or bruising
- History of nosebleeds or previous operative procedures
- History of transfusions
- Family history
- Medications taken

One of the more common patient complaints is the occurrence of nosebleeds. Specific questions should be directed at the frequency, amount, site (one nostril or both), and date of the last event. The patient should also be questioned regarding previous operative procedures and whether any comments were made about excessive blood loss or the need for transfusion. A discussion of the family history usually distinguishes congenital from acquired hemostatic disorders.

One of the most common causes for acute bleeding disorders in the patient postoperatively is the self-administration of drugs that interfere predominantly with platelet function. These include aspirin and aspirin-containing compounds, and nonsteroidal antiinflammatory drugs. It is estimated that several hundred drugs contain aspirin. Therefore detailed questioning with regard to the specific medications the patient has taken in the recent past is required. Aspirin in particular has a profound inhibitory affect on the function of platelets by the inhibition of cyclooxygenase.[20] Platelet half-life is 5 days and therefore discontinuation is required approximately 2 weeks before an elective operation. Although this is the ideal situation, many urgent and emergent operations can be performed safely with minimal blood loss despite the administration of aspirin as recent as the day of the operation. In addition, the preoperative administration of dipyridamole and the combi-

Table 9-1 Commonly Used Tests to Determine Status of Hemostasis

Test	Description	Normal values
Bleeding time	Assesses platelet function by measuring formation of a hemostatic plug; used if patient has recently taken aspirin	Duke method (earlobe), <6 min; Ivy method (forearm), 2-9.5 min
Thrombin time (TT), thrombin clotting time	Measures time needed for plasma to clot when thrombin is added; used to diagnose hypofibrinogenemia	15 sec or control value ±5 sec (varies widely)
Prothrombin time (PT)	Detects abnormalities in extrinsic system; used to monitor anticoagulation therapy in patients taking warfarin	10-14 sec or 100% (varies)
Partial thromboplastin time (PTT) or activated partial thromboplastin time (APTT)	Detects deficiencies in intrinsic system; used to monitor anticoagulation therapy in patients taking heparin	PTT: 30-45 sec APTT: 16-25 sec
Platelet count	Measures degree of thrombocytopenia	150,000-350,000/mm^3
Clot retraction	Confirms platelet dysfunction	After 1 hr clot retracts from side of tube; nearly complete in 4 hr and definitely complete by 24 hr

Continued.

Table 9-1 Commonly Used Tests to Determine Status of Hemostasis—cont'd

Test	Description	Normal values
Plasminogen/plasmin	Determines plasminogen level and active enzyme plasmin; useful during streptokinase therapy	6.1 ± 2.3 CTA units
Fibrinolysis/euglobulin lysis time	Used in evaluating fibrinolytic crisis	No lysis of plasma clot at 37° C for 3 hr
Fibrin split products	To determine degree of consumptive coagulopathy in DIC, thromboembolic disorders, and renal diseases (degradation of split products are identified by letters S, Y, D, and E).	Negative 4 µg/ml
Platelet adhesion	Detects abnormalities in platelet adhesion; Indicated in persons with no aspirin exposure for 2-3 wks and prolonged bleeding time	50,000-18,000/mm³, 20%-60% retention, 25%-58% adherence
Platelet aggregation	Detects abnormalities in platelet aggregation	Platelet aggregates develop in <5 min
Fibrinogen	Investigates abnormal PT, APTT, and TT and screens for DIC, fibrinolysis, fibrinogenolysis	Semiquantitative TT: 200-400 mg/dl or 2.0-4.0 g/L
Heparin neutralization	Determines amount of circulating heparin and whether heparin is responsible for the prolongation of TT	Interpretative report of amount of circulating heparin (µg)
Fibrinopeptide A	Reflects amount of active intravascular blood clotting as in subclinical DIC	0.6-1.9 mg/ml

nation of dipyridamole and aspirin postoperatively does not result in increased bleeding.[4]

Although the physical examination in general does not contribute to the assessment of bleeding disorders in most patients preoperatively, observance of *petechia, ecchymoses,* and *spider angioma* should prompt further evaluation.

Laboratory Screening Tests

Initial evaluation generally includes: Prothrombin time, Deactivated partial thromboplastin time, Total platelet count, Bleeding time *if* there is a history of bleeding or recent ingestion of a platelet inhibitory medication.

Commonly used tests for the determination of the status of hemostasis are summarized in Table 9-1. A listing of the known coagulation factors appears in Table 9-2.

The *partial thromboplastin time* (PTT) is effective in identifying abnormalities in the intrinsic system (Fig. 9-1). Prolongation may be due to a deficiency of factors VII, X, or V, prothrombin, or fibrinogen; presence of a circulating anticoagulant such as heparin; or a defect in the common pathway, because the end point for the PTT test is the development of a fibrin clot.

Table 9-2   Coagulation Factors

Factor	Description
I	Fibrinogen
II	Prothrombin
III	Tissue thromboplastin
IV	Ca^{2+}
V	Platelet phospholipids and calcium ions
VI	No longer a distinct part of coagulation
VII	Coenzyme (stabilizing factor)
VIII	Antihemolytic globulin
IX	Christmas factor (hemophilia)
X	Stuart-Prower factor
XI	Plasma thromboplastin antecedent
XII	Hageman factor
XIII	Fibrin stabilizing factor

Proteins present in blood plasma in an inactive form.
Platelets.

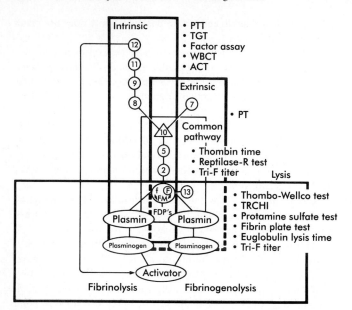

Fig. 9-1 Schematic representation of coagulation lysis and coagulation function studies. Fibrinogen; *F,* fibrin; *FDP,* fibrin degradation products; *FM,* fibrin monomer. Rapid and specific evaluation of postperfusion coagulation abnormalities requires selection and evaluation, usually of a combination of some of these commonly used tests. (From Young JA: Coagulation abnormalities with cardiopulmonary bypass. In Utley JR, ed: *Pathophysiology and techniques of cardiopulmonary bypass,* vol 1, Baltimore, 1982, Williams & Wilkins.)

If PTT is normal, it can be assumed that no defects are in the intrinsic or common pathway systems of coagulation. Further tests are necessary to differentiate abnormalities in the intrinsic and common pathway systems if the result is abnormal.

The *prothrombin time* (PT) is used to detect abnormalities in the extrinsic system. The test is prolonged if a deficiency of factors (XII, XI, IX, VIII, V, II, or I), a circulating anticoagulant, or a break in the common pathway is present. With these two tests differentiation can potentially be made between abnormalities in the intrinsic or extrinsic system.

The *thrombin time* can be used to identify defects in the lower portion of the common pathway. This test is performed if both the

PT and PTT are abnormal. A prolonged thrombin time is caused by fibrinolysis, accumulation of fibrin degradation products, or the presence of heparin.

Total platelet count should be more than 100,000 cells/mm^3. The quantitative platelet count does not measure the ability of platelets to adhere and form a hemostatic plug, however. This action can be assessed only by the *bleeding time*. Prolongation of the bleeding time (>6 minutes) generally occurs in thrombocytopenia (<100,000 platelets/mm^3), as a result of aspirin ingestion, or more specific functional platelet defects. A variety of more specific tests (Table 9-1) can be employed to help differentiate the particular defect in the coagulation system.

However, for practical purposes the patient's history plus the PT, PTT, and platelet count can be effective for screening purposes and identification of a postoperative coagulation defect.

Pathophysiology

Influence of Concomitant Diseases

Occasionally bleeding disorders go undetected by the patient's history and standard screening coagulation tests. If the condition is unrecognized, these patients may have significant bleeding problems in the postoperative period. Table 9-3 lists those conditions

Table 9-3   Disease States with Normal Coagulation Screening Tests but which Predispose to Bleeding Disorders

Disorder	Tests
Mild hemophilia	Prolonged PTT if factor VII is <20% or factor IX is <15%
Multiple myeloma	Occasional presence of heparin-like inhibitor
Amyloidosis	Association with acquired factor X deficiency
Systemic lupus erythematosus	Occasional presence (10%) of serum anticoagulant
Corticosteroid excess, sub-acute bacterial endocardi-tis, Waldenstrom's macro-globulinemia, renal failure	Nearly 20% of patients may have bleeding problems despite having normal coagulation screening results

which should alert the caregiver to the fact that bleeding might be a significant postoperative problem. If by history or physical examination signs or symptoms are observed that lead to the suspicion that one of these disease states is present, a hematologic consultation should be requested and concomitant further testing should be performed.

Other Predisposing Disease States

Hepatomegaly resulting from congestive heart failure reduces the effectiveness of hepatocytes to produce coagulation factors (Table 9-4). *Splenomegaly,* an occasional feature in these patients, produces thrombocytopenia. Preoperative treatment usually includes the administration of vitamin K. *Continued bleeding* generally results in a dilution and/or consumption of coagulation elements, compounding the existing bleeding. *Polycythemia* vera does not usually present a major problem to cardiopulmonary bypass (CPB) or contribute to postoperative bleeding. On occasion, however, these patients can exhibit bleeding or a tendency toward thrombosis. The hematocrit level and platelet count should be kept in the normal range preoperatively. Postoperatively, warfarin can be used without problems in these patients. Although splenectomy before CPB is preferable in patients with *idiopathic thrombocytopenic purpura,* successful operations have been achieved in patients without splenectomy.[16]

Occasionally a patient with a hemoglobulinopathy is referred for operative intervention, necessitating the need for CPB.[6] In most cases these patients can undergo the procedure with minimum difficulty if special preparations are carried out. Patients with *sickle cell disease* require special techniques during CPB to minimize the risk of sickling.[30] An increased amount of hemoglobin A_2 is

Table 9-4   Other Disease States Predisposing the Patient to Postoperative Bleeding

Hepatic congestion
Renal failure
Continued bleeding
Polycythemia vera
Sickle cell disease
Thalassemia
Spherocytosis
Glucose-6-phosphate dehydrogenase deficiency

seen in patients with *thalassemia*. However, other than the presence of anemia, this condition does not result in any major problems during operation or in the postoperative period. Patients with *spherocytosis* have undergone successful CPB without resultant hemolysis.[22] If possible, splenectomy should be performed before open heart surgery. This generally corrects the shortened half-life of red cells observed in this disease. *Glucose-6-phosphate dehydrogenase deficiency* is fairly rare in the United States but does affect approximately 10% of the black male U.S. population. Certain antibiotics and other drugs can potentiate hemolysis. However, because the mechanical and osmotic fragility are nearly normal, CPB has been successful.[30]

Effects of CPB

CPB can be associated with severe hematologic and coagulation abnormalities. The following advances in CPB have minimized these deleterious effects:

- Improvements in oxygenators[7,12,31]
- Improvements in pumps and tubing
- Better understanding of the effects of hemodilution and hypothermia
- More precise monitoring of the metabolic status of the patient
- More refined methods of heparinization and reversal with protamine

Heparin

Postoperative bleeding can be due to overheparinization or underestimation of the protamine dose required to reverse the effects of heparin. Heparin binds to the lysyl group of antithrombin III, inducing a change that increases the rate of binding and deactivation of factors XII, XI, X, and IX, and of thrombin. Therefore antithrombin III deficiency leads to heparin insensitivity.[27]

Activated Clotting Time Test

Most centers use the activated clotting time (ACT) test to modulate heparin dose.[2,3,22] The ACT test is a modification of the whole blood coagulation time. The mechanism of the test depends on the activation of the coagulation system when blood comes in contact with a glass surface. It is accelerated in the ACT tube 10-fold by the addition of diatomaceous earth. The initial heparin dose is calculated on the basis of the formula of 300 units heparin per kilogram of body weight. The ACT target value is 480 seconds. A two-point dose-response curve is then constructed, and subsequent maintenance heparin doses are then calculated for a maintenance ACT of 450 to 500 seconds.[2,3,32]

Protamine

Protamine sulfate binds heparin in a 1:1 ratio, thereby preventing heparin from enhancing the anticoagulant effect of antithrombin III. Protamine affects only circulating heparin. Therefore initial reversal may be inadequate if heparin reenters the vascular system from tissue deposition, the so-called heparin rebound.[25] Excess protamine can be a weak anticoagulant. Side effects of protamine administration include pulmonary vasoconstriction and systemic hypotension with resultant cardiac decompensation.[5,8,15]

Protamine Titration Curve

After cessation of bypass, neutralization of heparin is accomplished with the addition of protamine. The conventional method for determining the dose of protamine was the classic Bull heparin dose–activated clotting time curve, which is determined before bypass.[2,3] More recently a protamine titration curve, constructed with the ACT, has resulted in a significant reduction in amount of protamine administered.[26] This method seems to reduce markedly the patient's exposure to protamine and thereby may diminish the potential for protamine-associated side effects.

Mechanism of Coagulation

An understanding of the coagulation process is helpful in identifying the appropriate therapeutic intervention. Fig. 9-1 schematically demonstrates the coagulation process, and Table 9-1 lists a variety of tests that can be used to elucidate the particular defect that may be contributing to postoperative bleeding. Thrombus can be formed by two pathways. They are referred to as the intrinsic pathway or intravascular system, and the extrinsic pathway or extravascular system.

Intrinsic Pathway

Factor XII is activated when it interacts with a nonendothelial surface such as the extracorporeal circuit used in CPB or exposed collagen after vascular trauma. A cascade of events leads down the pathway to the eventual formation of a stabilized and insoluble fibrin clot.

Extrinsic Pathway

Factor X can also be activated by a shorter method, the extrinsic pathway. Tissue thromboplastins including tissue factor and tissue phospholipid can activate factor VII, which in turn activates factor X in the common pathway.

Fibrinolysis

Lysis of a thrombus occurs when plasminogen is activated to plasmin, which then can lyse both fibrin and fibrinogen. This activation can be coagulation dependent (fibrinolysis), meaning that activation (by factor XII) occurs after the initiation of the coagulation process. The activators in this system may be thromboplastic tissue substances, ischemia, or peripheral vasoconstriction. These processes can also occur during CPB if anticoagulation is not complete or can occur independently of anticoagulation.

Disseminated Intravascular Coagulation

Disseminated intravascular coagulation is a term used in many settings and can occur during CPB. Essentially hypercoagulability and bleeding occur as a result of coagulation factor consumption and secondary fibrinolysis, which are initiated by the intravascular hypercoagulability. Initial treatment involves administration of heparin and fresh-frozen plasma. Ultimately the primary stimulus for the intravascular thrombosis must be eradicated.

Management of Postoperative Hemorrhage

Surgical Considerations

Prevention of postoperative hemorrhage starts in the operating room (OR). There is no subsitute for meticulous operative technique (beginning with the sternotomy itself) and hemostatic control after cessation of CPB. A detailed and regimented protocol should be used to identify potential sources of bleeding before chest closure. Typical sites for bleeding include the following:

- Sternal periosteum
- Sternal notch
- Mammary bed

- Mammary pedicle
- Superior mediastinal fat pad
- Cut edge of the pericardium
- Diaphragmatic surface
- Anastomoses
- Cannulation and vent sites
- Incisions in the heart and great vessels

Adequate chest drainage should be implemented (see Chapter 4). After closure of the chest, chest tubes are immediately connected to a chest drainage system. The cardiotomy reservoir from the CPB setup is used at The Johns Hopkins Hospital.

Initial Assessment and Stabilization in the Intensive Care Unit

Management of bleeding in the postoperative period requires the diligent attention, communication, and cooperation of all persons involved in care of the patient. The responsible surgeon can often guide the management of bleeding by relating to the staff specific concerns he or she might have had in the OR.

The most common factors associated with (nonsurgical) bleeding after protamine administration are inadequate reversal of heparin; preoperative administration of heparin, aspirin, nonsteroidal antiinflammatory drugs, and thrombolytic agents; and previous median sternotomy.

On arrival in the intensive care unit (ICU) the team (physicians, nurses, respiratory therapists) works toward stabilizing the patient. The chest tubes, previously connected to a cardiotomy reservoir in the OR, are placed to suction at 20 cm H_2O. Although the chest tubes are not stripped, if clots develop, they are mechanically broken up to allow passage of blood. An initial recording of the chest tube output is made, and subsequent hourly measurements are taken (Fig. 9-2).

	Blood / & Driv.														
Chest Tubes	Hourly / present					60/10	100/10	110/10	120/10	50/10	40/10	30/10	20/10		
	24°/ total					60	160	270	390	440	520	550	570		
ATS	Hourly / 24° total					50/50	100/150	110/260	120/380	40/470	d/c'd				

Fig. 9-2 Documentation of chest tube output and autotransfusion system *(ATS)*.

The occurrence of postoperative bleeding is closely interrelated with blood pressure control, metabolic stability, maintenance of normothermia, the resultant effects of the operation and CPB and significant medical history. These issues are common to all patients and should be addressed upon the patient's arrival in the ICU (Table 9-5).

The initial therapeutic measure for the control of hypotension (after sedation) is the use of nitroprusside (Chapter 7). In addition to its well-known side effects of thiocyanate toxicity, it has also been shown to inhibit platelet aggregation.[17]

Treatment of Bleeding

Treatment of a postoperative patient who is bleeding requires an organized approach. Obvious blood loss requires constant blood replacement. This is done through banked blood or with autologous transfusion. In the ICU the cardiotomy reservoir is used as a reinfusion device (Fig. 9-3). The nurse manually returns the collected blood through a peripheral vein with a syringe or by an infusion pump. If multiple units of blood are infused, it is desirable to warm the blood in advance. Calcium chloride may be administered when clinically indicated at a dose of 250 mg when blood with i citrate-phosphorous-dextrose preparation is given.

With today's emphasis on blood conservation, moderate bleeding (75 to 150 ml/hr) is tolerated for a longer period of time before coagulation products are administered. Initial treatment includes normalization of the ACT with protamine sulfate (25 to 50 mg IV), and increase of positive end-expiratory pressure (PEEP) to 10 cm H_2O if systolic blood pressure and cardiac output are not compromised.

The use of DDAVP for the control of bleeding in patients with uremic and secondary platelet dysfunction has been reported.[19] In addition, its use has been reported in patients with heart disease undergoing reoperation. However, its role in the management of bleeding in patients undergoing cardiac surgery remains ill defined presently. Although its effective use has been reported, anecdotal experiences have reported a temporal relationship with the administration of the drug and saphenous vein graft occlusions.[18,29] A recent report shows no reduction in postoperative bleeding in patients undergoing uncomplicated cardiac surgery who received DDAVP.[10]

DDAVP's exact mechanism of action has not been elucidated.

Table 9-5   Therapeutic Adjuncts Used to Reduce Postoperative Bleeding

Condition	Therapeutic adjunct	Specific intervention
Intraoperative	Good technique	—
Blood pressure control (sBP <100 mm Hg)	Normalization of ACT	≤prebypass level
	Sedation	Morphine sulfate (2-5 mg IV q1-2 hr), midazolam (2-5 mg IV q1-2 hr), pancuronium (0.04-0.1 mg/kg IV) (if shivering occurs)
	Antihypertensive therapy	Nitroprusside (0.5-10 μg/kg/min IV), nifedipine (10 mg sublingually q2 hr), nitroglycerin (0.5-2.0 mg/kg/min IV)
Metabolic stability	Hemodynamics Cardiac index (>2 L/min/m²) Urine output (>0.5 ml/kg/hr) pH control during shivering	Optimize preload and inotropes
Temperature regulation	Maintain normothermia	Hyperthermia blanket, warming of blood and blood products if multiple units given
Coagulation status	Obtain routine lab tests	PT, PTT, platelet count; hematocrit, hemoglobin on admission and in 6-8 hr

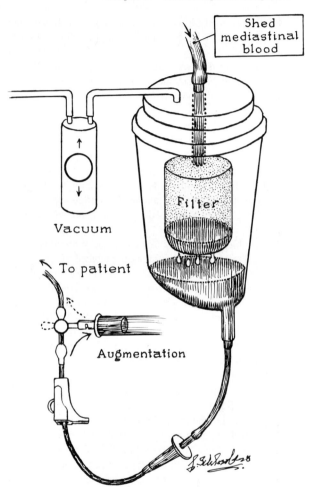

Fig. 9-3 Schematic representation of use of cardiotomy reservoir as autoperfusion system.

Its effect on the coagulation is to increase serum levels of factor VIII coagulum activity and to alter the properties of factor VIII (von Willebrand factor). The usual dose is 0.3 μg/kg diluted in 50 ml of normal saline solution and infused intravenously during a 15- to 30-minute period. At this time desmopressin is used sparingly in the ICU.

Although the use of PEEP is controversial in the role of reducing postoperative bleeding, a baseline level is applied (5 cm H_2O) to all patients to augment oxygenation.[11,21,23] The use of factor concentrates (Proplex and Konyne) are also not used in the OR and ICU because of the increased incidence of hepatitis after their use.[28]

If the PT or PTT is prolonged, fresh-frozen plasma (2 to 4 U) should be administered (Fig. 9-4). A platelet count less than $100,000/mm^3$ is an indication for platelet transfusion in a patient with persistent bleeding. Platelets are administered at approximately 1 U/10 kg body weight. If the platelet count, PT, and PTT are all moderately abnormal, we prefer to administer platelets first followed by fresh-frozen plasma only if bleeding persists. Because of platelet dysfunction after CPB, platelets are often administered as the initial coagulation products despite the apparently normal platelet count.

Persistence of bleeding beyond this initial use of blood products prompts repeated coagulation tests including a bleeding time (Fig. 9-4) and testing for fibrinogen and fibrin degradation products.[14]

If the fibrinogen level is less than 100 mg/dl, cryoprecipitate (1 U/10 kg) is administered (Fig. 9-4). Occasionally patients exhibit fibrinolysis manifested by a combination of a low fibrinogen level and a high level of fibrin degradation products. If bleeding is present with a markedly high level of fibrin degradation products, a low fibrinogen level, and decreased clot lysis time, ϵ-aminocaproic acid (Amicar) should be administered. This is a competitive binder to plasminogen that then blocks its activation. Clinical suspicion of fibrinolysis is prompted if, after the appearance of initial clot formation, recurrent bleeding through suture holes or through the pores of a prosthetic graft develops. The initial dose of 25 mg/kg IV is administered over 1 hour. It is followed by a dosage of 1 to 2 gm/hr for 4 to 5 hours. In our experience this drug is rarely indicated, but use of ϵ-aminocaproic acid can occasionally result in control of postoperative bleeding that is resistant to other more standard measures. Indications for mediastinum reexploration are the following:

- Bleeding rate of 200 ml/hr for 4 to 6 hours
- More than 1500 ml blood lost during a 12-hour period
- Sudden increase (300 to 500 ml) in chest tube output
- Evidence of pericardial tamponade

It is generally believed that bleeding at a rate of 200 ml/hr for 4 to 6 hours despite administration of coagulation products is an

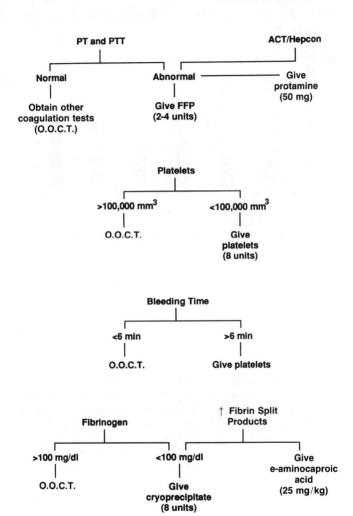

Fig. 9-4 Algorithms for evaluation and specific therapy for coagulation defects.

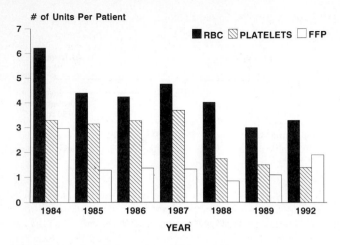

Fig. 9-5 Blood product use from 1983 to 1988.

indication for reexploration. Another criterion for reoperation is the loss of more than 1500 ml blood during a 12-hour period. A sudden increase (300 to 500 ml) of chest drainage requires immediate exploration and occasionally the performance of open thoracotomy in the ICU. Evidence of acute cardiac tamponade is also an indication for reexploration.

Blood product use has significantly decreased since 1984 in our cardiac surgery unit at The Johns Hopkins Hospital (Fig. 9-5). This decrease is a result of both a philosophical change and technical advances. The extent of postoperative hemorrhage in the ICU has progressively declined as manifested by the number of reoperations for bleeding. The incidence of return to the operating room for excessive bleeding is <2%. In addition, the use of the intraoperative cell saver, more precise management of heparin and protamine intraoperatively, autotransfusion, and allowance of the hematocrit to drift to approximately 25% have all contributed to this decrease in blood product usage.

Complications of Hemorrhage

Pericardial Tamponade

Although pericardial tamponade is more comprehensively discussed in Chapter 7, it is included here because it can be a life-threatening problem. The following statements address some of the issues of pericardial tamponade.

- Opening a pleural space contiguous with the pericardium is beneficial but not an absolute preventive measure against tamponade
- Tamponade can occur with the pericardium opened or closed
- A small thrombus strategically placed in the posterior portion of the pericardium compromising the left atrium or pulmonary veins will lead to symptoms of tamponade
- Tamponade should always be suspected if chest tube drainage abruptly decreases

The usual signs of tamponade are enlargement of the cardiac silhouette, equalization of atrial and ventricular diastolic pressures, pulsus paradoxus, and acute hypotension. Equalization of atrial and ventricular diastolic pressures and enlargement of cardiac silhouette are not reliable and seldom observed because a patient is receiving ventilatory support and the pericardium has been opened. Pericardial tamponade is a *clinical diagnosis*. Treatment of pericardial tamponade includes maintenance of blood pressure with volume administration and inotropes, immediate thoracotomy in the ICU if hemodynamics deteriorate despite supportive measures, and an immediate return to the OR.

Infection

Patients who are returned to the OR or who have received multiple transfusions are subject to an increased risk of infection in the postoperative period. In addition, retained blood in the pericardium or pleural space in patients who are not taken back to the OR carries a potential for infection. It is recommended that patients with unevacuated large pleural effusions resulting from bleeding be returned to the OR for evacuation even if the patient has stopped bleeding, to prevent subsequent problems of infection and lung entrapment compression. Viral infections caused by transmission through blood products include hepatitis and acquired immunodeficiency syndrome; the risk of developing hepatitis or AIDS from a unit of transfused blood is $1:200$ and $1:50,000$ to $1:1 \times 10^6$ respectively.

Complications of Transfusion

A reaction to blood or blood products occurs in 0.5% of transfusions. The severity of a reaction ranges from fever to anaphylaxis with occasional hemolysis. Anaphylaxis therapy consists of the following:

- Antihistamines are administered intravenously (diphenhydramine, 1 mg/kg) as an H_1-receptor antagonist
- Aminophylline (2 to 3 mg/kg IV infusion) is administered for bronchospasm
- Corticosteroids are given (methylprednisolone, 30 mg/kg IV)
- Hemolysis is treated with alkali administration and hydration to promote diuresis

Patients may also have noncardiogenic pulmonary edema usually attributable to a reaction to blood products or protamine administration. Treatment includes the previously mentioned therapies and vigorous diuresis. Less innocuous but still a postoperative problem is the weight gain that develops in a patient after the administration of multiple blood products. This is treated with gradual diuresis.

References

1. Bachmann F et al: The hemostatic mechanism after open-heart surgery, *J Thorac Cardiovasc Surg* 70:76, 1975.
2. Bull BS et al: Heparin therapy during extracorporeal circulation. I. Problems inherent in existing heparin protocols, *J Thorac Cardiovasc Surg* 69:674, 1975.
3. Bull BS et al: Heparin therapy during extracorporeal circulation. II. The use of a dose-response curve to individualized heparin and protamine dosage, *J Thorac Cardiovasc Surg* 69:685, 1975.
4. Chesebro JH et al: A platelet-inhibitor-drug trial in coronary-artery bypass operations, *N Engl J Med* 307:73, 1982.
5. Culliford AT, Thomas S, Spencer FC: Fulminating noncardiogenic pulmonary edema, *J Thorac Cardiovasc Surg* 80:868, 1980.
6. deLeval MR et al: Open heart surgery in patients with inherited hemoglobinopathies, red cell dyscrasias and coagulopathies, *Arch Surg* 109:618, 1974.
7. Edmunds LH et al: Platelet function during cardiac operation: comparison of membrane and bubble oxygenator, *J Thorac Cardiovasc Surg* 83:805, 1982.
8. Fiser WB et al: Cardiovascular effects of protamine sulfate are dependent on the presence and type of circulating heparin, *J Thorac Cardiovasc Surg* 89:63, 1985.
9. Gomes MM, McGoon DC: Bleeding patterns after open-heart surgery, *J Thorac Cardiovasc Surg* 60:87, 1970.
10. Hackmann T et al: A trial of desmopressin (1-desamino-8-D-arginine

vasopressin) to reduce blood loss in uncomplicated cardiac surgery, *N Engl J Med* 321:1437, 1989.

11. Hoffman WS, Tamasello DN, MacVaugh H: Control of postcardiotomy bleeding with PEEP, *Ann Thorac Surg* 34:71, 1982.

12. Hope AF et al: Kinetics and sites of sequestration of indium 111-labeled human platelets during cardiopulmonary bypass, *J Thorac Cardiovasc Surg* 81:880, 1981.

13. Kevy SV et al: The pathogenesis and control of the hemorrhagic defect in open heart surgery, *Surg Gynecol Obstet* 123:313, 1966.

14. Lambert CJ, et al: The Tri-F Titer: a rapid test for estimation of plasma fibrinogen and detection of fibrinolysis, fibrin(ogen) split products and heparin, *Ann Thorac Surg* 18:357, 1974.

15. Latson TW, Kickler TS, Baumgartner WA: Pulmonary hypertension and noncardiogenic pulmonary edema following cardiopulmonary bypass associated with an antigranulocyte antibody, *Anesthesiology* 64:106, 1986.

16. Lenardo D et al: Coronary artery bypass in idiopathic thrombocytopenia without splenectomy, *Ann Thorac Surg* 48:721, 1989.

17. Levin RI, Weksler BB, Jaffe EA: The interaction of sodium nitroprusside with human endothelial cells and platelets: nitroprusside and prostacyclin synergistically inhibit platelet function, *Circulation* 66:1299, 1982.

18. Mannuccio PM, Lusher JM: Desmopressin and thrombosis, *Lancet* 1:675, 1989.

19. Mannuccio PM et al: Deamino-8-D-arginine vasopressin shortens the bleeding time in uremia, *N Engl J Med* 308:8, 1983.

20. Michelson EL et al: Relation of preoperative use of aspirin to increased mediastinal blood loss after coronary artery bypass graft surgery, *J Thorac Cardiovasc Surg* 76:694, 1978.

21. Mills N: Postoperative hemorrhage after cardiopulmonary bypass, *Ann Thorac Surg* 34:607, 1982.

22. Moyes DG, Rogers MA, Coleman AJ: Cardiopulmonary bypass in hereditary spherocytosis: a case report, *Thorax* 26:131, 1971.

23. Murphy DA, et al: Effect of positive end-expiratory pressure on excessive mediastinal bleeding after cardiac operations, *J Thorac Cardiovasc Surg* 85:864, 1983.

24. Paul J et al: In vivo release of a heparin-like factor in dogs during profound hypothermia, *J Thorac Cardiovasc Surg* 82:45, 1981.

25. Pifarre R et al: Management of postoperative heparin rebound following cardiopulmonary bypass, *J Thorac Cardiovasc Surg* 81:378, 1981.

26. Rivard DC, Thompson SJ: *Demonstration of heparin reversal with protamine administration using an automated protamine dose assay: a comparison of two methods,* Proceedings of the 26th international conference of the American Society of Extra-Corporeal Technology, March 1989.

27. Rivard DC, Thompson SJ, Cameron DE: *The role of antithrombin 3 in heparin resistance*. Proceedings of the 27th international conference of the American Society of Extra-Corporeal Technology, April 1990. (in press).

28. Rossiter SJ et al: Hepatitis risk in cardiac surgery patients receiving factor IX concentrates, *J Thorac Cardiovasc Surg* 78:203, 1979.

29. Salzman EW et al: Treatment with desmopressin acetate to reduce blood loss after cardiac surgery: a double-blind randomized study, *N Engl J Med* 314:1402, 1986.

30. Szentpetery S, Robertson L, Lower RR: Complete repair of tetralogy associated with sickle cell anemia and G-6-PD deficiency, *J Thorac Cardiovasc Surg* 72:276, 1976.

31. van Oeveren W et al: Deleterious effects of cardiopulmonary bypass, *J Thorac Cardiovasc Surg* 89:888, 1985.

32. Verska JJ: Control of heparinization by activated clotting time during bypass with improved postoperative hemostasis, *Ann Thorac Surg* 24:170, 1977.

33. Young JA: Coagulation abnormalities with cardiopulmonary bypass. In Utley JR, ed: *Pathophysiology and techniques of cardiopulmonary bypass,* vol 1, Baltimore, 1982, Williams & Wilkins.

Arrhythmias

10

Patrick DeValeria and Bruce A. Reitz

Postoperative cardiac arrhythmias are common after cardiac surgery and can be grouped into two general categories: ventricular (early, most common) and supraventricular (often seen 24 hours to 5 days postoperatively). The hospital course of 3.7% to more than 50% of patients are complicated by the occurrence of a postoperative arrhythmia.[13,23,31,36,41,44,51,60] The key to treatment of arrhythmias is making the proper diagnosis. Once the diagnosis has been properly made, the underlying cause must be considered and an appropriate therapy chosen.

The first section of this chapter deals with making the proper electrocardiographic diagnosis of the arrhythmia. Subsequent sections discuss the use of epicardial pacing electrodes in diagnosis and therapy, antiarrhythmic medications, and finally management of specific arrhythmias.

Electrocardiographic Diagnosis of Arrhythmias

Basic Electrocardiography

Although a complete review of electrocardiogram (ECG) interpretation is beyond the scope of this manual, we will review some basic principles of ECG recording and interpretation. The reader is referred to the excellent text by Marriott[39] for a more thorough discussion.

The ECG machine is a voltmeter that records the electrical impulses produced by the heart. Myocardial cells are electrically charged and when stimulated depolarize and cause contractions. Fig. 10-1 represents a normal ECG. The electrical currents detected by the ECG leads are recorded on graph paper (1-mm rules) that

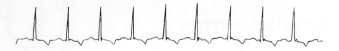

Fig. 10-1 Sinus tachycardia.

conventionally is run at 25 mm/sec. Thus each small box represents ⅟25 second or ⅟1500 minute, and each large box ⅕ second or ⅟300 minute.

With the preceding information one can use an ECG strip to determine rate. To identify the atrial rate, count the number of small boxes between P waves and then divide by 1500. The ventricular rate may be identified by counting the number of small boxes between R waves and dividing by 1500. Another method must be used if the rate is irregular. One can count the number of P-P or R-R intervals in a 6-second length of ECG tracing and multiply by 10 to obtain the heart rate. Six seconds of ECG paper is 30 large boxes when the paper is run at 25 mm/sec.

Once rate has been determined, the rhythm must be identified. The QRS complex should be identified and its duration determined. If the QRS complex is 0.1 seconds or less in duration, the rhythm is most likely generated from a supraventricular source. This determination must be done in several leads because some leads display the QRS clearer than others. The best leads are those with the greatest QRS voltage. A QRS complex that is widened is due to a supraventricular focus with aberrant ventricular conduction or ventricular ectopy. This diagnostic distinction is important to make because the conditions have different etiologies, consequences, and appropriate medical treatment strategies.

Certain points may be helpful in making this distinction:[22,62]

- QRS width in excess of 0.14 seconds is suggestive of ventricular tachycardia
- Conversion or slowing by vagal maneuvers is consistent with supraventricular source
- Atrioventricular (AV) dissociation is consistent with ventricular tachycardia
- A rapid ventricular rate (>200 beats/min) favors supraventricular source
- Fusion beats suggest ventricular origin
- Similar premature ventricular contractions before the tachycardia suggest ventricular source

- A preexisting bundle branch block (BBB) of the same configuration suggests a supraventricular source
- QRS configurations: (1) monophasic or biphasic QRS complex in lead V_1 suggests ventricular tachycardia; (2) right BBB pattern with a small R wave in V_1 favors supraventricular tachycardia; (3) left BBB pattern with QR or QS wave in V_6 suggests ventricular tachycardia

The third step in evaluating an ECG is to identify the P wave. The presence of a P wave and its morphology should be studied. An antegrade P wave (upright in lead II) or retrograde (down in lead II) should be noted. The atrial rate and duration of the PR interval also must be determined.

The next step is to assess the relationship between the P wave and its accompanying QRS complex. A PR interval of less than 0.10 seconds or greater than 0.40 seconds is unlikely to have a causal relationship. A one-to-one relationship between the P waves and QRS complexes and a consistent or lengthening PR interval must be sought.

Once these steps are taken, a diagnosis may be made and appropriate treatment instituted.

Causes of Perioperative Arrhythmias

A significant proportion of patients undergoing cardiac surgery have some type of postoperative arrhythmia. The cause can be difficult to pinpoint because several factors may be present in a patient simultaneously. Treatment should be aimed to remove or correct as many predisposing factors as possible.

In general, inhaled anesthetics (especially halothane) can sensitize the myocardium to catecholamines. Halothane also has a depressive effect on automaticity in the sinoatrial (SA) node. A major cause of arrhythmias relating to anesthesia with current techniques is the narcotic-induced respiratory suppression and hypoxia that occurs if the patient receives inadequate ventilation. A correlation has been shown between the severity of the patient's cardiac disease and the extent of perioperative arrhythmia.[2] A variety of medications and potential drug interactions can either decrease contractility, causing hypotension and hypoxia, or increase the arrhythmia potential of the myocardium.

Hypercalcemia, hypocalcemia, hypokalemia, hypomagnesium, and other electrolyte disturbances can increase the arrhythmia potential of the myocardium. Acidosis, uremia, and other metabolic alterations can cause arrhythmias. Pheochromocytoma (elevated catecholamine states), hyperthyroidism, and other abnormalities increase the likelihood of cardiac arrhythmias.

Changes in respiration can lead to hypercarbia, which causes acidosis and increased premature ventricular contractions with decreased contractility. Hypoxia also predisposes to arrhythmias. Pain, anxiety, or inadequate sedation can cause an elevated catecholamine level and increased cardiac arrhythmias.

Reversible surgical trauma from tension or pulling on the heart during surgery can cause myocardial irritability and atrial or ventricular arrhythmias. Hemorrhage, ischemia, or edema also can occur in surgery and create short-lived cardiac irritability. Irreversible trauma to the conduction tissue can occur in certain procedures, especially the closure of septal defects and operations for congenital heart conditions. BBBs can be caused by suture placement or valve debridement during valve replacement procedures. Hypothermia in the immediate postoperative period can cause bradycardia and ectopic atrial and ventricular arrhythmias.

Temporary Epicardial Wire Electrodes

Epicardial electrodes are wires placed in the atrial (and ventricular) epicardium at the completion of open heart surgery. These wires can be used postoperatively both diagnostically and therapeutically.[15,42,60] At The Johns Hopkins Hospital typically two stainless steel atrial wires are placed, one ventricular electrode and one skin (ground) electrode.

Atrial wire

Two atrial electrodes are placed high in the right atrium approximately 1 cm apart. By so doing, a bipolar atrial tracing can be obtained that has minimal ventricular electrical activity superimposed on it. Bipolar atrial pacing also has less artifact and is more readily interpreted than unipolar pacing.

Ventricular wire

One or two ventricular electrodes can be placed in the anterior or diaphragmatic wall of the right ventricle. As with atrial electrodes, an advantage to the use of two ventricular wires is the ability of bipolar pacing to create less ECG artifact, making determination of capture easier. However, the need for ventricular ECG recording is rare and unipolar ventricular pacing works well, so a single ventricular wire can be placed. If a single ventricular wire is used then a skin (ground) electrode should be placed.

Technique of Placement and Care

Wires are placed after cardiopulmonary bypass and attainment of hemostasis. We routinely use wires that have atraumatic curved needles wedged onto one end and a Keith needle at the other. The wire has a Teflon coating that ends approximately 2 cm before the curved needle.

Atrial wires are placed approximately 1 cm apart, then brought out through the anterior part of the chest to the right of the sternum. Ventricular wires can be placed with the atraumatic needle to embed the noncoated portion of the wire intramyocardially. The curved needle is cut off, and the straight needle is used to bring the wire to the anterior part of the chest, left of the sternum. If two ventricular wires are not used, a skin electrode is placed subcutaneously and brought out to the left of the sternum. All wires are secured to the skin with a 2-0 Tevdek suture. The Keith needle tip is broken off with a Halsted clamp, leaving a straight stainless steel shaft to use as a pacing electrode.

Pacing wires should be protected from inadvertent electrical contact. The nursing staff at The Johns Hopkins Hospital routinely dress wire sites with sterile gauze. The noninsulated steel shafts are protected in nonconductive material (either cut-off fingertips of surgical gloves or plastic caps from hypodermic needles). The protected ends are taped above the gauze dressing for ready access.

We routinely remove wires on the evening before anticipated hospital discharge. This task is readily accomplished by cutting the Tevdek stay sutures and gently pulling on the wires with the patient in a reclining position. This causes minimal discomfort and little to no morbidity. If a wire cannot be removed, it should be prepared in a sterile manner, pulled taut, and cut at the skin so it retracts below the surface.

Recording ECGs with Temporary Wire Electrodes

ECGs using temporary wires are useful in the postoperative period, especially in trying to differentiate tachydysrhythmias. It is helpful to have a multichannel recorder when obtaining atrial ECGs, but a single channel can be used by sequentially changing channels. Connect the leg leads to the patient in the usual fashion and connect the arm leads to each of the two atrial electrodes with alligator clips. A bipolar atrial tracing can then be obtained by running a conventional lead I tracing. Lead I normally records the voltage between the right and left arm: because these leads have been connected to the atrial wires, the lead I tracing records the voltage *between* atrial electrodes. By switching to lead II or III a unipolar tracing is recorded between a single atrial electrode and the left foot. Unipolar atrial tracings can also be obtained by connecting the atrial wire to the V lead and running V_2 on the ECG machine. Bipolar atrial tracing records primarily atrial activity; unipolar atrial tracing demonstrates both atrial and ventricular activity. By switching between lead I (bipolar) and leads II or III (unipolar), atrial electrical activity and atrial-to-ventricular association can be evaluated.

Pacing with Temporary Epicardial Wires

Temporary atrial and ventricular wires can be used to pace the heart postoperatively. Asynchronous, demand, and AV sequential pacing may all be accomplished.

Asynchronous pacing (rate fixed and no sensing of intrinsic cardiac electrical activity) is generally used only for atrial pacing. A Q-on-T phenomenon can be created by asynchronous ventricular pacing, precipitating ventricular fibrillation.

Demand pacing sets the pacing rate but allows the pacer to "sense" spontaneous electrical activity. The pacer fires only if no intrinsic beat occurs in a preset interval determined by the pacer rate setting. This is the mode used for most forms of ventricular pacing, because Q-on-T phenomenon should be avoided. The atrium cannot be demand-paced because atrial electrical activity cannot be adequately sensed by most current external pacers.

AV sequential pacing is a form of pacing that requires a more sophisticated external pacer. This allows coordinated atrial and ventricular paced beats so that the atrial "kick" is delivered before ventricular contraction. AV sequential pacing is most useful post-operatively for patients with AV heart block.

Atrial–sensing–ventricular demand pacing uses a sophisticated pacer that can sense the atrium, then, after preset delay, activate ventricles to contract if no ventricular electrical activity is seen. This is useful for sinus rhythm with complete AV block.

A further option is *atrial pacing–ventricular pacing*. If one does not have a pacer that can sense the atrium, the atrium can be asynchronously paced and the ventricles demand-paced. The atrium then contracts at a preset rate, and if after a delay no ventricular response occurs, a demand pacer discharges stimulating ventricular contraction coordinated to the paced atria.

Suggested Pacemaker Variable Settings

A wide variety of external battery-charged pacemakers are available. Most models of standard pacers are adequate for typical cardiac pacing. Certain arrhythmias may be treated with rapid overdrive pacing requiring rates up to 800 pulses/min. Special pulse generators are required to perform this function. The following are general instructions. The individual manufacturer's instruction manuals should be consulted for specific detailed instructions.

1. Ventricular demand (e.g., Medtronic 5375) pacemaker
   a. Connect distal electrode (ventricle) to the negative ($-$) lead.
   b. Connect ground (skin) to the positive ($+$) lead (may use the atrial wire as ground).
   c. Output (milliamperes): Start at 1 mÅ and slowly increase until evidence of electrical capture is seen with arterial pulse or ejection in arterial line. May increase up to twice threshold level.
   d. Sensitivity (millivolts): Start with 1 mV and slowly increase until the sensing function is lost. (This is the sensing threshold.) Then turn down to half the sensing threshold.
   e. Rate (pulses per minute): Set at desired physiologic rate.
2. Atrial pacing (asynchronous pacing): Use bipolar if possible to create fewer stimulation artifacts.
   a. Connect positive lead to one atrial wire electrode.
   b. Connect the other lead to the atrial wire electrode.
   c. Output (milliamperes) is determined as discussed previously. (Atria cannot generally be demand paced.)
   d. Sensitivity to asynchrony.
   e. Rate (pulses per minute): Set at desired physiologic rate (usually 90 to 100 pulses/min).
3. AV sequential pacing
   a. Connect the atrial and ventricular wires to the appropriate contacts on the pacemaker box.
   b. Adjust setup as discussed.
   c. Adjust sensitivity as discussed.
   d. Adjust rate as discussed.
   e. AV interval (PR interval) is set in milliseconds. Hold the

rate constant and start at 100 to 125 milliseconds, then slowly increase, checking the cardiac output by Swan-Ganz catheter, if possible, to maximize the atrial contribution to the cardiac output.

Technique of Overdrive Atrial Pacing

When attempting rapid overdrive pacing, an ECG should be continuously monitored in lead II. The patient should be reclining in bed. Attach each atrial wire to the positive and negative leads of a rapid-rate external pacer box. Set the pacer rate at 1.5 times the atrial flutter rate and turn the box on for 20 to 30 seconds until the atrial capture is observed (the atrial complexes flip from negative to positive in the lead II ECG tracing), then quickly shut off the pacer box. An alternative technique is called the "ramp technique." The pacer is set up as previously noted, but the rate of overdrive pacing is slowly increased until the atrial complexes are seen to flip from negative to positive in the lead II ECG. Once this capture has been identified, the pacer box is quickly shut off.

Antiarrhythmic Medications

Cardiac arrhythmias result from abnormalities in impulse conduction, abnormal automaticity (initiation of the impulse), or a combination of both mechanisms.[27] Electrical activity in the heart is produced by the movement of ionized particles across the polarized membrane. When cardiac muscle tissue is stimulated, an action potential is produced (Fig. 10-2). The standard cardiac muscle action potential can be described in five phases.

The Action Potential

Phase 0 occurs with activation of the myocardial cell when an impulse from the sinus node causes sodium-specific fast channels

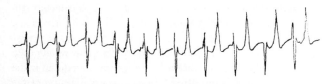

Fig. 10-2 PSVT on atrial ECG.

and calcium-specific slow channels to open. This allows movement into the cell of positively changed ions, and depolarization occurs, with the membrane potential rising to threshold potential (approximately -60 mV) and generating an action potential. The rapidly conducted depolarization of all ventricular muscle produces the QRS complex seen in the surface ECG.

Phase 1 is a rapid reestablishment of a new steady-state plateau, *phase 2*. During phase 2 the slow calcium channels and fast sodium channels are open, keeping a relatively long plateau (approximately 100 milliseconds). The phases are represented by the ST segment on the surface ECG.

Phase 3 is composed of a rapid repolarization to a negative transmembrane potential by the opening of potassium channels and the efflux of positively charged potassium ions. This is represented by the T wave on the surface ECG.

Phase 4 is the resting membrane potential maintained by an energy-dependent sodium-potassium ion pump system. Phase 4 is represented by the flat baseline on the ECG between the prior T wave and the following QRS complex. Ordinary atrial and ventricular muscle cells have stable phase 4 membrane potentials. Impulse-generating cells have a slow rise of the resting membrane potential toward -60 mV (threshold potential), at which point active depolarization occurs. Under normal conditions the rate of rise of the phase 4 transmembrane potential is steepest in the sinus node, making it the pacemaker of the heart. When conditions occur that increase the rate of spontaneous diastolic depolarization in other cardiac tissues, these cells supercede the SA node pacemaker function and create an ectopic beat. This is the abnormal automaticity associated with ectopic rapid cardiac arrhythmias.

Electrophysiologic Classification of Antiarrhythmic Medications

A wide variety of antiarrhythmic medications is currently available, with newer agents continually being evaluated and approved for clinical use. Several good texts[43] and recent review articles[8,17,37,59,62] discuss the pharmacology of these agents in greater detail than the scope of this chapter allows. The most widely used system for classifying antiarrhythmic agents was introduced in the early 1970s[54] and is based on the primary mode of action of the antiarrhythmic drug.

Class I Drugs

Drugs with class I action are all local-anesthetic type agents. These drugs depress the fast inward sodium current by inhibiting the fast sodium channel and thereby slowing the rate of rise of phase 0 depolarization. The amplitude of the action potential is diminished, and the conduction velocity is slowed. This class of agents can be further categorized with regard to their effect on cardiac muscle cell repolarization.

Class IA drugs (quinidine, procainamide, disopyramide) prolong the action potential duration and the effective refractory period by direct membrane effects, thereby delaying a repolarization. These drugs have an additional indirect anticholinergic effect.

Class IB drugs (lidocaine, phenytoin, mexiletine, tocainide) shorten the action potential duration and effective refractory period by accelerating repolarization and protecting against QT interval prolongation.

Class IC drugs (encainide, flecainide, and propofenone) are in a relatively new subcategory.[29] They inhibit conduction in the His-Purkinje system, causing a widening of the QRS complex with marked slowing of the polarization. These drugs have little or no effect on repolarization. They cause a moderate to marked prolongation of the PR interval and QRS complex. It should also be noted that all these drugs are extremely potent antiarrhythmics generally used for reentry ventricular tachycardias. They do have a significant proarrhythmic effect.

Class II Drugs

Class II drugs encompass all agents that are β-adrenergic–blocking medications. They act primarily through their β-blocking effect, thereby decreasing impulse formation (automaticity) in cardiac tissue.

Class III Drugs

Class III drugs (amiodarone and bretylium tosylate) do not affect automaticity or conduction velocity but delay phase 2 and 3 repolarization and cause a prolonged effective refractory period. They are effective for reentry-type arrhythmias and act by causing the ectopic focus to be unexcitable when the impulse reenters the circuit.[28]

Class IV Drugs

These agents (e.g., verapamil) block the slow calcium channels but have little or no effect on the fast sodium channels.[49] The SA and AV nodes are slow-response fibers that are activated through the calcium channels,[3] making class IV agents effective at slowing conduction velocity through the AV node and prolonging the AV node refractory period. This assists in keeping supraventricular impulses from being conducted into the ventricles.

Class V Drugs

These drugs have been added as a modification of the original classification system and include digitalis. At clinical doses, digitalis acts as an antiarrhythmic agent by vagal effects.[50] Vagal activation acts primarily on the atria and AV and SA nodes.

Specific Medications

The clinical uses, route of administration, pharmacokinetics, side effects, cautions, and drug interactions of specific medications are listed in Tables 10-1 to 10-7. All the class IA, IB, and IC, and class II, drugs in current clinical use are summarized.

Other Agents

Adenosine[1,10,45,52,63-65]

Adenosine is a naturally occurring nucleoside recently approved in the United States for the treatment of supraventicular tachycardia (SVT). At currently recommended doses, adenosine slows AV nodal conduction with prolongation of the PR segment. The drug can cause a brief, high-degree AV nodal block. Adenosine is used clinically to terminate reentry SVT. Adenosine also aids diagnostically by causing a brief, high-degree AV block, aiding in the differential diagnosis of ventricular tachycardia versus an SVT with aberrancy.[64]

For adults, an initial dose of 6 mg intravenously (IV) as a bolus injection is given; if no response occurs after 30 seconds, a second dose of 6 mg may be given. Again, if no response in 1 minute a third dose of 9 mg may be tried. Infants receive 0.05 mg/kg every 2 minutes to a maximum dose of 0.25 mg/kg.[52] Adenosine is rapidly metabolized with a half-life of approximately 10 seconds. Side effects include flushing, headache, bronchoconstriction, and

Text continued on p. 218

***Table* 10-1** Class IA Agents

Name	Clinical use	Administration	Pharmacokinetics
Quinidine sulfate	Suppression of ectopic atrial and ventricular arrhythmias	325 mg PO q 4-6 hr to maximum daily dose of 2 g	Hydroxylated in liver; $T_{1/2}$ = 7-9 hr; therapeutic blood levels, 2.3-5 mg/ml
Procainamide	Suppression of ventricular arrhythmias	IV: 100 mg loading dose then up to 1 g in the first hr (maximum rate 20 mg/min), then continuous infusion of 1-6 mg/min Oral: 1000 mg loading dose, then 375 mg PO q 4 hr or 500 mg PO q 6 hr of slow-release procainamide	Procainamide is acetylated in plasma with renal excretion; $T_{1/2}$, 3-4 hours; Drug is metabolized to NAPA, an active metabolite with $T_{1/2}$ of 6-8 hr; therapeutic blood level, 4 to 8 µg/ml for procainamide and 7-15 µg/ml for NAPA[47]
Disopyramide	Suppression of ventricular arrhythmias, especially if other class IA agents have failed	100-200 mg PO every 6 hr (also available in longer-duration formula)	Partially dealkylated plasma excreted in urine; $T_{1/2}$, 6-10 hr; therapeutic blood level, 2-4 µg/ml

GI, Gastrointestinal; *NAPA,* N-acetylprocainamide; *PO,* orally; *q,* every; $T_{1/2}$, half-life.

Side effects	Cautions	Drug interactions
Multiple; includes GI upset, headache, dizziness, and cardiovascular effects; drug can be very proarrhythmic, especially in patients with prolonged QRS duration and torsades de pointes	Precaution should be used in patients with intraventricular conduction defects, AV blockade, or BBB; also contraindicated in patients with myasthenia gravis; in treating atrial flutter one can see increased ventricular response (1 : 1 from 2 : 1) by slowing atrial rate; patient with atrial flutter should be adequately digitalized before starting quinidine therapy	Multiple; include increased serum digoxin levels; significant incidence of digitalis toxicity seen in patients receiving simultaneous digoxin and quinidine[46]; enhanced warfarin effect (by hepatic interaction); drugs that induce hepatic enzymes, e.g., phenobarbital and rifampin, can alter quinidine blood levels[53]; cimetidine can reduce hepatic metabolism of quinidine, raising blood levels[16]; interactions with Ca channel blocking agents
Hypotension if given as rapid IV infusion, rash, lupuslike syndrome (in slow acetylators), pleural and pericardial effusions and GI upset; duration of drug usefulness is often limited by adverse reactions[33]	Renal failure, heart failure, myasthenia gravis, heart block, prolonged QT, or torsades de pointes	Renal clearance inhibited by cimetidine; possible enhanced immune effects with captopril
Potent myocardial depressant with anticholinergic effects (can precipitate urinary retention), QT prolongation, and torsades de pointes; often drug has fewer GI side effects than quinidine	Absolutely contraindicated in patients with congestive heart failure; caution in patients with myasthenia gravis, glaucoma, or urinary retention; marked drop in cardiac output is seen in patients with prolonged QT interval	Marked reduction of cardiac output when patient is taking other negative inotropes (e.g., β-blockers, Ca channel blockers, or other type IA antiarrhythmic agents)

Table 10-2 Class IB Agents

Name	Clinical use	Administration	Pharmacokinetics
Lidocaine	Ventricular arrhythmia suppression	1 mg/kg IV loading dose (may repeat 2× over 10 min to maximum of 200-300 mg in 1 hr), then IV infusion of 20-40 μg/kg/min	Rapid first-pass hepatic deethylation so dosage must be ordered accordingly[26]; $T_{1/2} = 15$ min (for bolus) to 2 hr (for constant infusion); therapeutic blood level, 1.4-6 μg/ml
Tocainide	Suppression of ventricular arrhythmias (oral lidocaine analogue)	Dose must be individualized to patient's response/tolerance; recommended starting dose of 400 mg PO q 8 hr	40% excreted unchanged in urine; $T_{1/2} = 8$-15 hr with peak plasma level in ½-2 hr; therapeutic blood level, 4-10 μg/ml
Mexiletine	Suppression of ventricular arrhythmias (oral lidocaine analogue)	Dose is individualized; recommended starting dose of 200-300 mg PO q 8 hr	90% hepatic metabolism; $T_{1/2}$, 10-17 hr; therapeutic blood levels, 1-2 μg/ml with peak plasma levels at 2-4 hr
Phenytoin	Digitalis-induced arrhythmias and arrhythmias after pediatric cardiac surgery[57]	10-15 mg/kg IV over 1 hr, then 100 mg IV q 8 hr or 2-4 mg/kg/day PO (may be given in divided dose q 8 hr	Hepatic metabolism with $T_{1/2} = 10$-15 hr; therapeutic blood level; 10-18 μg/ml

GI, Gastrointestinal; *PO,* orally; *q,* every; $T_{1/2}$, half-life.

chest discomfort. With the very short half-life of this drug, all side effects are brief. However caution should be taken because the drug may worsen bronchospasm in patients with preexisting bronchospastic disease.

Drug interactions are yet to be defined, but dipyridamole (Persantine) enhances the pharmacologic effects of adenosine. Theophylline and methylxanthines antagonize the effects of adenosine.

Digitalis Toxicity

Digoxin is a commonly used medication in the postoperative period. It has a narrow therapeutic margin and is often administered

Side effects	Cautions	Drug interactions
Unlike IA agents, generally safe, with prolonged QT interval; drowsiness, numbness, speech disturbances at higher infusion rates, especially in elderly	Blood levels higher in patients with poor hepatic blood flow (e.g., congestive heart failure or β-blockade)	Elevated blood levels with cimetidine, decreased blood levels with liver enzyme enhancement (e.g., phenytoin or barbiturates)
Frequent nervous system and GI reactions, skin rash; rare pulmonary fibrosis and agranulocytosis[55]	Blood cell counts should be followed, drugs contraindicated in 2nd or 3rd-degree heart block	Few significant interactions; does not change digoxin levels
Neurologic (dizziness, disorientation), GI	2nd-3rd degree heart block, cardiogenic shock, liver failure	Decreased levels with hepatic enzyme inducers
May include cardiovascular collapse, neurologic, GI, and blood dyscrasias	Do not exceed infusion rate of 50 mg/min or hypotension can occur; contraindicated in high-degree AV block	Induces hepatic enzymes so alters blood levels and dosage requirements of variety of medications; drug levels affected by warfarin and phenobarbital

with other agents that can alter its own pharmacokinetics. Additionally, many patients after cardiac surgery receive potassium-wasting diuretics, which may predispose these patients to hypokalemia. Hypokalemia can cause an increased myocardial digoxin uptake and predispose patients to digoxin-induced cardiac arrhythmias. Additionally, many cardiac surgical patients are elderly with a prolonged digoxin half-life and often have chronic pulmonary disease and some degree of reduced renal function. These all can cause elevated serum digoxin levels. Although a detailed discussion of digitalis toxicity is beyond the scope of this text, certain keypoints need to be discussed. The reader is referred to

Table **10-3**   Class IC Agents

Name	Clinical use	Administration	Pharmacokinetics
Encainide	Suppression of resistant ventricular ectopy and suppression of variety of atrial arrhythmias	25-75 mg PO q 8 hr (start at low dose for 3 to 5 days and increase over several days if necessary)	Hepatic metabolism with 2 phenotypes for metabolism, extensive metabolizers, and poor metabolizers; extensive metabolizers produce 2 active metabolites with activities resembling class IA agents; $T_{1/2}$ range, 2-11 hr depending on patient's metabolic profile; therapeutic blood levels not known
Flecainide	Life-threatening, resistant atrial and ventricular ectopy and tachyarrhythmias	100-400 mg/day PO divided q 12 hr	Both hepatic and renal metabolism; $T_{1/2} = 12$-27 hr; therapeutic blood levels, 200-800 ng/ml

GI, Gastrointestinal; *PO,* orally; *q,* every; $T_{1/2}$, half-life.

the excellent review article by Bhatia and Smith[7] for further information.

The cellular mechanism of digitalis toxicity is multifactorial. A combination of excessive vagal stimulation, which causes AV blockade with increased levels of intracellular calcium, predisposing the patient to increased ventricular automaticity, together with a direct blockade of AV nodal tissue by digoxin may account for the manifestations seen in patients with toxic reactions to digitalis.

Table 10-7 summarizes the prominent clinical toxic effects of digitalis. The arrhythmias associated with digitalis toxicity are varied. Toxic reactions to digitalis must be considered in any patient receiving digoxin in whom a neurologic, gastrointestinal, or cardiac rhythm change develops.

The extent of treatment is guided by the severity of the patient's presenting symptoms. Twelve-lead ECG, serum digoxin level, and serum electrolyte levels (including potassium and magnesium) should be determined. The patient should also be moved to a monitored setting if not already there. Digoxin administration should be stopped. Serum potassium level should be normalized;

Side effects	Cautions	Drug interactions
Significant risk of proarrhythmic side effects; neurologic (visual changes, dizziness) and GI disturbances may also occur	Proarrhythmic effects of this drug require careful monitoring[61]; has little negative inotropic effect at recommended doses	Simultaneous administration of cimetidine causes increased encainide drug levels
Significant negative inotropic side effect[34]; significant proarrhythmic effect with neurologic (dizziness, visual changes) and GI disturbances (nausea)	Contraindicated in patients with reduced left ventricular function, caution with renal disease	Other negative inotropes (e.g., β-blockers); elevate digoxin levels; cimetidine can increase flecainide levels

however, potassium is contraindicated in patients with high-degree AV block because potassium may worsen AV blockade. Other medications that elevate serum digoxin levels (e.g., verapamil, quinidine) should be discontinued.

Symptomatic bradyarrhythmias should be treated with atropine (0.5 mg IV, repeated to a maximum dose of 2 mg). Bradyarrhythmias resistant to atropine should be treated by emergent transvenous pacemaker insertion (if temporary pacing wires are not already in place). AV pacing is preferable to decrease the chance of pacemaker-induced ventricular arrhythmias. An isoproterenol infusion may worsen ventricular ectopy, predisposing the patient to ventricular tachycardia and ventricular fibrillation.

Tachyarrhythmias are treated with lidocaine or phenytoin. Both these antiarrhythmic drugs have the advantages of not worsening AV blockade when present, and neither is a significant negative inotrope. Lidocaine is administered in 100 mg IV loading doses for adults to a maximum of 300 mg. This may be followed by a 2 to 4 mg/min maintenance IV infusion.

Phenytoin has the benefit of reducing AV blockade in addition to suppressing ventricular tachyarrhythmias. Ten to 15 mg/kg

Table 10-4 Class II Drugs

Name	Clinical use	Administration	Pharmacokinetics
Propranolol	To prevent supraventricular arrhythmias, treatment of sinus and SVT, tachycardias associated with thyrotoxicosis, decreasing ventricular response to atrial tachyarrhythmias and in digitalis intoxication	IV: 1.0 mg over 5 min, then 0.5 mg/min to response; maximum dose of 0.1 mg/kg. Oral: 10 mg q 6 hr, increased as necessary to maximum dose of 80 mg PO q 6 hr	Hepatic metabolism with $T_{1/2}$ = 1-6 hr; therapeutic blood levels are dependent
Esmolol	See propranolol; Ultra-short-acting β-adrenergic blocker	IV: 500 µg/kg as infusion loading dose over 1 min, then infuse at 50 µg/kg/min; continue to load q 1 min and increase infusion 25-50 µg/kg/min until desired heart rate and blood pressure tolerance is achieved, up to maximum infusion rate of 200 µg/kg/min	Hepatic metabolism of this ultra-short-acting β-adrenergic blocker gives it very short $T_{1/2}$ (9 min with complete reversal of hemodynamic and electrophysiologic effects at 30 min); therapeutic blood levels are patient dependent

This class of agents includes all β-adrenergic blocking agents. The antiarrhythmic properties of these drugs are due primarily to their β-blocking effects. A detailed description of all agents is not possible here, but a few selected drugs are discussed.

should be administered for 1 hour (maximum rate of administration should not exceed 50 mg/min in adults or 1 to 3 mg/min in infants or children) to a loading dose of up to 1g. An oral maintenance dosage of 400 to 600 mg/day may then be continued until the toxic arrhythmia has resolved.

Supraventricular Arrhythmias

Supraventricular arrhythmias are a common complication after cardiac surgery, occurring as frequently as 40% of the time.[2,40]

Side effects	Cautions	Drug interactions
Multiple; include cardiac (negative inotrope, bradycardia, heart block), bronchospasm, depression, decreased peripheral blood flow	Multiple contraindications including poor left ventricular function, bradycardia, heart block, asthma or bronchospastic disease, depression, severe peripheral vascular disease	Many; include reserpine-like drugs (hypotension), elevated blood levels with cimetidine, decreased blood levels with hepatic enzyme induction (phenytoin), AlOH gels reduce intestinal absorption
See propranolol	See propranolol	See propranolol; 10%-15% increase in serum digoxin levels when given with esmolol

Management includes treatment of any concomitant disease state and removal of any precipitating factors such as hypoxia, hypokalemia, hypovolemia, hypoglycemia, or drug interactions.

Sinus Tachycardia

Sinus tachycardia is defined as a sinus node–initiated heart rate greater than 100 beats/min. Spontaneous depolarization rate of the SA node is primarily determined by the tone of the autonomic nervous system. Either vagal blockade or β-adrenergic stimulation can generate sinus tachycardia. The heart rate is generally less

***Table* 10-5** Class III Drugs

Name	Clinical use	Administration	Pharmacokinetics
Amiodarone	Prevention of atrial and ventricular tachyarrhythmias	Loading doses are required; 800-1600 mg/day 1× to 3 wk as oral load followed by 100-600 mg/day maintenance dosage	Slow absorption with extremely slow elimination due to high lipid solubility; hepatic metabolism; $T_{1/2}$ = 25-110 days; therapeutic blood levels 1-2.5 μg/kg
Bretylium tosylate	Refractory ventricular tachycardia and defibrillation; may aid defibrillation without DC cardioversion[4]	5 mg/kg IV loading dose, may repeat 1× if patient tolerates (hypotension may be problem); then constant infusion of 2-4 mg/min	Renal excretion with $T_{1/2}$ = 7-9 hr in patients with normal renal function; therapeutic blood levels not defined

$T_{1/2}$, Half-life.

***Table* 10-6** Class IV Agents

Name	Clinical use	Administration	Pharmacokinetics
Verapamil	To slow AV conduction in atrial fibrillation-flutter and to prevent recurrent SVT; especially useful in management of SVT after open heart surgery[20,21,29,42]	1 mg test dose IV followed by 5-10 mg IV infusion over 2 min; drug may be given 80-120 mg PO q 8 hr	IV: Peak hypotensive effect in 5 min with peak AV nodal blockage in 10-15 minutes lasting approximately 4-6 hr; therapeutic blood level, 80-400 ng/ml; undergoes hepatic metabolism with renal excretion of active metabolites and $T_{1/2}$ = 3-7 hr

GI, Gastrointestinal; *PO*, orally; *q*, every; $T_{1/2}$, half-life.

than 140 beats/min but can go as high as 220 beats/min or greater in the pediatric population. Sinus tachycardia is most often an appropriate response to some underlying physiologic stimulus such as pain, fever, or hypovolemia, or other causes that generate an increased sympathetic tone. The main clinical concern is that the

Side effects	Cautions	Drug interactions
Multiple adverse reactions including skin changes, skin discoloration, neurologic abnormalities, hepatic abnormalities, pneumonitis[48]; pulmonary fibrosis, proarrhythmic effects	Many severe side effects including pulmonary fibrosis and thrombocytopenia; should therefore be restricted to use in serious life-threatening refractory arrhythmias	Additive proarrhythmic effect with other antiarrhythmics; can prolong prothrombin time (caution with warfarin)[22]; increases plasma digoxin levels
Hypotension, nausea, vomiting	Early transient hypertension and worsening arrhythmias caused by norepinephrine release from terminal neurons	Can aggravate digitalis toxicity; can potentiate pressor effects of other catecholamine agents (dopamine)

Side effect	Cautions	Drug interactions
Hypotension, heart block, dizziness, headache, and GI disturbances	Can be fatal in patients with preexisting AV blockade or β-blockade; myocardial depression may occur and can be improved by infusion of calcium gluconate	Patients with congestive heart failure or β-blockade with concomitant verapamil administration can have serious hypotensive or heart block interactions; may increase serum cyclosporine levels; raises serum digoxin levels

rapid heart rate can precipitate myocardial ischemia by increasing oxygen demand and reducing diastolic coronary filling time.

The key feature in ECG diagnosis of sinus tachycardia is a regular rhythm with a steady, constant relationship between P waves and the QRS complex that follows it. The P wave should

Table 10-7 Class V Agents

Name	Clinical use	Administration	Pharmacokinetics
Digoxin	When used for its antiarrhythmic properties, causes sinus slowing and AV nodal blockade; used to slow ventricular response rate in atrial fibrillation and flutter and to prevent SVTs	For adults, 0.5 mg IV followed by 0.25 mg IV q 4 hr for 2 doses, for total of 1 mg loading dose over 8 hr; a daily maintenance dose, 0.125-0.5 mg PO depending on patient's age, renal function, and drug interactions; most common daily adult dose is 0.25 mg	Partially metabolized in liver, with majority of drug excreted renally; $T_{1/2}$ = 1-2 days; therapeutic blood levels, 1-2 ng/ml; drug levels are affected by renal status, weight, and other medications being concurrently administered; higher serum levels may be necessary in controlling SVTs whereas certain other patients may be susceptible to toxic side effects at lower blood levels

GI, Gastrointestinal; *PO,* orally; *q,* every; $T_{1/2}$, half-life.

be upright in leads II, III, and aVF consistent with antegrade atrial depolarization (Fig. 10-1).

The treatment of sinus tachycardia is first considering and correcting any underlying causes. This includes normalizing intravascular volume, correcting hypoxia, and providing for adequate anesthesia and sedation, particularly for intubated patients who cannot communicate their needs adequately.

In patients with a significantly elevated cardiac index (hyperdynamic state) and in whom all underlying causes of the tachycardia have been treated, β-blockade can be initiated if there are no other contraindications, as follows:

- Esmolol, 500 μg/kg IV for 1 minute followed by incremental IV infusions (Table 10-4)
- Propranolol, 0.5 to 1.0 mg IV for 5 minutes, then 0.5 mg/min infusion (dose to response) to a maximum dose of 0.1 mg/kg (Table 10-4)

In appropriate patients we have increasingly used esmolol IV infusion for hyperdynamic states. We believe the ultra-short half-life (9.5 minutes) and rapid reversal of β-blockade make it an ideal drug for use in the intensive care unit (ICU).

Side effects	Cautions	Drug interactions
GI (nausea, vomiting), neurologic (headache, dizziness), cardiac (bradycardia, heart block, arrhythmias) (see digitalis toxicity)	Hypokalemia, chronic pulmonary disease, and renal failure can predispose patients to digitalis toxicity; acute hypoxemia can also sensitize patients to toxicity; contraindicated in serious heart block; drug not removed by hemodialysis	Multiple interactions include elevated blood levels with simultaneous use of quinidine, verapamil, quinine, and amiodarone; hypokalemia can sensitize patients to digitalis toxicity so serum K levels must be followed when diuretics are being administered concurrently with digoxin; certain antibiotics (tetracycline) can cause increase in serum digoxin levels through changes induced in intestinal flora

Paroxysmal Supraventricular Tachycardia

Paroxysmal supraventricular tachycardia (PSVT) is often due to reentry phenomena occurring within the AV node. Although it is not a common arrhythmia after cardiac surgery, it can often be confused with atrial flutter. In patients with aberrant ventricular conduction the arrhythmia can be confused with ventricular tachycardia.

The ventricular response rate in PSVT is extremely regular and generally ranges from 140 to 220 beats/min. It can often be broken by maneuvers that increase vagal tone. Atrial ECG tracings can be extremely helpful in diagnosis. The key finding is a 1:1 conduction and a consistently reproducible relationship between the atrial and ventricular deflections on the atrial ECG tracings (Fig. 10-2).

PSVT often demands immediate therapy because of the rapid ventricular response rate and hypotension that it often induces. The key to therapy for PSVT in the cardiac surgical patient population is that it is often responsive to the rapid atrial overdrive pacing techniques discussed previously.

In patients that do not have temporary atrial pacing wires in place or where capture of the atrium is not possible, the recently approved drug adenosine can be used for both diagnostic and therapeutic purposes. Adenosine causes a transient, high-degree blockade of AV conduction. The drug is extremely short acting (half-life <10 seconds) and acts by slowing AV conduction time, thereby interrupting reentry-type pathways. It is administered as a 6 mg IV bolus injection, with subsequent incremental doses 1 minute apart as necessary. Diagnostically adenosine slows or breaks PSVT, completely unmasking atrial flutter (Fig. 10-3), and does not affect ventricular tachycardia.

Therapeutically adenosine slows conduction in PSVT, breaking the reentry pathway and converting the rhythm. Hypotension generally does not occur, although a prolonged pause and short-lived bradycardia can be observed after cardioversion (Fig. 10-4).

Other therapeutic options for PSVT include the following:

- *Verapamil,* 5 to 10 mg IV for 10 minutes, has been effective in slowing the rapid ventricular response rate or converting the PSVT to sinus rhythm in the majority of cases. Verapamil has several contraindications including congestive heart failure, hypotension, high-degree AV blockade, or previously administered IV β-blockers (Table 10-6).

- β-Blockers, such as IV esmolol or propranolol are often effective at breaking the reentry rhythm and possibly preventing recurrence (Table 10-4).

- Digoxin, given as IV loading and oral maintenance doses, can be used to slow AV nodal conduction and to assist in rate control, but prompt termination of the PSVT is not likely. Digoxin alone or in combination with quinidine can be very effective in preventing recurrent PSVT. The parenteral agents

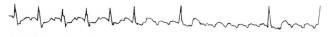

Fig. 10-3 Atrial flutter after administration of adenosine.

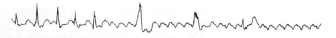

Fig. 10-4 Prolonged pause after adenosine.

adenosine, verapamil, and esmolol are probably the drugs of
first choice for acute treatment of this SVT (Table 10-7).

If atrial overdrive pacing is not available or has failed, and the
previous measures were also unsuccessful, or if the patient is highly
unstable and the arrhythmia is life threatening, immediate direct-
current cardioversion should be undertaken.

Ectopic Atrial Tachycardia

Ectopic atrial tachycardias are SVTs caused by a region of abnormal automaticity somewhere other than the SA node. They are
generally a less common cause of SVT than reentrant mechanisms.
They can be seen acutely in cases of digitalis toxicity, metabolic
abnormalities, myocardial infarction, or chronic lung disease.

The diagnosis of this arrhythmia depends on the demonstration
that the P wave during the episodes of tachycardia is different
from the sinus P wave. The ectopic P wave can be upright or
inverted, and the ventricular rate can vary widely (100 to 240
beats/min). Periods of AV block are often observed during this
type of SVT. The ectopic activity can have a single focus or
multiple foci.

As with all arrhythmias, treatment of any underlying causes
such as digitalis toxicity or hypoxia is paramount. Generally, ectopic atrial tachycardia does not respond well to overdrive pacing
techniques. The arrhythmia can be resistant to antiarrhythmic therapy that blocks AV nodal conduction. Options include *adenosine,*
a safe initial agent; *verapamil,* which often reduces the ventricular
response rate and can cause conversion to sinus rhythm, and *digoxin,* which also can slow the ventricular response, but large
doses may be required and digitalis toxicity is a risk. In addition,
electrical cardioversion may be necessary in highly symptomatic
patients.

Atrial Fibrillation

Atrial fibrillation is the most common supraventricular arrhythmia
observed after cardiac surgery. It is characterized by totally dis-
organized atrial depolarizations without any evidence of coordinated atrial contractions. The possible mechanism is a reentry
pattern of multiple excitation patterns with a variety of recovery
periods.[16]

Atrial fibrillation is recognized on ECG as irregular baseline
undulations of varying morphologies. These undulations ("F"

waves) are not always detectable on standard ECG leads. Lead V_1 and the inferior limb leads (II, III, and aVF) are the best leads to search for atrial activity. Unipolar and bipolar atrial ECGs often can show the atrial activity better than the conventional ECG leads (Fig. 10-5). The atrial rate in atrial fibrillation is generally between 350 and 600 beats/min. The hallmark of atrial fibrillation is the irregularly irregular ventricular response rate, usually between 110 and 180 beats/min.

The urgency of therapy is dictated by the ventricular response rate and the patient's hemodynamic tolerance of the arrhythmia. The atrial kick, or boost, to cardiac output created by a synchronized atrial contraction can contribute 10% to 20% of a patient's cardiac output. The loss of this addition to cardiac output can have extremely serious consequences in certain patients, particularly those with congestive heart failure or mitral stenosis.

The first line of therapy, unless contraindicated by hypotension (systolic blood pressure ≤80 mm Hg), is verapamil by IV injection. This calcium channel–blocking agent slows AV conduction and has mild to moderate negative inotropic effects, so it must be used with caution. When IV verapamil is given it is best to have the patient attached to a ventricular-demand pacemaker, if temporary wires are present. Verapamil is given as a test dose of 1 mg, to allow observation (3-5 minutes) for undesirable side effects such as hypotension. If hypotension does occur, calcium chloride, 200 to 500 mg IV, is often the appropriate treatment. Once the test dose has been tolerated, 5 to 10 mg of IV verapamil is administered for approximately 5 minutes with constant monitoring of the ECG, heart rate, and blood pressure. This may be repeated in 30 minutes if necessary.

The major therapeutic benefit of verapamil is a rapid slowing

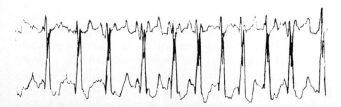

Fig. 10-5 Atrial fibrillation; atrial ECG; unipolar; bipolar.

of the ventricular response rate. Reversion to a sinus rhythm occurs in a minority of patients without the use of other medications such as digoxin.

Digoxin is administered IV in this setting because oral absorption can be extremely slow. The patient's serum potassium level should be checked and corrected. A loading dose of 0.5 mg IV can be given to adult patients, followed by 0.25 mg IV every 4 hours for two additional doses. An additional 0.125 to 0.25 mg IV may need to be administered, provided the patient has normal renal function and electrolyte status and no signs of toxic reaction to digitalis.

The onset of action of IV digoxin is approximately 30 minutes, with a peak effect at 3 hours. Once loading has been accomplished, the maintenance oral dose of digoxin varies between 0.125 mg and 0.5 mg depending on the patient's size, age, renal status, and concurrent medications. Serum digoxin levels are not reliable until a steady state has been achieved, about 4 hours after IV administration and 6 to 7 hours after oral administration.

Digoxin generally is effective in controlling the ventricular response rate in atrial fibrillation; whether it promotes conversion to sinus rhythm is a point of controversy in the literature. Digoxin, although having a slower onset of action than verapamil or esmolol, is generally the first drug of choice for hemodynamically stable patients because it is safe for patients with poor left ventricular function. Digoxin is also safe in patients with asthma.

With its rapid onset of action and brief duration (20 to 40 minutes), esmolol is probably the safest IV *β-blocker* to use in the ICU. Both esmolol and propranolol are effective at controlling the ventricular response rate of atrial fibrillation. β-blockers can cause a high-degree heart block when given within 1 hour of IV verapamil. When giving IV β-blockers it is appropriate to have a ventricular demand pacemaker connected for safety. For details on the administration of IV esmolol and propranolol see the discussion under Sinus Tachycardia.

Once the ventricular response rate has been controlled, it can be maintained by giving oral doses of either the aforesaid medications, or type IA antiarrhythmics.

DC cardioversion should be performed immediately for atrial fibrillation with a rapid ventricular response rate in patients with marked hypotension or myocardial ischemia. Some groups suggest procainamide, 100 mg IV, be administered before emergent DC cardioversion for atrial fibrillation.[5]

Anticoagulation therapy should be considered in patients who have had atrial fibrillation for several days before planned cardioversion. This is especially true in patients with a history of embolism, recurrent atrial fibrillation, or mitral valve disease with left atrial dilatation. Digoxin should be withheld for 24 hours before elective DC cardioversion to avoid postconversion arrhythmias induced by digoxin. The initial DC countershock should start at low energy levels (50 watt-seconds) and increase in increments of 10 watt-seconds as necessary.

Atrial Flutter

Atrial flutter is a relatively common supraventricular arrhythmia occurring 24 to 36 hours after open heart surgery. Uniform flutter waves can be observed on the ECG tracing at rates between 250 and 350 beats/min. The mechanism of atrial flutter is probably a reentry pattern within the atrium.[35]

Atrial flutter generally is diagnosed by presence of a sawtoothed atrial wave pattern on ECG, with rates of 250 to 350 beats/min. The regularity of the atrial rhythm may often be lost on a standard ECG tracing because flutter waves can be hidden in the QRS complex. Ventricular conduction is often 2:1 with a ventricular rate in the range of 150 beats/min. AV block can be variable, giving an irregular response rate. With the use of temporary atrial electrodes, the atrial ECG reveals the regular atrial flutter waves (Fig. 10-6) and a regular beat-to-beat variability.

As with all SVTs, atrial flutter can give rise to a very rapid ventricular response, resulting in hypotension and myocardial ischemia. Urgent therapy is required for patients with compromised vital signs (systolic blood pressure <80 mm Hg or heart rate >160 beats/min) or evidence of myocardial ischemia.

Atrial flutter is often responsive to rapid atrial overdrive pacing techniques. If overdrive pacing does not convert the tachycardia to sinus rhythm, atrial flutter often reverts to atrial fibrillation by

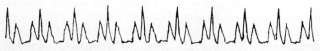

Fig. 10-6 Atrial ECG of atrial flutter.

overdrive pacing. The rapid ventricular response of atrial fibrillation is then often more readily controlled than atrial flutter rates.

Adenosine can be used to terminate the reentry circus movement of atrial flutter in patients not responsive to overdrive pacing techniques or without atrial electrodes in place (see previous discussion in this chapter under Paroxysmal Supraventricular Tachycardia).

Other therapeutic options are aimed at slowing the rapid ventricular response rate to the atrial flutter. These include the administration of verapamil, digoxin, esmolol, and propranolol. The indications, doses, and precautions are the same as for the treatment of atrial fibrillation.

Sinus Bradycardia

Sinus bradycardia is a sinus heart rate of less than 60 beats/min. It is not uncommon postoperatively and may be due to drugs (e.g., narcotics or β-blockers) or intrinsic sinus node disease.

Sinus bradycardia is diagnosed by a sinus mechanism (upright P wave in ECG leads I, II, or aVF) with normal morphology and relationship to the QRS complex with a rate less than 60 beats/min.

The first line of therapy in the postoperative period is to begin atrial pacing at a rate of 90 to 110 beats/min to improve cardiac output. Atrial pacing allows for the atrial kick of atrial contraction to boost cardiac output. This would not occur in ventricular pacing. The Swan-Ganz catheter may be used to follow improvements in cardiac output as the rate is increased. AV sequential pacing must be used if high-degree AV block is present. Ventricular pacing is the next temporary pacing technique that can be used in sinus bradycardia for patients without atrial wires.

Atropine (0.5 mg/dose to total dose of 2.0 mg in adults) may be administered IV if pacing techniques fail or are unavailable. An isoproterenol infusion can be used to increase chronotropic activity of the heart. Isoproterenol is both a β₁- and β₂-adrenergic agonist and is administered as a continuous IV infusion (1.0 to 5.0 μg/min).

Persistent bradycardia unresponsive to other therapy may require placement of either a temporary or permanent pacemaker.

Ventricular Arrhythmias

Postoperative ventricular arrhythmias are principally ectopic and must be taken seriously because they can be harbingers of potentially fatal ventricular tachycardia or fibrillation. Ventricular ectopy can develop in patients without a history of ectopy; it may also be improved postoperatively by revascularization of previously ischemic zones of myocardium.[6]

The possible etiology of ventricular arrhythmias has previously been listed. An accurate data base should be quickly acquired in the evaluation of any case of ventricular arrhythmias. This includes determination of arterial blood gas and serum potassium level. Both of these laboratory tests can be rapidly obtained, and, if abnormal, are common causes of ventricular ectopy that can be readily treated. A 12-lead ECG should also be obtained for the patient and compared with earlier tracings to evaluate for myocardial ischemia as a source of newly developed ectopy.

Premature Ventricular Contractions

Premature ventricular contractions (PVCs) are defined as impulses of ventricular origin that occur earlier than the next normally conducted sinus beat. Generally they arise from an actopic focus of ventricular myocardium, or they can be caused by reentry pathways in the His-Purkinje tissue.

A PVC has a wide (>0.12-second) QRS complex because the normal conduction pathways are not used. The ST and T waves have the appropriate polarity from the widened QRS complex. The PVC is followed by a compensatory pause before the next sinus beat. PVCs can be either unifocal, meaning each PVC has an identical morphology, or multifocal with a variety of QRS morphologies and intervals.

Any postoperative patient demonstrating six or more PVCs per minute, bigeminy, coupling, or R-on-T phenomena should be treated with an IV bolus of lidocaine unless contraindicated. Lidocaine is administered as a 1 mg/kg bolus and started as an infusion, 20 to 40 μg/kg/min. An additional 1 mg/kg bolus may be given for recurrent ectopy. Lidocaine is cleared by the liver, and this clearance is slowed by cimetidine and propranolol, requiring dosage adjustment in liver failure or in the presence of these medications.

Most early postoperative arrhythmias are due to metabolic disturbances. Patients with ventricular ectopy should have a serum potassium concentration maintained greater than 4.5 mEq/L and an arterial oxygen pressure of 75 mm Hg or greater. Correcting the serum potassium concentration alone may eliminate ventricular ectopy; additionally, lidocaine is more effective in patients with a high serum potassium level.

Potassium is administered as an IV potassium chloride infusion or "run." Each potassium run consists of 10 to 15 mEq infused for approximately 30 to 60 minutes. One can expect a 0.1 mEq/L rise in the serum potassium concentration of an average adult for every 2 mEq administered IV. The dosage should be in the range of 0.1 to 0.15 mEq/kg/hr in the pediatric population. The physician must be certain of adequate renal function before the administration of potassium-containing medications.

Magnesium sulfate may be given for low serum magnesium levels (<1.3 mEq/L) and presence of ventricular ectopy. One to 4 g diluted in a 0.9% sodium chloride solution given for 2 to 4 hours will return the magnesium level back to a normal range of 1.3 to 2.1 mEq/L. Caution should be used because serum potassium levels increase as magnesium levels increase.

In patients with atrial pacing wires in place, ventricular ectopy can be suppressed by overdrive pacing the atria at a rate 10 to 20 beats/min greater than the patient's sinus rate. This can be done only when the patient does not have an existing sinus tachycardia.

In patients with PVCs treated and responding to lidocaine therapy we generally maintain the drip infusion for approximately 12 to 24 hours. The infusion may then be stopped and the patient monitored an additional 3 to 6 hours without medication. If the ventricular ectopy recurs, lidocaine may be reinstituted and the patient will need to be begin oral medication. We frequently start therapy with procainamide, 500 mg orally every 6 hours, and discontinue the lidocaine drip after the third dose of procainamide.

The next line of therapy for PVCs not responding to lidocaine therapy is IV procainamide therapy. The IV use of procainamide is initiated with a 100 mg IV bolus for 2 minutes. This may be repeated every 5 minutes up to a maximum dose of 1 g, to suppress ventricular ectopy. A constant drip infusion may then be started at 20 µg/kg/min. The physician must be aware that procainamide has a short half-life (3.5 hours) in patients with normal renal function. The active metabolite N-acetylprocainamide (NAPA) has a longer half-life, in the range of 6 to 9 hours. Serum levels for both procainamide and NAPA should be followed because NAPA accumulates disproportionally in patients with impaired renal function. In these patients the dosage may need to be decreased by as much as 50%.[14]

Bretylium tosylate is the next line of therapy for patients resistant to procainamide therapy. This drug is usually begun as a 5 mg/kg IV loading bolus and may be repeated once as the patient tolerates. A constant infusion of 2 to 4 mg/min is then begun. Bretylium is a class III antiarrhythmic agent with a mechanism of activity different from lidocaine or procainamide. One must remember that bretylium can aggravate digitalis toxicity and cause significant suppression of ventricular function.

Ventricular Tachycardia

Ventricular tachycardia is generally due to a reentry cycle in the His-Purkinje system.[35] Ventricular tachycardia is defined as three successive ventricular-originated ectopic beats (QRS >0.12 seconds) at a rate greater than 100 beats/min.

Any wide QRS tachycardia must be presumed to originate from the ventricle until otherwise proved. The differential diagnosis of such a wide QRS tachycardia includes SVT with preexisting BBB or SVT with aberrant ventricular conduction. Some ECG features that may be useful in making this differentiation have previously been discussed. SVTs may have aberrant ventricular conduction because the premature supraventricular impulse enters a refractory region of the ventricular conducting tissue. The right bundle branch has a longer refractory period than the left bundle branch; thus SVT with aberrant ventricular conductions often take the configuration of a right BBB pattern. Such ECG distinctions may be useless when the patient's hemodynamic status is severely compromised by the tachycardia. When the patient's hemodynamic status is severely compromised, all wide complex QRS tachycardias must be treated as a ventricular tachycardia until otherwise proved.

As with all arrhythmias initial treatment includes identifying and removing any predisposing factors contributing to the arrhythmia. The method of treatment for ventricular tachycardia depends on both the duration of the arrhythmia and the degree of hemodynamic compromise it induces in the patient. Patients with short periods of ventricular tachycardia without severe compromise of hemodynamic parameters should be started on lidocaine therapy as done for PVCs. Procainamide should be tried for persistent runs of ventricular tachycardia not responsive to lidocaine therapy. Ventricular overdrive pacing at a rate greater than the ventricular tachycardia may also convert the patient to a normal sinus rhythm. If these therapies fail, IV amiodarone can be life-saving.

The patient who has persistent ventricular tachycardia, or ventricular tachycardia with hemodynamic compromise (hypertension, shock, congestive heart failure, or myocardial ischemia) must be treated with immediate DC cardioversion while simultaneously beginning pharmacologic therapy. Pulseless ventricular tachycardia or ventricular flutter are treated as ventricular fibrillation.

Ventricular Fibrillation

Ventricular fibrillation is a devastating ventricular rhythm generated by multiple ectopic foci within the ventricle. There is no organized electrical activity, no coordinated depolarization, and therefore no ventricular contraction. Cardiac resuscitation protocols and immediate nonsynchronized DC cardioversion are the treatment for this dysrhythmia. Cardiopulmonary resuscitation should be instituted while the defibrillation equipment is prepared. The argument can be made to withhold cardiopulmonary resuscitation when the defibrillation equipment is immediately available. External cardiac compressions in patients after sternotomy can rupture the sternal closure, damage bypass grafts, or produce myocardial injury. Patients not responding to attempts at electrical and pharmacologic intervention should be considered candidates for reopening of the sternotomy and internal cardiac compressions and defibrillation and placement of selected patients on percutaneous cardiopulmonary bypass.

Defibrillation and DC Cardioversion

The unit of energy on most defibrillators is the joule (1 J = 1 watt-second). Defibrillation is accomplished when sufficient current is transferred through the chest to depolarize a critical mass of the myocardium. Current delivery is affected primarily by the strength of the shock and the transthoracic impedance. Some of the factors affecting transthoracic impedance include electrode size, electrode-skin interface, time interval between shocks, the phase of ventilation, transelectrode distance, and the pressure applied on the paddles.[9,15,19,32] Other variables that can affect the success of defibrillation include hypoxemia, medications, and the acid-base status of the patient.

Nonsynchronized shocks are used for wide-complex ventricular tachycardia and ventricular fibrillation. The proper energy level to use for defibrillation is still somewhat controversial. Myocardial damage increases as the energy applied in cardioversion is increased. Therefore the lowest effective energy level should be used during cardioversion. In pulseless ventricular tachycardia or ventricular fibrillation the current guidelines recommend an initial defibrillation of 200 J. If unsuccessful, a second shock of 200 to 300 J should be delivered. If these are not successful, the next shock should not exceed 360 J. A recurrence of fibrillation should then be treated with a shock at the previously effective energy level.[66] The risk of too low an energy level is that it will be inefficient and prolong myocardial ischemia whereas too high an energy level risks myocardial injury.[10,15,19]

References

1. DiMarco JP: Adenosine for paroxysmal supraventricular tachycardia: dose ranging and cyanosis with verapamil—assessment in placebo-controlled multicenter trials, *Ann Intern Med* 113:104, 1990.
2. Angelini P et al: Cardiac arrhythmias during and after heart surgery: diagnosis and management, *Prog Cardiovasc Dis* 16:469, 1974.
3. Antman EM et al: Calcium channel blocking agents in the treatment of cardiovascular disorders. I. Basic and clinical electrophysiologic effects, *Ann Intern Med* 93:875, 1980.
4. Arcidiacono R: Use of bretylium tosylate in ventricular fibrillation, *Clin Ter* 84:253, 1978.
5. Aronow WS: Management of supraventricular tachyarrhythmias *Comp Ther* 15:11, 1989.
6. Aronow WS: Management of ventricular arrhythmias, *Comp Ther* 14:25, 1988.
7. Bhatia JJS, Smith TW: Digitalis toxicity: mechanisms, diagnosis and management, *J Cardiac Surg* 2:453, 1987.
8. Bigger TJ Jr: Antiarrhythmic treatment: an overview, *Am J Cardiol* 53:8B, 1984.
9. Connel PN, Ewy GA, Dahl CF et al: Transthoracic Impedance to Defibrillator Discharge. Effect of Electrode Size and Electrode—Chest Wall Interface, *J Electrocardiogr* 6:313, 1973.
10. Conti CR: Editors note: adenosine: clinical pharmacology and applications, *Clin Cardiol* 14:91, 1991.
11. Cooper TB et al: Overdrive pacing for supraventricular tachycardia: a review of theoretical implications and therapeutic techniques, *Pace* 1:196, 1978.
12. Cosio FG et al: Electrophysiologic studies in atrial fibrillation: slow condition of premature impulses: a possible manifestation of the background for reentry, *Am J Cardiol* 51:122, 1983.
13. Daudon P et al: Prevention of atrial fibrillation or flutter by acebutolol after coronary bypass grafting, *Am J Cardiol* 58:933, 1986.
14. Davis D: Diagnosis and management of cardiac arrhythmias in the postoperative period, *Surg Clin North Am* 63:1091, 1983.

15. Ewy GA, Hellman DA, McClung BS et al: Influence of ventilation phase on transthoracic impedance and defibrillation effectiveness, *Crit Care Med* 8:164, 1980.
16. Farringer JA et al: Cimetidine-quinidine interaction, *Clin Pharmacol* 3:81, 1984.
17. Federman J et al: Clinical pharmacology: series on pharmacology in practice, 2. Antiarrhythmic drug therapy, *Mayo Clin Proc* 54:531, 1979.
18. Garcia R, Lee TG: Broad QRS tachycardia: electrocardiographic diagnosis and management, *Am J Emerg Med* 334-341, 1983.
19. Geddes LA, Tacker WA, Cabler P et al: The decrease in transthoracic impedance during successive ventricular defibrillation trials, *Med Instrum* 9:179, 1975.
20. Gronzalez R, Scheinman MM: Treatment of supraventricular arrhythmias with intravenous and oral verapamil, *Chest* 80:465, 1981.
21. Gray RJ et al: Role of intravenous verapamil in supraventricular tachyarrhythmias after open heart surgery, *Am Heart J* 104:799, 1982.
22. Hamer A et al: The potentiation of warfarin anticoagulation by amiodarone, *Circulation* 65:1025, 1982.
23. Hammon JW Jr et al: Perioperative beta blockade with propranolol: reduction in myocardial oxygen demands and incidence of atrial and ventricular arrhythmias, *Ann Thorac Surg* 38:363, 1984.
24. Harken AH et al: Cardiac dysrhythmia in the acute setting, *J Emerg Med* 5:129, 1987.
25. Harrison DC: Antiarrhythmic drug classification, New Science and practical applications, *Am J Cardiol* 56:185, 1985.
26. Harrison DC: Should lidocaine be administered routinely to all patients after acute myocardial infarction? *Circulation* 58:581, 1978.
27. Hoffman BF, Rosen MR: Cellular mechanisms for cardiac arrhythmias, *Circ Res* 49:1, 1981.
28. Deleted in galleys.
29. Iberti TJ et al: Use of constant-infusion verapamil for the treatment of postoperative supraventricular tachycardia, *Crit Care Med* 14:283, 1986.
30. Ivey MF et al: Influence of propranolol on supraventricular tachycardia early after coronary artery revascularization: a randomized trial, *J Thorac Cardiovasc Surg* 85:214, 1983.
31. Josephson ME, Horowitz LN et al: Recurrent sustained ventricular tachycardia, *Circulation* 57:431, 1978.
32. Kerber RE, Grayzel J et al: Transthoracic resistance in human defibrillation. Influence of body weight, chest size, serial shocks, paddle size, and paddle contact pressure, *Circulation* 63:676, 1981.
33. Kosowsky BD et al: Long-term use of procainamide following acute myocardial infarction, *Circulation* 47:1204, 1973.
34. Legrand V et al: Hemodynamic effects of a new antiarrhythmic agent,

flecainide (R-818), in coronary heart disease, *Am J Cardiol* 51:422, 1983.

35. Leier CV et al: Prolonged atrial conduction: a major predisposing factor for the development of atrial flutter, *Circulation* 57:213, 1978.

36. Leitch JW et al: The importance of age as a predictor of atrial fibrillation and flutter after coronary artery bypass grafting, *J Thorac Cardiovasc Surg* 100:338, 1990.

37. Liem LB et al: Update: cardiac antiarrhythmic drugs, *Comp Ther* 15:17, 1989.

38. Malcolm ID et al: The use of temporary atrial electrodes to improve diagnostic capabilities with Holter monitoring after cardiac surgery, *Ann Thorac Surg* 41:103, 1986.

39. Marriott HJL: *Practical electrocardiography,* ed 8, Baltimore, 1988, Williams & Wilkins.

40. Michelson EL et al: Postoperative arrhythmias after coronary artery and cardiac valvular surgery detected by long-term electrocardiographic monitoring, *Am Heart J* 97:442, 1979.

41. Mohr R et al: Prevention of supraventricular tachycardia with low-dose propranolol after coronary bypass, *J Thorac Cardiovasc Surg* 81:840, 1981.

42. Murphy CE, Wechsler AS: Calcium channel blocks and cardiac surgery, *J Cardiac Surg* 2:299, 1984.

43. Opie LH, ed: *Drugs for the heart,* ed 3, Philadelphia, 1991, WB Saunders.

44. Parker FB Jr et al: Supraventricular arrhythmias following coronary artery bypass: the effect of preoperative digitalis, *J Thorac Cardiovasc Surg* 86:894, 1983.

45. Pinski SL, Maloney JD: Adenosine: a new drug for acute termination of supraventricular tachycardia, *Cleve Clin Med* 57:383, 1990.

46. Polish LB et al: Digoxin-quinidine interaction: potentiation during administration of cimetidine, *South Med J* 74:633, 1981.

47. Roden DM et al: Antiarrhythmic efficacy, pharmacokinetics and safety of *N*-acetyl procainamide in human subjects, comparison with procainamide, *Am J Cardiol* 46:463, 1980.

48. Rotmensch HH et al: Possible association of pneumonitis in amiodarone therapy, *Am Heart J* 100:412, 1980.

49. Sinah BN et al: Electrophysiologic and hemodynamic effects of slow channel drugs, *Prog Cardiovasc Dis* 25:103, 1982.

50. Smith JW, Haber E: Digitalis, *N Engl J Med* 289:945, 1973.

51. Stephenson LW et al: Propranolol for prevention of postoperative cardiac arrhythmias: a randomized trial, *Ann Thorac Surg* 29:113, 1980.

52. Till J et al: Efficacy and safety of adenosine in the treatment of supraventricular tachycardia in infants and children, *Br Heart J* 62:204, 1989.

53. Twum-Barima Y, Carruthers SG: Quinidine-rifampin interaction, *N Engl J Med* 304:1466, 1981.

54. Deleted in galleys.

55. Volosin K et al: Tocainide associated agranulocytosis, *Am Heart J* 109:1392, 1985.

56. Waldo AL, McLean WAH: *Diagnosis and treatment of cardiac arrhythmias following open heart surgery: emphasis on the use of atrial and ventricular epicardial wire electrodes,* Mount Kisco, NY, 1983, Futura Publishing.

57. Webb Kavey RE et al: Phenytoin therapy for ventricular arrhythmia occurring late after surgery for congenital heart disease, *Am Heart J* 104:794, 1982.

58. Wellens HJ: The electrocardiogram 80 years after Einthoven, *J Am Coll Cardiol* 7:(3)484, 1986.

59. Weng JT et al: Antiarrhythmic drugs: electrophysiological basis of their clinical usage, *Am Thorac Surg* 41:106, 1986.

60. Williams JB et al: Arrhythmia prophylaxis using propranolol after coronary artery surgery, *Ann Thorac Surg* 34:435, 1982.

61. Winkle RA et al: Malignant ventricular tachyarrhythmias associated with the use of encainide, *Am Heart J* 102:857, 1981.

62. Woosley RL et al: Overview of the clinical pharmacology of antiarrhythmic drugs, *Am J Cardiol* 61:61A, 1988.

63. Viskin S, Belhassen B: Acute management of paroxysmal atrioventricular junctional reentrant supraventricular tachycardia: pharmacologic strategies, *Am Heart J* 120:180, 1990.

64. Sharma AD, Klein GJ, Yee R: Intravenous adenosine triphosphate during wide QRS complex tachycardia: safety, therapeutic efficacy, and diagnostic utility, *Am J Med* 88:337, 1990.

65. Belardinelli L, Linden J, Berne RM: The cardiac effects of adenosine, *Prog Cardiovasc Dis* 32:73, 1989.

66. Standards and guidelines for CPR and ECC, *JAMA* 255:2905, 1986.

Nutritional Support   11

Charles D. Fraser, Jr.

The correlation between malnutrition and increased morbidity and mortality after surgical stress is well established.[38,43,57-59,61,81] This relationship is equally important in patients undergoing cardiac surgery.[1,4,36] To date, however, no reports have been published that confirm a beneficial role for preoperative nutritional support in the patient with cardiac disease. In the recently published Veterans Affair Cooperative Study, perioperative (preoperative and postoperative) total parenteral nutrition was shown to reduce the incidence of postoperative infectious complications in severely malnourished general surgical patients.[85] Potentially these results may be applicable to patients undergoing cardiac surgery. The nature of cardiac illness, however, often makes preoperative nutritional assessment difficult and inaccurate. In practice, nutritional support in cardiac surgery has been relegated to the postoperative patient in the cardiac intensive care unit who has had an untoward complication as the result of underlying disease or the surgical procedure. These patients often present complex management problems stemming not only from requirements for nutritional support but also the provision of such support in the context of other major organ system dysfunction.

In this chapter the assessment of nutritional requirements in the patient after cardiac surgery is reviewed. Indications for nutritional support, modes of administration, evaluation of adequacy of support, and potential complications are discussed. Although not intended to be a complete review of surgical nutrition, this chapter should provide the reader with a practical reference guide for use in a cardiac intensive care setting.

Nutritional Status Assessment

Patients requiring support in the cardiac surgical intensive care unit can be placed into two general categories. The first includes patients in whom unexpected complications develop after cardiac surgery but who were well nourished before surgery. These patients are distinctly different from the second category of persons who have preoperative cardiac cachexia. This group of patients faces a substantially increased surgical risk because of preexisting malnutrition.[11,28]

Cardiac cachexia associated with severe congestive heart failure has long been recognized. These patients generally have poor appetites, a fact that may be compounded by the large doses of medication they often require. Clinically they characteristically demonstrate protein-calorie malnutrition with systemic manifestations of weakness, lethargy, anorexia, and poor wound healing.[14] Despite a relatively normal body weight, physical examination reveals signs of chronic malnutrition with temporal muscle wasting, thinness, fragile skin, loss of arm fat, and loss of muscle mass.[65] Anthropometric measurements may be useful in patients with cardiac cachexia because the arms are usually not affected by the massive changes in extracellular fluid involving the rest of the body. Thus losses of muscle and fat in the arm can be readily assessed. Laboratory evaluations may reveal decreased levels of albumin, folate, thiamine, potassium, calcium, magnesium, iron, and zinc.[65,66]

Cardiac cachexia is thought to have multiple causes including nephrotic syndrome, protein-losing enteropathy, fat malabsorption, and tissue edema.[65] This condition is often associated with valvular heart disease, especially rheumatic mitral disease.

In contrast, patients with acquired postoperative malnutrition are often relatively well nourished preoperatively. Nonetheless, in those patients with complications from open heart surgery, lack of nutrient intake and excessive losses associated with sepsis and multisystem organ failure can result in the rapid onset of nosocomial malnutrition.[5,8] This form of malnutrition may be more insidious in that patients may appear to be adequately nourished. This is especially true in the obese patient, where underlying muscle wasting and protein loss is masked by preserved adipose stores.[1] In these patients accurate, objective nutritional assessment is critical in early recognition of developing deficits and in the provision and evaluation of nutritional support.

Clinical Assessment

Weight loss

As noted previously, changes in body weight may be misleading in patients in the cardiac intensive care setting, especially in patients with classic cardiac cachexia and related hypoproteinemia. In these patients changes in weight are unreliable as predictors of nutritional status because of massive shifts in extracellular fluids. Weight changes in patients without cardiac cachexia, however, may provide some indication of nutritional deficit. It is generally recognized that a weight loss of 10% of ideal body weight is associated with increased morbidity.[73] Ideal body weight may be considered the patient's usual body weight or that obtained from standard references of age, height, and sex.[53]

Anthropometric data

Anthropometric measurements are used to estimate subcutaneous fat and skeletal muscle stores. This information is obtained in an effort to make an objective clinical assessment of a patient's nutritional deficits.[13,25,86] These data have inherent weaknesses that limit their usefulness in clinical practice. Static measurements need to be compared with normal values obtained from healthy control populations. Where an individual patient's measurements may compare to such control values can be extremely variable. For example, a patient starting with a greater than normal arm circumference may lose significant lean mass and still fall within standardized normal ranges. A potentially more useful indicator is temporal variation within a person. Such determinations, however, need to be made for extensive time intervals, thus limiting their usefulness. Unfortunately, several recent studies have demonstrated the lack of consistency of anthropometric data as a reliable predictor of clinical malnutrition.[7,60]

Biochemical markers

Because levels of plasma proteins depend on synthesis and thus on availability of substrate precursors, they may be considered to be markers of nutritional status. Other factors affect plasma protein levels, however, including rates of catabolism and volume of distribution. Nonetheless, acute decreases in protein intake may rapidly affect synthesis, thus making determinations of plasma proteins potentially useful.

The commonly measured proteins are albumin, prealbumin, and transferrin.

Albumin is the major protein synthesized by the liver, and approximately 40% of this protein mass is in the circulation. It has a half-life of approximately 18 days, which limits its usefulness as an acute marker of protein depletion. Albumin levels, however, have been correlated with clinical outcome in several studies. A serum albumin level of 2.8 to 3.5 g/dl represents mild protein depletion; 2.2 to 2.7 g/dl, moderate depletion; and less than 2.2 g/dl, severe depletion.[69,74]

Transferrin is a β-globulin that transports iron in plasma and has a half-life of 8 days. Serum levels are affected by protein balance and iron metabolism. Although the shorter half-life predicts more clinical utility in measurements of transferrin, this has not been demonstrated in a previous clinical study.[7]

Measurable changes in prealbumin, a thyroxine-binding protein, occur within 7 days of a change in nutrient intake. As with transferrin, however, this marker has not proven to be of greater clinical usefulness than albumin.[12,84]

Other objective measurements have been used in an effort to measure and predict the degree of protein-calorie malnutrition. Cell-mediated immunity and total lymphocyte counts are known to be affected by malnutrition.[52] However, as with biochemical measurements, these determinations are more suitably used in epidemiologic surveys than in individual patients. The problem of use for a patient lies in the separation of effects of actual nutrient deprivation from those of the disease process in altering the measurements. For example, hepatic disease, nephrotic syndrome, and protein-losing enteropathy may all combine to reduce serum protein levels in excess of existing nutritional deficits. Infection and multisystem organ failure may make measurements of delayed hypersensitivity unreliable.[51] *To date no objective measurement or combination of objective data has proven more reliable in predicting malnutrition in the individual patient than careful clinical evaluation.*[7,60]

Nutritional Requirements

The nutritional requirements of a patient after cardiac surgery are dictated in large part by the patient's age, body size, sex, and degree of activity. In patients with complications, however, the basal metabolic rate (BMR) may be greatly increased. The neuroendocrine response to such major stress as sepsis and single or multiple organ system failure has been well described.[8] In general mediators and hormones of catabolism (catecholamines, glucocorticoids, glucagon) are found in increased circulating levels whereas anabolic mediators (insulin and growth hormone) are relatively decreased. Thus the severely stressed patient may have marked hypermetabolism with increases in the BMR to 50% or greater than the nonstressed state. Patients with severe cardiac cachexia may also have a similar increase in metabolic demand. The basal energy requirement or BMR can be calculated from standardized nomograms or equations that have been derived in healthy persons. A commonly used formula is the Harris-Benedict equation[10]:

Men: Kcal per day = 66 + (137 × weight [kg]) + (5 × height [cm]) − (6.8 × age [yr])

Women: Kcal per day = 655 + (9.6 × weight [kg]) + (1.7 × height [cm]) − (4.7 × age [yr])

Determining the requirements in the patient with complications of surgery is clearly more complex and inexact. In general, estimated energy requirements should be 25% to 50% greater than the calculated BMR in cases of moderate to severe stress. Repletion of existing deficits requires an even greater caloric intake. Adequacy of support can be determined only by frequent monitoring of nutritional parameters (see following section).

After energy needs have been estimated, protein requirements must be assessed. As noted previously, there are no precise, consistent measurements to determine preexisting protein deficits. In general, the protein requirement for most adults is approximately 0.8 to 1.0 g/kg/day. Protein losses occur in urine and stool such that most healthy adults are in zero nitrogen balance (grams of protein × 6.25 = grams of nitrogen). Critically ill patients, including patients with complications after cardiac surgery and patients with cardiac cachexia, may require 1.5 to 2.0 g/kg/day of protein.[1,65] In summary, protein requirements are 0.8 to 1.0 g/kg/day for normal persons and 1.5 to 2.0 g/kg/day for stressed patients. Most standard enteral and parenteral formulas provide this increased protein requirement if the patient can tolerate increased volumes of formula. This is because most standard mixtures provide nutrients in a fixed protein/calorie ratio. The standard nitrogen/calorie ratio for most prepared formulas is 1:150 (1 g nitrogen per 150 kcal). This increased intake of protein may be poorly tolerated in patients with hepatic, renal, or multisystem organ failure. Considerations for nutritional support in these patients are discussed subsequently.

Patients with severe cardiac cachexia may have fat malabsorption. In these patients special consideration should be given to the dietary fat source. Because approximately 80% of medium-chain triglycerides are absorbed directly into the portal circulation, this source may be preferable to long-chain triglycerides, which require bile salt solubilization and chylomicron transport. However, in patients receiving medium-chain triglycerides as the fat source the essential fatty acid linoleic acid must be provided.[9,34,50]

Fluid and sodium requirements in the patient undergoing cardiac surgery should be minimized, especially in patients with preexisting or ongoing congestive heart failure. In general, most patients require 1 ml water for every ingested kilocalorie, usually 1500 to 2500 ml/day of water. This value should be limited to 0.5 ml/kcal/day for patients with congestive heart failure.[37,46] In summary, water requirements are 1 mg/kcal/day for persons with normal heart function and 0.5 mg/kcal/day for those with congestive heart failure. As with all therapeutic manipulations, frequent clinical and laboratory assessments are mandatory in guiding treatment modifications. Serum values for major electrolytes (sodium, potassium, chloride, calcium, magnesium, phosphate) should be frequently measured, especially during the initiation phases of therapy. Trace element supplementation must also be included in nutritional support. Recommended dietary allowances for various trace minerals and vitamins have been determined and should be provided in standard intravenous and oral preparations[3,75] (Table 11-1).

Considerations in Multisystem Organ Failure

Renal Failure

Unfortunately, a significant percentage of patients with complications in cardiac surgery have some degree of acute renal impairment. This dysfunction may range from mild elevations in blood urea nitrogen (BUN) and creatinine to complete renal shutdown with anuria and azotemia. Patients with acute postoperative renal failure have been demonstrated in an experimental study to have increased energy expenditure by as much as 130% to 190% of basal values.[75] Muscle protein degradation is increased and protein synthesis is diminished as a result of increased insulin resistance and increased glucagon and catecholamine levels seen in acute renal failure (ARF).[47] Carbohydrate metabolism is also abnormal as a result of the insulin resistance of ARF, resulting in hyperglycemia and increased insulin requirements. Serum lipid clearance is also affected by the peripheral tissue resistance to insulin.[54] Diminished clearance of nitrogenous wastes with increased protein breakdown results in increasing levels of BUN and creatinine. Electrolyte regulation may be compromised with elevations in potassium, phosphorus, and magnesium. With severe impairment volume overload occurs, necessitating fluid restriction or dialysis.

The multiple metabolic derangements of ARF make standard measures of nutritional status unreliable. Alterations in protein metabolism and fluid balance limit the usefulness of plasma transport proteins as markers of nutritional status. Changes in body weight and anthropometric data are also difficult to interpret for the same reasons.[87] Nonetheless, consistent and frequent assessment of nutritional status in these patients is mandatory. Measurements of energy expenditure by indirect calorimetry are essential in the individualization of nutritional support in patients with ARF[82] (see discussion of therapeutic monitoring in this chapter). Excessive caloric administration of these persons may produce hepatic steatosis, excessive carbon dioxide production, increased catecholamine release, and production of fat over muscle. Inadequate caloric intake may carry the risk of further protein depletion. In general, recommended caloric intake should be equal to measured total energy expenditure (TEE) if weight maintenance is desired and up to 130% of TEE if weight gain is desired.[24]

Amino acid requirements and composition are designed to achieve a positive nitrogen balance. In highly catabolic patients up to 2 g/kg/day of protein may be required. This level of intake may be difficult unless dialysis is considered. A recent study revealed that optimal nitrogen utilization is achieved by a mixture of essential and nonessential amino acids.[44] Metabolism of muscle protein and a portion of parenteral amino acids result in increased blood urea. Those amino acids used for muscle protein synthesis are not catabolized and thus do not increase BUN. If muscle protein

Text continued on p. 252.

Table 11-1   Vitamin and Mineral Requirements

Vitamin/mineral	Units	RDA for daily oral intake	Daily requirement of moderately injured	Daily requirement of severely injured	Amount provided by 1 pill	Daily amount provided by standard IV preparations	Suggested daily IV intake	Daily amount provided by commercially available mixture
A (retinol)	IU	1760 (F)-3300 (M)	5000	5000	10,000	3300 (retinal)		
D (ergocalciferol)	IU	200	400	400	400	200		
E (tocopherol)	mg	8-10	Unknown	Unknown	15	10 IU*		
K (phylloquinone)	µg	20-40 †	20	20	0	0‡		
C (ascorbic acid)	mg	60	75	300	100	100		
Thiamine (B$_1$)	mg	1.0-1.5	2	10	10	3.0		
Riboflavin (B$_2$)	mg	1.2-1.7	2	10	10	3.6		

Nutrient	Unit						
Niacin	mg	13-19	20	100	100	40	
Pyridoxine (B₆)	mg	2.0-2.2	2	40	5	4.0	
Pantothenic acid	mg	4-7 (adults)†	18	40	20	15	
Folic acid	mg	0.4	1.5	2.5	0	0.4	
B₁₂	μg	3.0	2	4	5	5	
Biotin	μg	100-200⁻	Unknown	Unknown	0	60	
Zinc	mg	15				2.5-5.0§	5.0
Copper	mg	2-3†				0.5-1.5	1.0
Manganese	mg	2.5-5.0†				0.15-0.8	0.5
Chromium	mg	0.05-0.2†				0.01-0.015	0.1
Iron	mg	10 (M)-18 (F)				3	

F, Female; *M*, male; *RDA*, Recommended Dietary Allowance.

*Equivalent to RDA.

†Estimated to be safe and adequate dietary intakes.

‡Must be supplemented in peripheral venous solutions.

§Burn patients require an additional 2 mg.

catabolism decreases with nutritional support, BUN may actually decrease.[83]

Close serial measurement of serum electrolytes is necessary to direct ongoing requirements. As noted, phosphorus, potassium, and magnesium clearance may be deranged and thus levels of these electrolytes need close observation.

Nutritional administration in critically ill patients with ARF may take the form of enteral or parenteral supplementation. Although the enteral route may appear preferable, this may not be practical in most postoperative cardiac patients with ARF. In general, appetites are depressed and in patients with severe uremia, alterations in bowel function including ileus may result in poor tolerance of enteral feedings. If the enteral route is not tolerated or practical, total parenteral nutrition (TPN) should be instituted with concentrated glucose, lipid, and amino acid solutions to minimize volume loads. These high concentrations of nutrients necessitate central venous administration. (See Chapter 6 for technique of central line insertion.) In addition, dialysis can be modified for the provision of some nutrients. Patients receiving peritoneal dialysis can absorb 60% to 80% of dialysate glucose, providing 700 to 4000 kcal/day.[4] In addition, dialysate modified with 1.1% and 2% amino acid solutions have been well tolerated and result in significant amino acid absorption.[5,33] Slow continuous ultrafiltration and hemodialysis provide no protein supplementation and may be responsible for losses of 9 to 12 g/day of protein.[17-20] Moderate amounts of glucose used in dialysate baths are retained, resulting in up to 500 kcal/day. Thus hemodialysis may allow lower maintenance TPN and allow increased protein administration.

Hepatic Failure

Hepatic failure occurring in patients after cardiac surgery is an ominous condition resulting from impaired hepatic perfusion, malnutrition, sepsis, and a variety of other poorly understood factors. With severe liver failure hepatic glucose production, amino acid uptake, and ketogenesis are decreased.[8] Plasma levels of branched-chain amino acids (BCAA) are decreased whereas clearance of aromatic amino acids (AAA) is impaired, resulting in increased plasma concentrations. These in turn may be metabolized to false neurotransmitters, resulting in hepatic encephalopathy and coma. Patients dying of multisystem organ failure associated with sepsis and injury have been observed to have lower clearance of amino acids, lower BCAA, and higher AAA concentrations than those with similar illnesses who survived.

No specific countermeasures are known for preventing hepatic failure in the critically ill patient, aside from assuring adequate perfusion and providing sufficient substrate for hepatic metabolism. Once hepatic failure has been established, hypercatabolism and prevention of encephalopathy must be addressed by specially designed formulas. Standard nutrient solutions in such patients may aggravate neurologic symptoms. These patients should receive formulas with increased amounts of BCAA and decreased quantities of AAA (phenylalanine, tyrosine, and tryptophan) and the sulfur-containing amino acid methionine.[22,23,45]

Pulmonary Failure

Adult patients with acquired cardiac disease, especially coronary artery disease, often have some degree of compromised pulmonary function. On occasion postoperative pulmonary function disturbances together with preexisting lung disease make extended periods of mechanical ventilation necessary. Appropriate nutritional support in these patients is essential in allowing lung recovery and promoting eventual ventilator weaning.

Although successful nutritional support and repletion of preexisting deficits requires adequate caloric intake, the source of these calories plays an important role in the patient with ventilatory failure. In general, whether nutritional support is provided enterally or parenterally, it is recognized that excessive carbohydrate intake can result in increased oxygen consumption (V_{O_2}) and carbon dioxide production (V_{CO_2}).[8] Heymsfield et al. evaluated respiratory, cardiovascular, and metabolic changes during enteral alimentation in malnourished patients receiving either high-carbohydrate or high-fat solutions. They observed greater increases in V_{CO_2}, V_{O_2}, heat production, and minute ventilation in the patients receiving the high-carbohydrate formula.[37]

In fasting persons energy demands are met by metabolism of endogenous fat stores, which are oxidized at a *respiratory quotient* (RQ) (equivalent to CO_2 produced [in milliliters] divided by O_2 consumption [in milliliters]) of 0.7. Patients receiving standard parenteral nutrition solutions utilize glucose (RQ = 1.0) as their primary energy source. Askanazi et al.[6] examined stressed patients (sepsis, severe injury) receiving parenteral nutrition with glucose as the primary source of nonprotein calories. They observed a 21% increase in V_{O_2}, a 53% increase in V_{CO_2}, and a 121% increase in minute ventilation in these patients. Their explanation for this phenomenon stemmed from the fact that in patients receiving excess glucose calories, carbohydrate is converted to fat at the RQ of 8.0, resulting in a large increase in CO_2 production. In patients with compromised lung function, especially patients with chronic obstructive pulmonary disease with elevated resting CO_2 levels, there is an increased tendency toward CO_2 retention. Thus in the patient with difficulty in weaning from ventilatory support, administration of excessive glucose could result in CO_2 retention and failed weaning. Administration of fat as an alternate energy source is potentially beneficial in these persons because as fat is oxidized at an RQ of 0.7 and therefore is associated with lower CO_2 production.

Enteral Versus Parenteral Nutrition

No controlled, randomized studies have demonstrated a definite benefit of enteral over parenteral nutritional support in patients undergoing cardiac surgery. Nonetheless, recent experimental and clinical study into the central role of the gastrointestinal tract in surgical stress tend to favor enteral nutrition if no contraindications to this route are encountered.

Although previously believed to be a quiescent organ system during periods of severe illness, a recent study has reported the central role of the gastrointestinal tract during stress. Considerable information has been accumulated that demonstrates the important metabolic function of the intestine during stressed states and its role as a barrier to enteric microorganisms and their toxins.[21,78] During periods of significant stress and malnutrition, intestinal barrier function may be compromised, thus allowing significant ongoing bacterial contamination. Translocated intestinal flora are believed to be responsible for increased septic complications in critically ill patients, whereas absorbed bacterial endotoxin may contribute significantly to the multisystem organ failure syndrome.[32,41] Enteral feedings are known to be a highly effective method of maintaining intestinal integrity and function. The use of standard parenteral nutrition solutions, however, has been associated with gut mucosal atrophy and loss of brush border enzyme activity.[29,42,48,76,80] Clinical reports have also demonstrated reductions in septic complications after major surgical stress (major abdominal trauma) in patients receiving enteral nutrition early in their postoperative course.[56]

Administration of enteral nutrition may be difficult in the early postoperative course of a patient after cardiac surgery. Recent experimental interest, however, has focused on therapy capable of supporting the intestinal mucosa whether given by the enteral or parenteral route. *Glutamine* is a nonessential amino acid and is the most abundant amino acid in mammalian plasma. Experimental investigation by Windmueller and Spaeth[89] in 1974 revealed that glutamine is an important respiratory substrate for cells in the small intestinal mucosa.[68] Later studies by Windmueller[88] demonstrated that glutamine is the principal oxidizable fuel of the small intestine. During periods of major surgical stress, glutamine consumption by the small intestine is markedly increased. This phenomenon is also observed after administration of glucocorticoids, implicating the pituitary-adrenal axis as central to accelerated intestinal glutamine uptake during stress.[77,79]

Glutamine has been previously classified as a nonessential amino acid because it can be synthesized from other amino acids and precursors. However, during critical illness glutamine concentrations in blood and tissue decrease significantly as it is mobilized as a gut energy source. This leads to a situation of marked glutamine depletion. Although additional dietary glutamine is unnecessary during states of good health, supplementation appears to be beneficial when depletion is severe. In animal models enteral feedings enhanced with supplemental glutamine were associated with increased intestinal villus hyperplasia and increased cellularity.[87] Substituting glutamine for other nonessential amino acids in a glucose-based parenteral nutrition formula has been shown to result in significant increases in mucosal cellularity in the jejunum, ileum, and colon.[39,40]

In summary, most data support enteral over parenteral nutritional support, especially in terms of protecting intestinal mucosal barrier function. In circumstances under which the gastrointestinal tract cannot be used, parenteral nutrition enhanced with glutamine is associated with increased mucosal cellularity and protected barrier function.

Enteral Support

Indications

Most patients with complications after cardiac surgery require some form of nutritional support. In patients confined to the intensive care unit the oral route is usually not an option. Enteral feedings, however, are still preferable in these patients for the previously mentioned reasons. This should be the primary route considered in all patients unless they do not have a functioning gastrointestinal tract.

Access

Temporary access to the gastrointestinal tract is best obtained by nasogastric or nasoduodenal intubation. In patients with a clear sensorium and no increased risk of aspiration, nasogastric feeding may be acceptable. In patients with increased probability of aspiration, however, placement of a tube beyond the pylorus is essential. Previous study has demonstrated that the likelihood of gastroesophageal reflux is greatly diminished when tube placement is beyond the ligament of Treitz.[31] Small-bore silicone elastomer tubes can be passed into the stomach, and then the patient can be rotated to the right side in an effort to pass the tip through the pylorus and into the duodenum. If this is unsuccessful, metoclopramide can be administered (usual adult dose, 10 mg). Ultimately, proper placement may require fluoroscopic or endoscopic guidance. Correct positioning must be confirmed before the instillation of any solution. Plain radiology or aspiration of enteric contents may not always be adequate to determine gastric placement. In certain cases infusion of small amounts of contrast material (5 ml of dilute barium) may be necessary to confirm placement in the duodenum or proximal portion of the jejunum.

Long-term access to the gastrointestinal tract is probably best achieved by gastrostomy or jejunostomy. In patients who have undergone previous extensive surgery of the upper abdomen, open gastrostomy or jejunostomy may be necessary. In others percutaneous endoscopic gastrostomy, alone or with jejunostomy, is a more acceptable option. Endoscopic gastrostomy placement has been well described and is a safe and reliable technique.[27,68] In patients with increased risk of aspiration the percutaneous endoscopic gastrostomy technique has been modified for the simultaneous placement of gastric and jejunal tubes such that the stomach can be kept decompressed during ongoing small bowel feeding.[67]

Formula Selection and Administration

In patients with cardiac cachexia, especially those with ongoing or previous congestive heart failure, sodium (1 to 2 g/day) and fluid (1000 to 1500 ml/day) restriction may be necessary. *Os-*

molarities of administered formulas should be varied according to site of delivery:

- Gastric feeding: High osmolarity, bolus method
- Jejunal feeding: Lower osmolarity, continuous infusion

The stomach has a large reservoir capacity and can accept large osmotic loads. Therefore hyperosmolar gastric feeds are readily tolerated. For small bowel feeding large boluses of hyperosmolar solutions are poorly tolerated, resulting in cramping, diaphoresis, nausea, and diarrhea. Initiation of small bowel feeding should be by continuous infusion at a low rate of a dilute (hypoosmolar) solution. In time osmolarity and volume can be increased, but unlike the stomach, bolus feeding in the small bowel are not tolerated, so continuous infusion is mandatory.

Enteral formulas that are either fixed composition or modular (variable composition) can be selected.[36] Fixed-composition formulas selected for patients with cardiac disease usually are chosen on the basis of high caloric density (>1.5 kcal/ml), and low water and sodium content (see Table 11-2). Such formulas have carbohydrate as the main caloric source and are well tolerated when administered directly into the stomach. For patients on receiving small bowel feedings, fat-based balanced diets may be more easily tolerated.

Disease-specific formulas can be varied in composition according to patient need. Such modular solutions are prepared by varying amounts of protein, carbohydrate, fat, minerals, and vitamins to meet the patient's requirements. Thus in patients with absorption problems the nitrogen source can be altered to the form of peptides and amino acids to improve nitrogen retention. Fat in the form of medium-chain triglycerides is also more easily absorbed in such patients. In patients with diabetes complex sugars and starches may help reduce hyperglycemia. Varying carbohydrate loads may also be useful in patients with ventilator dependency and CO_2 retention. As noted previously, hepatic formulas with increased BCAA and decreased AAA are helpful in preventing hepatic encephalopathy. Patients with renal dysfunction benefit from formulas containing protein in the form of essential amino acids.

Complications

Several potential complications are possible in patients receiving enteral nutritional therapy. Aspiration of enteric contents can be a

Table 11-2 Composition of Balanced-Formula Diets

Caloric density (kcal/ml)	Protein (g/L)	Carbohydrate (g/L)	Fat (g/L)	Products
0.6	40	121	1.7	Citrotein
1.0	26-45	175-248	1.3-13.5	Criticare HN, Precision LR and High-Nitrogen diets,* Vital High Nitrogen,* Travasorb HN Peptide and Standard Diets
	28-49	123-159	30-44	Isocal‡, Ensure,* Enrich,† Precision Isotonic Diet, Osmolite,* Travasorb MCT Diet
	60	130	23	Sustacal
1.5	55-61	190-200	53-57	Ensure Plus,* Sustacal HC
	62-83	105-143	68-92	Pulmocare,* Traumacal‡
2.0	70-75	225-250	80-91	Magnacal¶, Isocal‡ HCN

Based on product literature.
*Ross Laboratories, Columbus, Ohio.
†Includes as a fiber source 21 g/L soy polysaccharide.
‡Mead Johnson
¶Organon

major source of morbidity and mortality in the critical care setting.[90] As mentioned previously, placement of a feeding tube beyond the pylorus reduces the risk of aspiration. All patients with altered sensoria should have frequent assessment of gastric residuals to assess for gastric retention. Elevating the head of the bed is another effective method of avoiding reflux. Patients with a history of previous aspiration or reflux are at increased risk, and small bowel feeding or parenteral therapy should be considered.

Metabolic monitoring must be routinely undertaken in all patients receiving enteral nutrition. Potential derangements include hyperglycemia, renal impairment, hepatic impairment, dehydration, and electrolyte disturbances.[16]

Gastrointestinal disturbances may include abdominal distention, cramping, diarrhea, and vomiting. Diarrhea is the most frequent disturbance and is defined as more than three loose stools in a 24-hour period. Many causes of diarrhea in enterally fed patients are possible including lactose intolerance, fat malabsorption, *Clostridium difficile* enterocolitis, and excessive infusion rates.

In general, reducing osmolarity and rate of infusion should be the initial maneuver while diagnostic studies are undertaken. Administration of antidiarrheal medication, especially opiates, should be avoided until clostridial toxin and bacterial overgrowth has been ruled out.

Parenteral Support

Indications

If caloric needs cannot be provided by the enteral route, some form of parenteral therapy is indicated. Parenteral venous nutrition may be administered through either the peripheral or central vein. Because peripheral veins are sensitive to high osmolar solutions, formulas administered by this route have lower caloric density. Thus adequate support requires larger-volume loads. As noted earlier, in patients with cardiac disease, excessive fluid administration may be undesirable. Thus the peripheral route is not generally preferable in the patient after cardiotomy. Centrally administered formulas have higher caloric density and thus can be given in lower volumes.

Central venous TPN is initiated only if the expected duration of therapy is 7 days or more. This situation may apply to postoperative cardiac patients with cardiac failure, pulmonary insufficiency, renal failure, neurologic injury, or other major organ system dysfunction.

Access

Acceptable access for TPN is provided only by cannulation of a central vein, preferably either the subclavian or internal jugular vein. Although femoral venous catheters are a possible short-term alternative, they are associated with a much higher incidence of catheter-related sepsis.[55]

Catheters used for TPN should be dedicated to that purpose only. Previous study has ascertained that infusing TPN through a central catheter used for other purposes is associated with an unacceptable rate of catheter sepsis.[30,72] Similarly, use of one port of a multilumen catheter for TPN also results in higher rates of sepsis.[63] Catheter care is best provided by hospital personnel specially trained in TPN line care.

The preferred site for central venous cannulation is the superior vena cava (SVC)–right atrial (RA) junction through a percutaneous puncture of either subclavian vein. Although several techniques for insertion are possible, the Seldinger method is vastly superior in terms of safety and reproducibility. In experienced hands this technique should result in a procedure-related complication rate of less than 1%. Briefly, the Seldinger method involves placing a flexible guide wire into the superior vena cava through the subclavian vein. This guide wire is inserted through an introducer needle inserted beneath the clavicle, parallel to the chest wall, and directed toward the suprasternal notch. The wire should pass easily and meet no resistance. The physician performing the cannulation must ensure that at all times the guide wire is accessible. The venous catheter is advanced over the guide wire and the wire removed. After any residual air is aspirated, the catheter is flushed with heparinized saline solution and secured in place, and a sterile dressing is applied. Immediate chest radiography is performed to ascertain catheter positioning at the SVC–RA junction. Positioning in the atrium or ventricle mandates repositioning because of risks of cardiac chamber perforation. Once radiographically confirmed, the catheter is ready for use.

A second option for cannulation of the superior vena cava is through either internal jugular vein. This may be acceptable in some patients but is to be avoided in patients with tracheostomies. In this situation prevention of direct catheter contamination by tracheal flora is virtually impossible.

Formula Selection and Administration

As noted previously, administration of central venous TPN requires careful ongoing clinical and laboratory assessment followed by appropriate formula modifications as needed. Ten percent dextrose in water should be run at a low rate (20 ml/hr) to initiate therapy immediately after line placement. This is to allow confirmation of line positioning before administration of high osmolar fluids, which could be potentially harmful if infused into a malpositioned catheter.

Starting TPN solutions vary somewhat but usually consist of administration of 1000 to 1500 ml/day in an average-sized adult. Fluid composition includes carbohydrate, usually 25% dextrose (250 g/1000 ml); amino acids, 5% (50 g/1000 ml); and electrolytes. Major electrolytes are added in concentrations appropriate to the particular clinical situation. Base needs are met by administration of acetate because bicarbonate is incompatible with nutrient solutions. Minor electrolytes and trace minerals are provided by commercially available mixtures but should be used with caution in patients with impaired elimination (ARF, hepatic failure). All patients should receive vitamin supplementation in the form of prepared mixtures added daily. Vitamin K (10 mg) is administered weekly. Patients undergoing prosthetic valve replacement, however, require long-term warfarin anticoagulation, and in these patients vitamin K is contraindicated.

Fats can be provided as either 10% or 20% solutions (usually 500 ml). Essential fatty acid requirements are fulfilled by weekly administration of 500 ml of 20% lipid. In patients with cardiac disease daily addition of lipid solutions to TPN provides additional calories without substantially increasing fluid administration. Fluids can be limited further by increasing concentrations of amino acids (up to 8.5%) and carbohydrate (70% dextrose) in so-called hi-cal formulations.

A standard TPN solution for a 70 kg person consists of the following:

- Solution: 1000 to 1500 mg/day
- Carbohydrate: 25% dextrose (250 g/1000 mg)

- Amino acids: 5% (50 g/1000 ml)
- Major and minor electrolytes
- Base needs: Acetate
- Trace minerals
- Vitamin mixtures (including vitamin K)
- Fat: 10% to 20% solution (500 ml)

TPN solutions containing the previously mentioned compositions of carbohydrate (25% dextrose) and protein (5% amino acids) provide 1 kcal/ml. Thus 1500 to 2500 ml/day is required for caloric needs. Addition of fats to the solution increases caloric density to 1.15 kcal/ml and thus somewhat limits obligate fluid administration. Additional measures include increasing glucose and protein concentrations and volumes as tolerated.

After therapy is initiated at 1000 to 1500 ml/day, TPN administration is gradually increased during the ensuing 2 to 3 days as tolerated. Again, frequent clinical examination is mandatory, to evaluate the patient's condition for signs of excessive fluid administration.

As discussed in this chapter in the section under Considerations in Multisystem Organ Failure, patients in the cardiac intensive care unit often have both multiple severe organ system dysfunction and diminished cardiac function. Provision of TPN in such patients demands individualization of solutions to meet their particular metabolic requirements and tolerances. Thus in patients with *pulmonary insufficiency* excessive carbohydrate loads may result in increased V_{CO_2} and V_{O_2} measurements. Provision of solutions with decreased glucose (12.5%) and increased lipids (10% daily) may be beneficial in limiting V_{CO_2} and improving ventilator weaning.[8]

In patients with *ARF* diminished clearance of nitrogenous wastes and increased protein catabolism have a severe impact on nitrogen balance.[44,83] Patients in this category benefit from TPN solutions with a high essential amino acid content (2% to 3%) and with primary energy requirements provided by glucose (25% to 40% dextrose). Thus nitrogen/calorie ratios are increased compared with the standard TPN formulation.

Patients with *hepatic failure* require some form of nutritional support, and TPN has been shown to increase the survival rate in these patients.[26] Nonetheless, these persons may have severely impaired ability to handle protein loads, especially AAA. In these patients amino acid formulations can be modified to provide BCAA while avoiding AAA.[22,23,45]

Complications

Complications related to TPN may be categorized as mechanical, septic, or metabolic. Mechanical complications are related to catheter placement and maintenance. As noted previously, the Seldinger method of line insertion has been proven a safe and reliable technique of catheter insertion in experienced hands. Thus the operator placing a central line for TPN should be either experienced or closely supervised by an experienced practitioner. During line insertion anatomic landmarks should be strictly observed, and catheter insertion should be smooth and without resistance. Any difficulty during insertion mandates aborting that approach. Patients undergoing line insertion should have normal coagulation parameters and adequate platelet counts ($>50,000/mm^3$). Line tips should be positioned at the SVC–RA junction. Line positioning in the right atrium and against the wall of the superior vena cava can result in perforation and cardiac tamponade. Other potential mechanical complications are similar to those possible with other central lines, namely air embolus and inadvertent catheter dislodgement.

Catheter sepsis is always a potential hazard in a patient in the intensive care unit receiving TPN. Catheter-related sepsis is the most common serious complication of TPN with reported rates in the range of 1% to 10%.[62,71] Catheter infection may result either from direct contamination through the insertion site or from blood-borne bacteria from a second septic source. Infection related to catheter site contamination can be markedly reduced by appropriate catheter and site care.[72]

In critically ill patients with cardiac disease, determining the source of sepsis can often be challenging. Pneumonia, urinary tract infections, wound infections, and other potential sources may make localizing the exact focus of the central venous catheter difficult. If peripheral blood cultures are positive, especially for organisms associated with direct skin contamination *(Staphylococcus aureus, Staphylococcus epidermidis),* the TPN line should be removed and the tip cultured. If blood cultures remain negative yet the patient has persistent fever and/or leukocytosis without a definite clinical source, line sepsis can be determined by a sterile line change over a guide wire and catheter tip culture. This method has proven effective in elucidating line sepsis in equivocal situations.[49,64] If the cultured tip is positive, the line should subsequently be removed.

Metabolic complications related to TPN are frequent but usually of minor concern, requiring only small adjustments in solution composition. Major and minor *electrolyte disturbances* may occur and require intermittent solution modification. Transient mild *hyperglycemia* is frequent. This problem is most commonly managed by small doses of subcutaneous insulin initially and later addition of insulin to the nutrient solution. Ten to 40 U/L of regular insulin may be needed in some patients. If refractory hyperglycemia remains a problem, patients may be given a separate continuous insulin drip and have frequent serum glucose determinations to regulate the insulin infusion. Additionally, solutions can be altered to provide more calories as fat rather than as glucose.

On occasion severe hyperglycemia can progress to a hyperosmolar state with dehydration and altered mental status. This usually is the result of inadequate monitoring, excessive administration, or decreased tolerance with sepsis. Treatment appropriate for hyperglycemia should be instituted in this situation, including cessation of TPN, frequent glucose monitoring, and rehydration.

Rebound hypoglycemia may also be observed after periods of long-term TPN support. This situation is believed to result from excessive endogenous insulin production caused by chronic pancreatic islet cell stimulation. Maintaining an infusion of 10% dextrose for 24 hours after ceasing TPN will avoid this potential problem.

As noted previously, increases in V_{CO_2} and V_{O_2} occur with administration of TPN in hypermetabolic patients. Although not always a problem, excessive CO_2 production may be particularly troublesome in long-term ventilator-dependent patients, and appropriate modifications in solution should be made.[6]

Numerous biochemical alterations are possible including liver function abnormalities. This may result from excessive glycogen and fat deposition in the liver and usually responds to decreasing TPN rates. A full discussion of all other potential complications is beyond the scope of this text. Diligent monitoring, however, will reveal existing and developing complications.

Metabolic and Therapeutic Monitoring

Protocols for metabolic monitoring vary depending on the clinical status of the patient. Postcardiotomy patients in critical condition require more frequent monitoring than less ill patients. Monitoring should consist of the following:

- Intake and output records
- Daily weight
- Urine tests for ketones and glucose every shift and, if necessary, blood glucose determination by glucometer
- Serum electrolytes, urea, creatinine, and glucose levels three times weekly
- Minor electrolyte determinations and liver function tests weekly

A standard measurement of adequacy of nutritional support is provided by *serial nitrogen balance determination*. This should be undertaken on a weekly basis while patients are receiving TPN therapy. To make this measurement a 24-hour collection of urine is made and kept cold (on ice at the patient's bedside). Volume and urea nitrogen concentrations can be measured from this sample. Under normal conditions urine urea nitrogen accounts for 70% to 80% of total urinary nitrogen.[65,70] Nitrogen intake is calculated from known protein intake by the following equation: grams of nitrogen $= 6.25 \times$ grams of protein. A rough estimate of fecal nitrogen loss is usually 2 g/day. Therefore total nitrogen loss can be estimated as follows:

Nitrogen loss (g/day) = urine nitrogen (g/day) + (0.3 × urine nitrogen [g/day]) + 2 g/day (feces)

A net negative nitrogen balance demands reassessment of TPN support to achieve ultimately a positive balance.

A more accurate assessment of energy balance in the severely ill patient can be provided by calculating energy expenditure from V_{O_2}. This value can be directly measured with a metabolic cart with a spirometer and a CO_2 absorber. From measured V_{O_2} the metabolic rate can be calculated with the following equation:[36]

Metabolic rate (kcal/hr) = V_{O_2} (ml/min) × 60 min/hr × (1 L/1000 ml) × 4.83 kcal/L

From these data more accurate estimates of energy demands can be made, potentially avoiding both underfeeding and overfeeding.

Conclusion

Nutritional support should be standard therapy in all patients unable to maintain adequate caloric intake after cardiac surgery. This is particularly true in the patient with complications such as organ system dysfunction and sepsis. Although enteral nutrition is the preferred approach, this route may not always be practical or feasible in this patient population. TPN is a satisfactory alternative and should be readily instituted if the clinical situation warrants.

References

1. Abel R et al: Malnutrition in cardiac surgical patients: results of a prospective, randomized evaluation of early postoperative parenteral nutrition, *Arch Surg* 111:45, 1976.
2. AMA Department of Foods and Nutrition: Guidelines for essential trace element preparations for parenteral use: a statement by an expert panel, *JAMA* 241:2951, 1979.
3. AMA Department of Foods and Nutrition: Multivitamin preparations for parenteral use: a statement by the Nutrition Advisory Group, 1975, *J Parenteral Enteral Nutr* 3:258, 1979.
4. Anderson G et al: Glucose absorption from the dialysis fluid during peritoneal dialysis, *Scand J Urol Nephrol* 5:77, 1971.
5. Arteen S et al: The nutritional/metabolic and hormonal effects of nine weeks continuous ambulatory peritoneal dialysis with a 1% amino acid solution, *Clin Nephrol* 33:192, 1990.
6. Askanazi J et al: Respiratory changes induced by the large glucose loads of total parenteral nutrition, *JAMA* 243:1444, 1980.
7. Baker J et al: Nutritional assessment: a comparison of clinical judgments and objective measurements, *N Engl J Med* 306:969, 1982.
8. Baue A: Nutrition and metabolism in sepsis and multisystem organ failure, *Surg Clin North Am* 71:549, 1991.
9. Berkowitz D, Croll M, Likoff W: Malabsorption as a complication of congestive heart failure, *Am J Cardiol* 11:43, 1963.
10. Blackburn G et al: Nutritional and metabolic assessment of the hospitalized patient, *J Parenteral Enteral Nutr* 1:11, 1977.
11. Blackburn G et al: Nutritional support in cardiac cachexia, *J Thorac Cardiovasc Surg* 73:489, 1977.
12. Borass M et al: Serum proteins and outcome in surgical patients, *J Parenteral Enteral Nutr* 6:585, 1982.
13. Burr M, Phillips K: Anthropometric norms in the elderly, *Br J Nutr* 51:165, 1984.
14. Carr J, Stevenson L, Walden J, Heber D: Prevalence and hemodynamic correlates of malnutrition in severe congestive heart failure secondary to ischemic or idiopathic dilated cardiomyopathy, *Am J Cardiol* 63:709, 1989.
15. Carrilo C et al: Multiple-organ-failure syndrome, *Arch Surg* 121:196, 1986.
16. Cataldi-Betcher E et al: Complications occurring during enteral nutrition support: a prospective study, *J Parenteral Enteral Nutr* 7:546, 1983.

17. Chanard J et al: Evaluation of protein loss during hemofiltration, *Kidney Int* 33:5114, 1988.
18. Clowes G et al: Survival from sepsis: the significance of altered protein metabolism regulated by proteolysis inducing factor, the circulating cleavage product of interleukin-1, *Ann Surg* 202:446, 1985.
19. Compher C, Mullen J, Barker C: Nutritional support in renal failure, *Surg Clin North Am* 71:597, 1991.
20. Davenport A, Roberts N: Amino acid losses during continuous high-flux hemofiltration in the critically ill patient, *Crit Care Med* 17:1010, 1989.
21. Deitch E, Winterton J, Li M, Berg R: The gut as a portal of entry for bacteremia, *Ann Surg* 205:681, 1987.
22. Dudrick P, Souba W: Amino acids in surgical nutrition, *Surg Clin North Am* 71:459, 1991.
23. Fischer J et al: The effect of normalization of plasma amino acids on hepatic encephalopathy in man, *Surgery* 80:77, 1976.
24. Forster J et al: Hypercalcemia in critically ill surgical patients, *Ann Surg* 202:512, 1985.
25. Frisancho A: New norms for upper limb fat and muscle areas for assessment of nutritional status, *Am J Clin Nutr* 34:2540, 1981.
26. Galambos J et al: Hyperalimentation in alcoholic hepatitis, *Am J Gastroenterol* 72:535, 1979.
27. Gauderer M, Ponsky J, Izant R: Gastrostomy without laparotomy: a percutaneous endoscopic technique, *J Pediatr Surg* 6:872, 1980.
28. Gibbons G et al: Pre and postoperative hyperalimentation in the treatment of cardiac cachexia, *J Surg Res* 19:439, 1976.
29. Gleeson M, Dowling R, Peters T: Biochemical changes in intestinal mucosa after experimental small bowel bypass in the rat, *Clin Sci* 43:743, 1982.
30. Goldman D, Maki D: Infection control in total parenteral nutrition, *JAMA* 223:1360, 1973.
31. Gustke R, Varma R, Soergel K: Gastric reflux during perfusion of the small bowel, *Gastroenterology* 59:890, 1970.
32. Hammer-Hodges D, Woodruff P, Cuevas P et al: Role of the intraintestinal gram negative bacterial flora in response to major injury, *Surg Gynecol Obstet* 138:599, 1974.
33. Hanning R, Balfe J, Zlorkin S: Effectiveness and nutritional consequences of amino acid–based vs glucose-based dialysis solutions in infants and children receiving CAPD, *Am J Clin Nutr* 46:22, 1987.
34. Helcamp G, Wilmore D, Johnson A et al: Essential fatty acid deficiency in red cells after thermal injury: correction with intravenous fat therapy, *Am J Clin Nutr* 26:1331, 1973.
35. Heymsfield B, Bleier J, Wenger N: Detection of protein-calorie undernutrition in advanced heart disease, *Circulation* 56(suppl III):102, 1977.

36. Heymsfield S, Smith J, Redd S, Whitworth H: Nutritional support in cardiac failure, *Surg Clin North Am* 61:635, 1981.

37. Heymsfield S et al: Respiratory, cardiovascular, and metabolic effects of enteral hyperalimentation: influence of formula dose and composition, *Am J Clin Nutr* 40:116, 1984.

38. Hickman D et al: Serum albumin and body weight as predictors of postoperative course in colorectal cancer, *J Parenteral Enteral Nutr* 4:314, 1980.

39. Hwang T, O'Dwyer S, Smith R, Wilmore D: Preservation of the small bowel mucosa using glutamine enriched parenteral nutrition, *Surg Forum* 37:56, 1986.

40. Jacobs D et al: Trophic effects of glutamine-enriched parenteral nutrition on colonic mucosa, *J Parenteral Enteral Nutr* 12:6, 1988.

41. Jarrett F et al: Clinical experience with prophylatic antibiotic bowel suppression in burn patients, *Surgery* 83:523, 1978.

42. Johnson L et al: Structural and hormonal alterations in the gastrointestinal tract of parenterally fed rats, *Gastroenterology* 68:1177, 1975.

43. Kaminski M et al: Correlation of mortality with serum transferrin and anergy, *J Parenteral Enteral Nutr* 1:27, 1977.

44. Klahr S, Purkeson M: Effects of dietary proteins on renal function and on the progression of renal disease, *Am J Clin Nutr* 47:146, 1988.

45. Latifi R, Killam R, Dudrick S: Nutritional support in liver failure, *Surg Clin North Am* 71:567, 1991.

46. Lee W, Packer M: Prognostic importance of serum sodium concentration and its modification by converting-enzyme inhibition in patients with severe chronic heart failure, *Circulation* 73:257, 1986.

47. Leonard C, Luke R, Siegel R: Parenteral essential amino acids in acute renal failure, *Urology* 6:154, 1975.

48. Levine G et al: Role of oral intake in maintenance of gut mass and disaccharidase activity, *Gastroenterology* 67:975, 1974.

49. Maki D, Weise C, Sarafin H: A semiquantitative culture method for identifying intravenous-catheter-related infection, *N Engl J Med* 296:1305, 1977.

50. Maynard A et al: Essential fatty acid deficiency with intravenous hyperalimentation, *Fed Proc* 31:717, 1972.

51. McLoughlin G et al: Correlation between anergy and a circulating immunosuppressive factor following major surgical trauma, *Ann Surg* 190:297, 1979.

52. Meakins J et al: Delayed hypersensitivity: indicator of acquired failure of host defenses in sepsis and trauma, *Ann Surg* 186:241, 1977.

53. Metropolitan Life Foundation: *Stat Bull Metrop Insur Co* 64:2, 1983.

54. Mitch W et al: Influence of insulin resistance and amino acid supply on muscle protein turnover in uremia, *Kidney Int* 32:510, 1987.

55. Moncrief J: Femoral catheters, *Ann Surg* 147:166, 1958.

56. Moore F et al: TEN versus TPN following major abdominal trauma: reduced septic morbidity, *J Trauma* 29:916, 1989.

57. Mullen J et al: Implications of malnutrition in the surgical patient, *Ann Surg* 114:121, 1979.

58. Mullen J et al: Prediction of operative morbidity and mortality by preoperative nutritional assessment, *Surg Forum* 30:80, 1979.

59. Nazari S et al: Cluster analysis of nutritional and immunological indicators for identification of high risk surgical patients, *J Parenteral Enteral Nutr* 5:307, 1981.

60. Neithercut W, Smith A, McAllister J, La Ferla G: Nutritional survey of patients in a general surgical ward: is there an effective predictor of malnutrition? *J Clin Pathol* 40:803, 1987.

61. Neumann C et al: Immunologic responses in malnourished children, *Am J Clin Nutr* 28:89, 1975.

62. Padberg F, Ruggiero J, Blackburn G, Bistrian B: Central venous catheterization for parenteral nutrition, *Ann Surg* 193:264, 1981.

63. Pemberton B, Lyman B, Lander V, Covinsky J: Sepsis from triple vs single lumen catheters during total parenteral nutrition in surgical or critically ill patients, *Arch Surg* 121:591, 1986.

64. Pettigrew R et al: Catheter-related sepsis in patients on intravenous nutrition: a prospective study of quantitative catheter cultures and guidewire changes for suspected sepsis, *Br J Surg* 72:52, 1985.

65. Pittman J, Cohen P: The pathogenesis of cardiac cachexia, *N Engl J Med* 271:403, 1964.

66. Pittman J, Cohen P: The pathogenesis of cardiac cachexia (concluded), *N Engl J Med* 271:453, 1964.

67. Ponsky J: Percutaneous endoscopic trauma, *Surg Clin North Am* 69:1227, 1989.

68. Ponsky J, Gauderer M, Stellato T, Ceszodi A: Percutaneous approaches to enteral alimentation, *Am J Surg* 149:102, 1985.

69. Reinhardt G et al: Incidence and mortality of hypoalbuminemic patients in hospitalized veterans, *J Parenteral Enteral Nutr* 4:357, 1980.

70. Rudman D et al: Elemental balances during intravenous hyperalimentation of underweight adult subjects, *J Clin Invest* 55:94, 1975.

71. Ryan J et al: Catheter complications in total parenteral nutrition, *N Engl J Med* 290:757, 1974.

72. Sanderson I, Deitel M: Intravenous hyperalimentation without sepsis, *Surg Gynecol Obstet* 136:577, 1973.

73. Seltzer M, Slocum B, Cataldi-Belcher E: Instant nutritional assessment: absolute weight loss and surgical mortality, *J Parenteral Enteral Nutr* 6:218, 1982.

74. Shetty P, Watrasiewicz K, Jung R, James W: Rapid-turnover transport proteins: an index of subclinical protein-energy malnutrition, *Lancet* 2:230, 1979.

75. Soop M et al: Energy expenditure in postoperative multiple organ failure with acute renal failure, *Clin Nephrol* 31:139, 1989.

76. Souba W, Scott T, Wilmore D: Intestinal consumption of intravenously administered fuels, *J Parenteral Enteral Nutr* 9:18, 1985.

77. Souba W, Smith R, Wilmore D: Effects of glucocorticoids on glutamine metabolism in visceral organs, *Metabolism* 34:450, 1985.

78. Souba W, Smith R, Wilmore D: Glutamine metabolism by the intestinal tract, *J Parenteral Enteral Nutr* 9:608, 1985.

79. Souba W, Wilmore D: Postoperative alterations of arteriovenous exchange of amino acids across the gastrointestinal tract, *Surgery* 94:342, 1983.

80. Steiner M, Bourges H, Freeman L, Grey S: Effect of starvation on the tissue composition of the intestine in the rat, *Am J Physiol* 215:75, 1969.

81. Studley H: Percentage of weight loss: a basic indicator of surgical risk in patients with chronic peptic ulcer, *JAMA* 106:458, 1936.

82. Studley H: Percentage of weight loss: a basic indicator of surgical risk in patients with chronic peptic ulcer, *JAMA* 106:458, 1935.

83. Toback F: Amino acid enhancement of renal regeneration after acute tubular necrosis, *Kidney Int* 12:193, 1977.

84. Tuten M et al: Utilization of prealbumin as a nutritional parameter, *J Parenteral Enteral Nutr* 9:709, 1985.

85. Veterans Affairs Total Parenteral Nutrition Cooperative Study Group: Perioperative total parenteral nutrition in surgical patients, *N Engl J Med* 325:525, 1991.

86. Wilmore J, Behnke A: An anthropometric estimation of body density and lean body weight in young women, *Am J Clin Nutr* 23:267, 1970.

87. Wilmore D et al: The gut: a central organ after surgical stress, *Surgery* 104:917, 1988.

88. Windmueller H: Glutamine utilization by the small intestine, *Adv Enzymol* 53:201, 1982.

89. Windmueller H, Spaeth A: Uptake and metabolism of plasma glutamine by the small intestine, *J Biol Chem* 249:5070, 1974.

90. Winterbauer R et al: Aspirated nasogastric feeding solution detected by glucose strips, *Ann Intern Med* 95:67, 1981.

12

Complications in Other Organ Systems

Alfred S. Casale *and* Susan Ullrich

Cardiac surgery with its attendant need for general anesthesia and cardiopulmonary bypass (CPB) (and usually hypothermia) can lead to dysfunction in any organ that has undergone perfusion through a variety of physical and biologic mechanisms (Table 12-1). Hypoxia, altered formed blood elements, disordered coagulation, microemboli of particulate matter or air, and vasoactive inflammatory mediators have all been implicated in organ injury after CPB. Global hypoperfusion during cardiopulmonary bypass can lead to multiple organ system dysfunction. Regional flow and pressure relationships are also affected by CPB, and hypoperfusion injury to individual organs can be seen. Intraoperative mechanical catastrophes such as aortic dissection, atheroembolism, or embolism of preformed thrombus can lead to obstructive hypoperfusion in any organ.

This chapter treats the more common manifestations of injury involving the neurologic, gastrointestinal, and renal systems.

Neurologic Dysfunction

Central and peripheral neurologic, and neuropsychologic, complications occur after open heart surgery. Stroke, a neurologic deficit lasting more than 24 hours and confirmed by computed tomographic scan, can be a devastating consequence of cardiac surgery and is usually related to hypoperfusion or embolic events. It is generally evident once the effects of anesthesia have dissipated

Table 12-1   Mechanisms of Organ System Injury
in Cardiac Surgery

Physical causes	Biologic causes
Hypoperfusion	Hypoxia
Inadequate CPB flow	Hematologic
Inadequate CPB pressure	Formed blood elements
Obstructed regional flow	Coagulation systems
Cannula placement	Immunologic phenomena
Arterial dissection	Inflammation
Embolus (microembolus	Drug effects
or macroembolus)	
Atheroma	
Air	
Particulate debris	
Thrombus	
Fat/marrow	
Hypothermia	

and can be characterized by focal motor and/or sensory defects, by cognitive or attention defects, or combined abnormalities. Occasionally massive brain trauma results in frank coma and a very poor prognosis.[4] Although most strokes occur intraoperatively, they can occur suddenly at any time in the early postoperative period. In a 7-year review of patients undergoing isolated coronary artery bypass grafting, there was a strong relationship between age and the incidence of stroke (Fig. 12-1). Other reported risk factors include previous stroke, carotid bruits, previous carotid endarterectomy, diabetes, and hypertension.

Neurologic consultation is appropriate to define the nature of the abnormality and to establish a baseline with which to compare changes. Computed tomographic scanning or magnetic resonance imaging is usually performed but rarely needs to be done emergently. Lumbar punctures are rarely done. Electroencephalograms can be useful to differentiate diffuse metabolic abnormalities from more focal structural lesions.

Prognosis for improvement is variable and depends on age, the degree of initial impairment, mechanism of injury, and area of brain involved. Expert neurologic advice is useful in determining prognosis. Vigorous physical and rehabilitation therapy optimizes recovery. In the short term we customarily employ hyperventilation

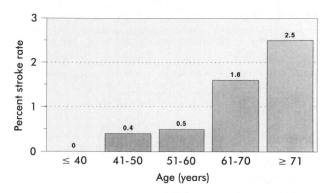

Fig. 12-1 Relationship of age to incidence of stroke after coronary artery bypass grafting *(CABG)*.

and at times bolus steroids administered intravenously but admit that no strong evidence exists of the efficacy in decreasing brain edema or in mitigating neurologic complications.

Transient deficits in cognitive abilities and/or alterations in mood occur almost uniformly after cardiac surgery. Subtle cognitive changes can persist for months, especially in computational ability. Nevertheless, most resolve completely. These changes are generally thought to be caused by CPB, because patients undergoing operations of similar magnitude but not requiring CPB have far fewer noted defects.[5]

Seizures can occur as a consequence of structural brain injury or of metabolic encephalopathic processes. Benzodiazepines, phenytoin, and phenobarbital are used to stop the acute seizure activity. Dosing is very patient specific and usually recommended by the neurologist. An aggressive search must be made for metabolic derangements that might be contributing to the seizures. An electroencephalogram is important in this setting, and neurologic consultation is in order.

Peripheral nerve injury occurs as a consequence of direct physical trauma to neural structures. The lower roots of the brachial plexus can be injured by a combination of stretch and compressive forces generated by the clavicle and highest ribs. This usually is a result of the sternotomy retractor being positioned high and opened widely.[6] The motor and sensory changes in the arms that result usually resolve in several months but in the meantime can be frustrating and distracting. Occasionally they persist as long-term problems. The most common complaint is numbness on the palmar aspect of the fourth and fifth fingers (ulnar n.)

Pressure injuries to the nerves of the hands and arms result from positioning on the operating table. Phrenic nerve injuries can occur as a result of direct injury during mobilization of the internal mammary artery, during division of the pericardium to allow positioning of the internal mammary artery, or from cold injury to the nerves by topical cooling solutions or ice. These injuries result in diaphragmatic weakness or paralysis and may lead to severe respiratory compromise. The prognosis for these problems depends on the mechanism of injury. Cold injury usually results in transient (<6 months) paralysis or weakness.

Gastrointestinal Dysfunction

Perioperative dysfunction of all organs of the gastrointestinal (GI) tract has been reported. Anesthetic drugs and analgesics can cause mild self-limited ileus and nausea. Persantine is another common offending agent. Discontinuance of all nonessential drugs, restriction of oral intake, intravenous (IV) administration of fluids, and ambulation usually lead to prompt resolution. If significant distention, pain, or signs of peritoneal irritation occur, gastric decompression and aggressive evaluation for surgical problems are mandatory. Total parenteral nutrition is initiated early. If an operation is required, a feeding jejunostomy and/or a gastrostomy are performed.

Gastroduodenal bleeding from either erosive mucosal lesions or from frank ulceration is the most common serious GI complication of open heart surgery.[2] It typically occurs in patients with a previous history of peptic disease. Elderly patients with perioperative hypotension, low cardiac output, or significant pressor requirements are especially susceptible. Aspirin, dipyridamole, warfarin, and heparin are often implicated in the pathogenesis of GI bleeding. As with all patients with an upper GI hemorrhage, nasogastric tube placement and lavage of the stomach are necessary, and prompt esophagogastroduodenoscopy with appropriate endoscopic therapy should be promptly undertaken. Prophylactic H_2 blockade is used with increasing frequency, as are antacids and cytoprotective agents like sucralfate. H_2-blockers include cimetidine hydrochloride, 300 mg IV every 6 to 8 hours, or ranitidine hydrochloride, 50 mg IV every 6 to 8 hours. Because of some of the cardiac effects reported in the literature with cimetidine hydrochloride, specifically hypotension and dysrhythmia, ranitidine hydrochloride is the drug used routinely in our institution. Operative intervention for upper GI bleeding is associated with a high mortality rate.

Mesenteric ischemia is a grave GI complication of open heart surgery and is usually caused by hypoperfusion, caused either by poor cardiac output or embolic obstruction of major abdominal arteries. Signs are often subtle, and these critically ill patients may be too ill to offer specific complaints. Vigilance and consideration of bowel ischemia in unstable patients with acidosis is important if early recognition of these complications is to occur. If an arterial blood gas determination demonstrates acidosis, a serum lactate determination may be beneficial in further assessment. If all diagnostic measures fail and the diagnosis is still not ruled out, abdominal exploration may be undertaken in the hope of finding a correctable problem such as necrotic bowel. We have from time to time, as an alternative to formal laparotomy, performed diagnostic peritoneal lavage and/or laparoscopy.

Cholecystitis, especially in its acalculous form, occurs after open heart surgery and requires prompt operative treatment. Antibiotics alone are rarely sufficient, and although these patients have a variety of atypical complaints, physical examination is usually unequivocal.

Mild elevations of hepatic enzymes are common after CPB and are usually innocuous. Severe hepatocellular injury reflected by massive increases of liver enzyme levels is usually a consequence of global hypoperfusion and hypoxia and carries a poor prognosis. Supportive measures with optimization of hemodynamics, avoidance of hepatotoxic agents, and adjustment of drug doses for hepatically metabolized agents are essential.

Diarrhea is usually related to either antibiotic-associated colitis or to quinidine therapy. Analysis of stool for *Clostridium difficile* toxins and appropriate antibiotic therapy should be initiated promptly. Rarely colitis can become fulminant and life threatening, and operative treatment is required to save these patients.

Frank symptomatic pancreatitis is uncommon after CPB, but elevations in serum amylase and lipase levels are frequently seen.[3] Conservative management, including limited oral intake and supportive care, and discontinuance of thiazide and other diuretics are all that is usually required for prompt resolution of symptoms and biochemical abnormalities.

Renal Dysfunction

Although mild alterations in glomerular filtration rate, as reflected in urine outputs of 0.5 to 1 ml/kg/hr, and mild elevation in serum creatinine level (1.5 to 2.0 mg/dl) can occur in as many as 30% of patients after CPB, severe oliguric acute renal dysfunction occurs in only about 1% to 2% of patients. Nevertheless, because the morbidity and mortality rates associated with acute renal failure may approach 50%, especially if sepsis complicates severe oliguric dysfunction, prevention of acute renal failure and aggressive management if it does occur, are very important.[1]

Any decrease in urine output to less than 0.5 ml/kg/hr and/or elevation in serum creatinine level should be evaluated by assessment of the hemodynamic state (usually with a pulmonary artery catheter and thermodilution cardiac output measurements), and by measurement of plasma and urine electrolytes and osmolality. It is often useful to subdivide acute renal failure into three classes, depending on daily production of urine. Anuric renal failure is defined as a production of less than 100 ml of urine per day. Patients with oliguric renal failure produce less than 400 ml of urine per day, and patients are considered nonoliguric if they produce more than 400 ml of urine per day. Five potential mechanisms for acute deterioration in renal function can be identified (Table 12-2).

Prerenal Azotemia

Prerenal azotemia can be defined as an alteration in renal function resulting from hypoperfusion of the kidneys without the development of renal parenchymal changes. This pathophysiologic state usually reverses rapidly on restoration of effective perfusion of the

Table 12-2 Mechanisms in Perioperative Renal Dysfunction

Prerenal azotemia (includes acute renovascular obstruction)
Acute tubular necrosis
Acute interstitial nephritis
Acute glomerulonephritis
Obstructive uropathy

kidneys. A prerenal state is characterized by a relatively benign appearing urinalysis, elevation of blood urea nitrogen (BUN) out of proportion to the elevation in serum creatinine (ratio >10:1), relatively low urine sodium levels (usually <20 mEq/L), and urine osmolality usually greater than 500 mOsm/L, suggesting preservation of renal parenchymal function (Table 12-3). The low urine output seen in prerenal azotemia is usually caused by decreased cardiac output or decreased intravascular volume. Intraoperatively it can be a consequence of low CPB flow rates or the use of potent arterial vasoconstrictors in large doses. Regardless of cause, hypoperfusion leads to nephron ischemia and decreased cortical blood flow, resulting in decrements in urine output and in excretory and filtration function. These effects can be worsened by nonsteroidal antiinflammatory drugs and adrenocortical extract inhibitors.

Acute obstruction of the renal arterial inflow to, or renal venous outflow from, a single functioning kidney, or bilateral vascular catastrophes affecting two kidneys, results in what can be seen as a specific type of prerenal azotemia. This hypoperfusion rapidly leads to irreversible acute tubular necrosis and is caused by either thrombotic, embolic, or mechanical obstruction of the renal vasculature. Atheroemboli can "trash" the kidneys. A malpositioned intraaortic counterpulsation balloon can interfere mechanically with renal blood flow or dislodge atheromatous debris. Dissection of the abdominal aorta can also lead to renal hypoperfusion.

Acute Tubular Necrosis

Acute tubular necrosis (ATN) is a consequence of an intrinsic structural abnormality in the kidneys, usually characterized by tubular cell damage from prolonged ischemia, hypoxia, or the presence of toxic agents. Together with prerenal azotemia, it accounts for 90% of perioperative acute renal dysfunction. The de-

Table 12-3   Differentiation of the Major Mechanisms of Renal Dysfunction

	Prerenal azotemia	Acute tubular necrosis
BUN/creatinine ratio	>10:1	<10:1
Urine sodium (mEq/L)	<20	>20-40
Urine osmolality (mOsm/L)	>500	~350*

*Equal to serum osmolality.

creased urine output and excretory abnormalities seen with ATN are not immediately reversible on restoration of renal blood flow or elimination of offending toxic agents. Toxins can include myoglobin, hemoglobin, various antibiotics and anesthetic agents, and IV contrast agents.

ATN is characterized by the findings of granular casts and tubular cells seen on microscopic examination of the urine. The BUN/creatinine ratio is usually less than 10:1, urine sodium concentration tends to be greater than 20 to 40 mEq/L, and serum osmolality is approximately equal to serum levels (approximately 350 mOsm/L).

Acute Glomerulonephritis

Acute glomerulonephritis is an uncommon cause of perioperative renal failure. It occurs when glomerular inflammation interferes with effective glomerular filtration. It can be seen in bacterial endocarditis and is difficult to manage. Renal consultation is always required.

Acute Interstitial Nephritis

Acute interstitial inflammation of the renal parenchyma can occur as a consequence of antibiotics, nonsteroidal antiinflammatory drugs, diuretics, or cimetidine. It is usually characterized by rash, fever, and the finding of eosinophils in blood and urine.

Obstructive Uropathy

Obstruction of urine drainage from either one functioning kidney or theoretically both kidneys, or obstruction of a Foley catheter, could lead to a postrenal form of acute renal failure. Ths is rare and generally easy to recognize when investigated. As an initial maneuver, the Foley catheter is irrigated. Renal ultrasonography can visualize the collecting system and rule out any obstruction.

Prophylaxis and Treatment

Obviously it is better to avoid renal failure than to treat it. Maintenance of normal or slightly elevated cardiac output minimizes acute renal failure unless this hemodynamic state is achieved with high doses of vasoconstricting pressor agents with their tendency to decrease renal blood flow. Nephrotoxic drugs should be avoided when possible.

We commonly administer diuretics and mannitol during CPB and in the immediate perioperative period to maintain a brisk urine output (>1 ml/kg/hr). Although this may not prevent the development of acute renal failure, it certainly seems to prevent oliguria and thus makes management of renal dysfunction, if it develops, much easier. Furosemide administration potentially leads to renal vasodilation and decreased oxygen consumption in the renal parenchyma, and the intratubular flow augmentation it creates can provide a salutary flushing of debris. Furosemide may, however, increase the risk of acute renal failure in patients concomitantly receiving aminoglycosides. Furosemide is administered in increasing doses (20 to 80 mg IV). If there is no response, bumetanide (5 to 10 mg IV) is given alone or as a constant infusion (2 mg/ cc to run at 1 to 5 mg/hr) or with chlorothiazide (250 to 500 mg IV in one or two doses daily) to initiate a diuresis. Dopamine at doses of 1 to 3 μg/kg/min increases renal blood flow and may be synergistic with diuretics in maintaining renal function.

If, despite these prophylactic measures, urine output remains low and serum BUN and creatinine levels continue to increase, we focus efforts at maintenance of fluid and electrolyte balance, minimize volume administration, and frequently check serum electrolytes. If severe oliguria or anuria occur, we discontinue use of the Foley catheter and catheterize the bladder twice a day. Urine cultures are also prepared.

A variety of support methods are now available to take over temporarily the excretory and filtration functions of the kidneys. Hemodialysis, peritoneal dialysis, intermittent or continuous ultrafiltration, and continuous arteriovenous hemodialysis can be used. We find peritoneal dialysis rarely useful in perioperative cardiac surgery patients because of the respiratory dysfunction it leads to and because of the often uncertain status of the abdominal viscera.

Arteriovenous hemodialysis, hemofiltration, continuous venovenous ultrafiltration, hemofiltration, or hemodialysis (Fig. 12-2), and slow continuous arteriovenous ultrafiltration, hemofiltration, or hemodialysis (Fig. 12-3) provide the clinician with alternative modalities for patients who do not tolerate hemodialysis. The specific technique used is based on the patient's prior dialysis history, hemodynamic status, and ability to tolerate intravascular/extravascular fluid shifts. It may also depend on the meth-

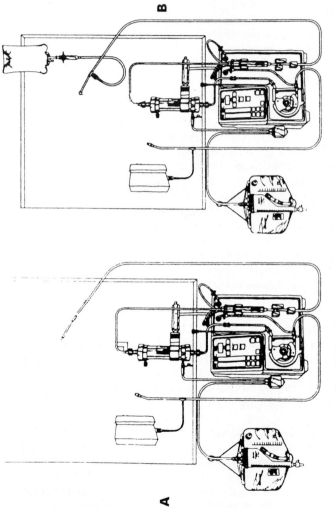

Fig. 12-2 A, CVV ultrafiltration. **B,** CVV hemofiltration.

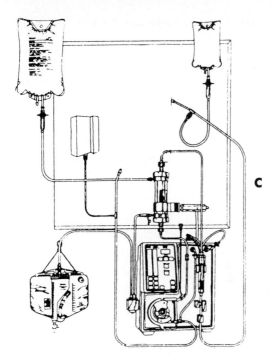

Fig. 12-2 *cont'd* C, CVV hemodialysis.

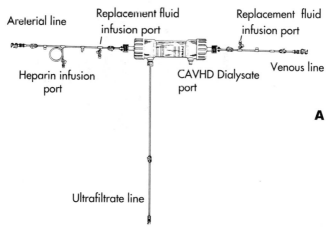

Fig. 12-3 A, Slow continuous arteriovenous ultrafiltration system *(SCUF).* *Continued.*

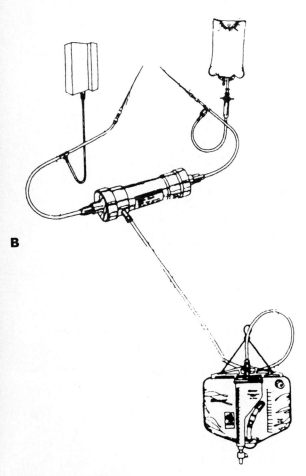

Fig. 12-3, *cont'd.* **B,** Continuous arteriovenous hemofiltration *(CAVH)* system.

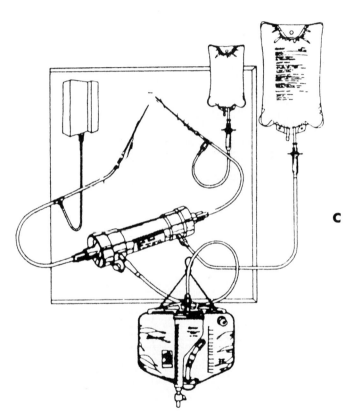

C

Fig. 12-3, *cont'd.* **C,** Continuous arteriovenous hemodialysis *(CAVHD)* system. (Courtesy of Mary Jo Holechek.)

ods available in the hospital and the experience of the nephrology staff. Continuous venovenous and arteriovenous methods are almost always limited to the intensive care unit (ICU) setting because of the frequent monitoring and documentation required (Figs. 12-4 and 12-5). Most frequently cannulas are placed in the subclavian vein for hemodialysis if the patient does not have an arteriovenous

```
GREENFIELD HEALTH SYSTEMS          MRN
CVVH/CVVH-D/CVVU TREATMENT PLAN
LOCATION-_____DATE -_____    NAME

DRS.ORDERS- PT/PTT FREQ._____    PATIENT ASSESSMENT-       TX DAY#_____
____D-20 ____D-30                   PRE-WEIGHT_____KGS     CPR STATUS_____
UF RATE-____ML/HR                   TEMP-_____(C)          VASOPRESSORS:
HEPARIN INFUSION RATE___UNITS/HR    BP-_____/_____
REPLACEMENT THERAPY_____
BLOOD FLOW RATE-_____ML/MIN.              signature-_____
```

					VEN	TOTAL	DIALYSATE	LOSS/	NET		CUM.	
TIME	BFR	AP	VP	ABD	LEVEL	OUTPUT	INFUSED	HOUR	LOSS	REPLC.	OUT	INITS

NOTES:_____

INITIALS	SIGNATURE

```
MACHINE PRECHECKS-

NO._____
MACHINE SELF TEST- PASS/FAIL
TREATMENT MODE-_____
VENOUS LINE IN DETECTOR-_____
VENOUS LINE IN CLAMP-_____
ALARM PARAMETERS AT 100mmHg-_____
ABD ARMED_____
SIGNATURE-_____
```

Fig. 12-4 Documentation flow record for continuous venovenous ultrafiltration *(CVVU)*, hemofiltration *(CVVH)*, and hemodialysis *(CVVHD)*.

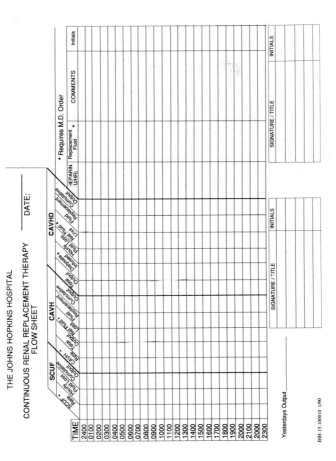

Fig. 12-5 Documentation flow record for slow continuous arteriovenous ultrafiltration (*SCUF*), hemofiltration (*CAVH*), and hemodialysis (*CAVHD*).

shunt from previous dialysis. If the subclavian vein cannot be used, cannulas may be placed in the femoral region. Continuous venovenous and arteriovenous catheters are usually placed femorally because the area is easily accessible and the cannulas are temporary. Nursing and physician personnel should be educated for each of the methods used in setup, maintenance, and troubleshooting. A resource person should be available to assist with troubleshooting the device. If patients are moved from the ICU for testing, it is recommended that the method be discontinued and the catheters flushed with a heparin solution (e.g., 1:1000) to maintain patency. The method may be restarted again when the patient has returned to the ICU.

Indications for dialysis include fluid overload that compromises the patient's pulmonary function, severe metabolic acidosis, hyperkalemia (K^+ >5.5 mEq/L), and uremic syndrome (e.g., altered mental status, asterixis, vomiting). Elevations of serum BUN to more than 100 mg/dl or of serum creatinine level to more than 10 mg/dl often lead to platelet dysfunction and can in and of themselves be indications for dialysis.

References

1. Abel RM, Buckley MJ, Austen WG, et al: Etiology, incidence, and prognosis of renal failure following cardiac operations: results of a prospective analysis of 500 consecutive patients, *J Thorac Cardiovasc Surg* 71(3):323–33, 1976.
2. Krasna MJ, Flancbaum L, Trooskin SZ, et al: Gastrointestinal complications after cardiac surgery, *Surgery* 104(4):773–80, 1988.
3. Leitman IM, Paull DE, Barie PS, et al: Intra-abdominal complications of cardiopulmonary bypass operations, *Surg Gynecol Obstet* 165(3):251–4, 1987.
4. Levy DE, Knill-Jones RP, Plum F: The vegetative state and its prognosis following nontraumatic coma, *Ann N Y Acad Sci* 315:293–306, 1978.
5. Shaw PJ, Bates D, Cartlidge NE, et al: Neurologic and neuropyschological morbidity following major surgery: comparison of coronary artery bypass and peripheral vascular surgery, *Stroke* 18(4):700–7, 1987.
6. Vander Salm TJ, Cereda JM, Cutler BS: Brachial plexus injury following median sternotomy, *J Thorac Cardiovasc Surg* 80(3):447–52, 1980.

Special Care Issues

13

Mary Lohmann-Edwards, Helen O. Michalisko, and Sharon G. Owens

The approach to the cardiac surgical patient during the perioperative period is multidisciplinary and goes far beyond the specific operation. As described in Chapter 1, during the patient's hospital stay a considerable number of issues involving physicians, nurses, and social workers, and the coordination of care among these disciplines, must be addressed for the optimal wellness of the patient and his or her family or significant other.

This chapter addresses the special care issues that are often overlooked in dealing with the critically ill patient but are nonetheless as important as respiratory and hemodynamic management. The responsibilities for the routine skin care of the patient, which incorporate the care of the surgical wounds and the normal wound healing process, are initially described. The management and restorative care of the breakdown of skin integrity caused by infection, ischemia, or decreased mobility during the perioperative period are then addressed.

Because of the nature of the median sternotomy approach and the harvesting of the saphenous veins, drains are used to facilitate the evacuation of irrigation fluid and blood. The types of drains and indications for use are discussed.

Finally, the psychosocial aspects of patient care, as importnat to patient healing and total wellness as any physical care given by the health care professional, are discussed. We discuss this focus of care as it relates to the social worker, family, and community and how each relates to the other and to the total care of the patient.

287

Skin Integrity

Wounds

Most surgical wounds, including those acquired during coronary artery bypass grafting, prosthetic valve replacement, and heart transplant operations, heal in a similar way, modified by a person's specific disease status. The human body's innate tendency to restore unhealthy tissue to its prewound condition is routinely expected in the otherwise healthy person with an intact immune system. Current patients, however, are older, are often hospitalized for several days before the operation, and have other disorders. These states often compromise the patient's ability to heal adequately. The hospitalized patient should therefore be carefully prepared for the operation so that the healing properties of the human body are afforded every chance to function optimally.

Physiology of Wound Healing

Wound healing has been described in three distinct phases based on physical symptoms and duration[1a,4]:

- Inflammatory phase, lasting up to 5 days
- Proliferative phase, lasting from 5 to 20 days
- Maturation phase, lasting from 21 days to 2 years

Inflammatory phase

The first phase of normal wound healing begins with the traumatic injury itself, either surgical or accidental, and the almost immediate vasoconstriction caused by capillary damage to the vessels surrounding the wound site.[4] Almost immediately the same vessels dilate with the release of histamine, prostaglandins, and complement.[1a,4,18] This vasodilation of the arterioles, venules, and capillaries expedites healing and results in the characteristic inflammatory response. The capillaries also become permeable, enabling water, plasma, and electrolytes to leak into the soft tissues; forming the inflammatory exudate; and causing edema.

Hematologic responses also play a primary role in the initial phase of normal wound healing. Platelets aggregate almost immediately to form a fibrin clot, a product of the conversion of fibrinogen.[18] As previously mentioned, the antibody response to the injury activates the complement system, which in turn attracts neutrophils.[18] The neutrophil count should be monitored closely during the postoperative course. The normal percentage of neutrophils to the total white blood cell count is 60% to 70%. However, if infection is present, immature neutrophils or bands proliferate at the wound site through chemotaxis.[1a] The neutrophils continue the inflammatory process by phagocytizing bacteria; therefore where a proportionate increase of neutrophils to the white blood cell count is present, one should be highly suspicious of wound infection and appropriate action should be taken by the team to identify the bacterial source and treat accordingly.

Proliferative phase

This second stage of normal wound healing is also referred to as the fibroblastic or connective tissue phase.[1a] The cells that dominate this phase are the fibroblasts, which produce collagen strands to initiate the groundwork for wound closure. Epithelialization of the wound takes place at this time. The horizontal process usually ends when the epithelial sheet of one edge of the wound meets the epithelial sheet of the other edge. Horizontal migration of epithelial cells continue until they completely fill the epidermal layer.[1]

Maturation phase

The final stage of normal wound healing is also known as the remodeling phase.[1a,4] This stage includes a dramatic decrease in vascularity of the scar, shrinking of the fibroblasts, and reorientation of the collagen network.[18] During this stage the wound gains strength and the person can return to normal activities of daily living. It should be noted, however, that only 50% of the wound's tactile strength is regained within the first 6 weeks.[18]

Median Sternotomy or Thoracotomy Incision

Preoperative preparation and care are discussed in Chapter 3.

Postoperatively the occlusive surgical dressing should be left intact for 18 to 24 hours after the operation and reinforced if saturated. When the operative dressing is removed, a dry, sterile dressing should replace it for another 24 hours. If the patient is extubated, the wound may be left open to air on postoperative day 2 as long as no sign of drainage is present. Any excessive drainage should be reported. If the patient is still intubated or if the patient has a tracheostomy, a dry, sterile dressing should cover the incision to prevent contamination with secretions. This dressing should be changed every 24 hours.

Saphenous Vein Procurement Incisions

Preoperative care

As in the case of the sternal wound, preoperative care begins the night before surgery (see Chapter 3).

Postoperative care

On the patient's return to the intensive care unit (ICU), the vascular status of the operative leg should be assessed. If a woven elastic bandage or antithromboembolic stocking has been placed in the operating room *(OR)* it should be removed and reapplied. If no vascular compromise is evident, the elastic bandage should be taken off and rewrapped 6 to 8 hours postoperatively, and the dressings assessed for excessive drainage and reinforced if necessary. The leg or legs are then rewrapped in elastic bandages.

On the first postoperative day the elastic bandages should be removed. The incision sites should be covered with a dry, sterile occlusive dressing and remain in place for a minimum of 24 hours.[3] On the second postoperative day, if there is no drainage, the graft sites may be left open to air. Further drainage from the graft site at this time should be evaluated, however, and a dry, sterile occlusive dressing should remain on the wound if drainage persists.

Other Care Sites

Chest tube sites

The chest tube dressing applied in the OR should be removed or changed on the first postoperative day. After the physician removes the chest tubes, the sites should be covered with petroleum jelly–coated gauze. An occlusive sterile dressing should be changed every 24 hours until the sutures are removed. The sites are then left open to air. As always, the chest tube sites must be assessed every 24 hours for signs of infection.

Pacing wire sites

Temporary pacing wires, placed in the patient during the operative procedure, remain in place until immediately prior to discharge. During this time the pacing wire sites should be cared for by application of a dry, sterile dressing every 24 hours.

Catheterization sites

If the patient was catheterized shortly before the operation, the catheterization site should be covered with a sterile dressing on admission to the ICU. The site must be assessed every shift for bleeding or hematoma formation. On postoperative day 2 the site should be left open to air if no bleeding or drainage is present.

Intraaortic balloon pump site

When an intraaortic balloon pump catheter is inserted in the OR or the ICU, it is essential that the insertion site be routinely monitored for bleeding and infection while the catheter is in place and after it is removed. After removal of the catheter, the site should be monitored for possible hematoma formation.

An occlusive sterile dressing is placed on the catheter site in the OR or in the ICU and should be changed every 24 hours while the balloon catheter is in place and after its removal.

Factors Affecting Wound Healing

The presence of age, nutritional state, diabetes mellitus, use of steroids, and obesity are risk factors that can affect wound healing in the postoperative period.[1a,4,6,18]

Age

The patient more than 65 years of age may have wound healing difficulties for various reasons, including dehydration or a poorly functioning immune system.[1a] Because a majority of patients undergoing cardiac surgery are more than 60 years of age, caregivers should expect to see these factors frequently.

Nutritional state

Malnutrition is a common problem in the cardiac surgical population. In a 1977 study Hill and colleagues confirmed previous studies regarding malnutrition of hospitalized patients, which indicated that approximately 35% of the hospital patient population showed evidence of nutritional depletion.[15] Depending on the severity and length of the cardiac illness, many of these patients may have been unable to take in an adequate amount of calories and nutrients. Because malnutrition is often associated with poor wound healing and increased risk of infection, a nutritional consultation should be obtained as soon as these patients are identified. Assessment should include determination of:

- Ideal body weight
- Creatinine clearance role
- Total protein

- Serum albumin
- Iron and transferrin levels
- Total lymphocyte count

Once the results have been correlated, the health care team should take immediate corrective action, usually in the form of high-calorie, protein- and fat-balanced hyperalimentation.

Diabetes

The diabetic patient is twice as likely to have poor wound healing and postoperative infection as a patient without a systemic illness.[4] Those with chronic disease and vascular compromise are at greatest risk. Because of the diabetic patient's limited wound-healing capacity, it is advisable to have the patient's serum glucose level controlled before surgery. Postoperative control of diabetes can be managed by an insulin sliding scale, continuous intravenous insulin administration, and serum glucose tests every 4 hours.

Use of steroids

Steroid use can alter normal wound healing, inhibiting the inflammatory response as a result of a reduction in the migration of macrophages and neutrophils.

Obesity

Excess adipose tissue surrounding the surgical wound contains decreased vasculature, which limits the transport of oxygen and reparative nutrients to the wound site.[11]

Wound approximation in overweight patients can be difficult to achieve in the OR and to maintain in the postoperative period. Skin closure is usually accomplished with staples. The female patient who is obese or who has pendulous breasts is issued a mammary support, which should be worn throughout the postoperative period to avoid wound dehiscence. A sterile gauze dressing is often placed over the incision between the breasts to reduce moisture accumulation. This area of the skin incision should be checked frequently because it is the site most prone to breakdown.

Postoperative Complications

Mediastinitis

Despite the precautions taken by the health care team throughout the perioperative period, the rare case of mediastinitis still occurs. Incidence of mediastinitis has been reported to be between 1% and 2%.[13,16] Patients with mediastinitis are known to have increased rates of morbidity and mortality, and increased hospital costs.[6,7] The mediastinum is the area located in the center of the thorax. It encompasses the heart, great vessels, and esophagus. It is bound anteriorly by the sternum, posteriorly by the vertebral column, and laterally by the pleura.[6] The mediastinum is virtually avascular in that the major vessels pass through it but do not supply the area.[16]

Risk factors

Risk factors that have been associated with the development of mediastinitis include:
- Patient factors (diabetes, obesity)
- Postoperative hemorrhage
- Prolonged cardiopulmonary bypass and operative time
- External cardiac massage
- Harvesting of bilateral mammary arteries
- Low cardiac output
- Tracheostomy or prolonged artificial ventilation[5,8,13,14,16]

Nursing considerations

Early recognition of signs of infection during assessment of the patient can significantly reduce patient morbidity. Prevention of infection is an important consideration in the care of the patient. Emphasis should be placed on handwashing between caring for different patients, sterile technique during dressing changes, adequate nutritional support, and emotional support.

The patient's ability to heal and fight infection is directly related to his or her nutritional state.[12] Because high-calorie, high-protein diets are required to deliver the additional nutrition required by the infected patient, an early consultation with the nutritional support service is advisable.

Postoperative infection often significantly increases length of stay in the ICU and overall hospitalization. Patients may require additional emotional support and attention to financial situations. Body image is occasionally altered if reconstructive surgery is necessary, and the patient should be allowed to ventilate feelings of concern and anger regarding the additional surgery. Consultation with the social worker is occasionally recommended for these patients.

If postoperative hemorrhage occurs and subsequently a mediastinal hematoma develops, the risk of mediastinitis is increased.[14] Prolonged cardiopulmonary bypass and operative time increases the patient's potential exposure to contaminants.

External cardiac massage has been reported to be associated with sternal wound complications. Sternal approximation can be disrupted during compressions, potentially allowing bacteria to enter the sternal wound. Although the infection generally begins in the mediastinum, cardiopulmonary resuscitation can result in this complication.[6]

Conflicting reports linking increased infection with the use of a single mammary artery have appeared in the literature. The use of bilateral mammary arteries, especially in the diabetic patient, is associated with an increase in sternal wound complications. The internal mammary artery is the major source of vascular supply to the sternum. More complicated dissections leading to extended operative time, and its use for grafting, would decrease the major blood supply to the medistinal area and hinder wound healing.[14]

Patients with a low cardiac output during the postoperative period run a higher risk of mediastinitis.[13,14,17] These patients are usually more ill and require longer ICU stays, which are also associated with a higher incidence of infection.

If the patient requires long-term ventilatory support or a tracheostomy during hospitalization, the risk of mediastinitis is increased. The proximity of the sternal wound and the tracheostomy wound allows for entry of bacteria into the mediastinal space.[14] Frequent endotracheal suctioning with potential spillage adds to the risk of sternal infection. As mentioned previously, an occlusive dressing should be applied to the sternal wound until the epidermis is sealed.

Diagnosis

Mediastinitis can develop as early as 3 days after the surgical procedure and as late as 60 days postoperatively.[14,16] The nurse and physician should be alert to excessive incisional pain during this period. Any drainage from the incision during this time, regardless of its characteristics, should warrant further evaluation.

An unstable sternum may be associated with mediastinitis. Its presence should increase the awareness of the health care team. The nurse or physician may test for an unstable sternum by holding a hand over the sternum and asking the patient to cough. Any clicking or movement of the sternum is evidence of instability requiring further observation. An unstable sternum may simply require rewiring; however, laboratory results must be reviewed to determine more serious developments.[14]

Mediastinitis is sometimes difficult to diagnose. The following symptoms and signs may be associated with sternal wound problems:

- Chest pain
- Fever
- Leukocytosis
- Sternal click
- Erythema and/or tenderness
- Drainage

The presence of a fever and elevated temperature is variable. A temperature of 38.5° C 3 to 4 days after operation should heighten awareness. The occurrence of increasing sternal pain seems to be a reliable predictor of infection.

A definitive diagnosis of mediastinitis must be made by positive cultures and gram stains of drainage from the mediastinum. Needle aspiration may be required. The two approaches recommended include the subxiphoid and retrosternal technique.[14] The latter technique requires ultrasound guidance.

Chest x-ray films and computerized axial tomographic scans may be used in determining the extent of the infection.[6]

Treatment

Once the diagnosis of mediastinitis is made, treatment should be initiated immediately. Antibiotic therapy consisting usually of vancomycin is begun. Consultation with the plastic surgeon is also usually made at this time and a method of approach is determined.

If reexploration is necessary, the cardiac surgeon and the plastic surgeon work together to perform the necessary operations. The cardiac team inspects the mediastinum, debrides the necrotic tissue, and drains any purulent fluid.[6] The mediastinum is then irrigated with diluted antibiotic (cefamandol) solution. Muscle interposition flaps (pectoralis, rectus, latissimus dorsi) are then used to close the wound.[6,9]

Because of its size and vascularity, the pectoralis major muscle frequently is used to obliterate the mediastinal cavity. The muscle is stretched and approximated to the sternum.[6,9]

The rectus abdominus muscle is used if a significant portion of the lower sternum is involved; however, if the internal mammary artery was used for revascularization during the initial surgery, the corresponding rectus abdominus cannot be used, because the internal mammary artery is the main blood supply for this muscle.[6,9,10] If both internal mammary arteries have been used, alternative methods of closure should be discussed with the plastic surgeon.

If infection is extensive, a primary closure may not be made and the wound is left open and packed with povidine-iodine–soaked gauze.[6] Closure is delayed until all signs of infection are no longer evident. The patient is then returned to the OR and closure is performed. Because it requires the patient's return to the OR, delayed closure is not the treatment of choice. Every effort should be made to close the wound after initial debridement and drainage of the mediastinum. Antibiotic therapy is continued postoperatively until all drains are removed. Choice of antibiotics is determined by culture obtained at time of operation and by subsequent sensitivity results.

Pressure ulcers

All patients undergoing cardiac surgery are at risk for pressure ulcers. It has been reported that in 17% to 20% of hospitalized patients in the United States some stage of a pressure ulcer develops.[1] All patients should be carefully assessed according to a standard protocol throughout the hospital stay for disruption of skin integrity and the development of pressure ulcers. Prophylactic interventions are used for all patients undergoing operations (see Chapter 3). Preoperative considerations include application of egg-crate foam mattress in the surgical ICU, arrangement for specialty bed if needed, and proper use of hypothermia blanket.

The ICU bed is prepared with an egg-crate foam mattress for relief of pressure in the immediate postoperative period. If the patient is already using a specialty bed or air mattress, arrangements are made for the patient to return to the same bed postoperatively. The hypothermia blanket is placed on top of the foam mattress and covered completely with a full-size bath blanket. This allows separation of the patient from direct contact with the hypothermia blanket. To minimize risk of skin breakdown, the hypothermia blanket should be removed from the bed as soon as the patient's temperature approaches 37° C.

Certain patients are at increased risk for this complication. The following factors have been associated with development of pressure ulcers after cardiac surgery:

- Immobility
- Malnutrition
- Diabetes
- Altered sensation
- Poor circulation
- Age greater than 65 years
- Altered mental status
- Obesity
- Edema
- History of pressure ulcers
- Chronic disease
- Paralysis
- External devices such as restraints

The nurse should assess all patients on admission and throughout the hospital stay, especially those with any risk factors. Preoperative and ICU admission assessment identifies these factors. A Pressure Sore Risk Assessment Sheet is then completed by the nurse as a guideline for the patient's risk level and appropriate intervention (mattress and bed preparation).

The following skin care protocols used in the Johns Hopkins Cardiac Surgical ICU can be used when potential or actual skin care problems are identified. Pressure, friction, shear, moisture, and nutrition have been assessed as factors contributing to impaired skin integrity. Protocols have been designed to ensure early diagnosis and intervention. (Table 13-1).[1]

Drains

Chest Tubes

Postoperative drainage of the mediastinum is essential. The evacuation of blood and irrigation solution is necessary to prevent clot formation and fluid collection around the heart, which may cause life-threatening cardiac tamponade.

Prophylactic drainage of the mediastinum is accomplished generally by placement of a mediastinal tube and a pleural tube (the left side of the chest is usually opened with takedown of the internal mammary artery) before sternal closure. A Y-connector is used to connect both tubes to the chest drainage system. The system em-

Text continued on p. 302.

Table 13-1 Skin Care Protocols at Johns Hopkins Cardiac Surgical ICU

2.0 Nursing interventions regarding pressure and immobility
2.1 Mobility
   2.1.1 Request physician order for physical therapy consultation as needed
   2.1.2 Encourage maximum mobility
2.2 Positioning
   2.2.1 Ensure patient turns or shifts in bed every 2-4 hr
   2.2.2 Position pillows behind upper part of back and thighs (not buttocks), and between knees
   2.2.3 Ensure patient shifts in chair every 20 min-3 hr
2.3 Use pressure-relieving devices
   2.3.1 Mattress
      2.3.1.1 Egg-crate foam for moderate-risk patients
      2.3.1.2 Use of intermediate-level modality (e.g., Gaymar SofCare, Gaymar Industries, Inc, Orchard Park, NY) for high-risk patients and partial-thickness ulcers <8 cm^2
      2.3.1.3 Use of low-air-loss or air-fluidized bed for significant ulcers (approval of [ET] nurse required.
   2.3.2 Other
      2.3.2.1 Egg-crate foam in chair
      2.1.2.2 Pillows under calves or foam heel elevators (special order)
2.4 Massage areas of risk q shift and prn
3.0 Nursing interventions regarding friction and shear
3.1 Use means to facilitate mobility (e.g., draw sheet or trapeze)

3.2 Keep head of bed at or below 30° angle if possible, and reposition patient when necessary to raise higher (Note: Head of bed must be elevated at 45° if patient is receiving tube feedings)

3.3 Position in bed or chair to minimize sliding (e.g., knee gatch)

3.4 Use sheepskin pad under heels

3.5 Use cornstarch powder judiciously on skin in contact with metal or plastic surfaces (except on immunosuppressed patients)

4.0 Nursing interventions regarding moisture control

4.1 Incontinence management

4.1.1 Provide for elimination at frequent intervals

4.1.2 Institute measures to contain fecal and/or urinary incontinence (e.g., condom catheters, Foley catheters, fecal bags, diapers, and cloth underpads); minimize use of plastic pads (if used, avoid direct contact with skin)

4.2 Maintain clean dry skin

4.3 Apply products to protect skin integrity (e.g., protective barrier, film wipes, Pericare products)

4.4 Consider need for specialized bed providing aeration (e.g., air or fluidized air beds)

4.5 Request medical evaluation of incontinence

5.0 Nursing interventions regarding nutrition

5.1 Consider dietary consultation for calorie and protein assessment

5.2 Institute nursing measures to maximize patients' nutritional status (e.g., feeding patients, offering supplements and high-calorie beverages instead of water if appropriate)

5.3 Request physician order for multivitamin and vitamin C supplements

6.0 Management of impaired skin ulcer

Continued.

Table 13-1 Skin Care Protocols at Johns Hopkins Cardiac Surgical ICU—cont'd

Protection of intact but reddened skin (stage I ulcer) with any of following:

Product	Frequency of change	Indications for use
Moisture barrier ointment	q8 hr and prn	Excessive diaphoresis
Protective barrier film	q24 hr	Incontinence drainage under fecal bag area surrounding adhesive dressing
Hydrocolloid dressing	≤q4 days (discontinue if unable to adhere) ≥24 hr	Good tissue turgor
Film dressing	≤q5 days	Good tissue turgor outside sacral area

7.0 Wound care of partial-thickness ulcers or blisters (stage II)

7.0.1 Obtain MD order for RN/ET nurse to choose dressings per pressure ulcer protocol or to follow physician's orders.

Stage	Wound color	Dressing	Frequency of change	Cleansing	Indications
II	Red	Film	q3-4 days and prn for leakage	NSS	Minimal drainage Minimal leakage
		Hydrocolloid	q3 days and prn leakage or fever	NSS	Intact skin, limited friction, no diabetes or immunosuppression
		Topical antibiotic	q8 hr	NSS	Friable skin

II	Yellow	Film	q3 days and prn for leakage	NSS	Minimal drainage, minimal friction
		Hydrocolloid	q3 days and prn leakage or fever	If no red areas, may use ½ strength H_2O_2 and rinse with NSS	Intact skin
		Topical antibiotic	q8 hr		Friable skin, high infection risk
		Wet-to-dry gauze with NSS	q6-8 hr		Friable skin

7.1 Wound care of full-thickness ulcers (stages III and IV)
   7.1.1 Request physician order for plastic surgery consultation for stage IV ulcer
   7.1.2 Obtain specific physician orders for treatment
8.0 Teaching patient and family
8.1 Teach basic cause of patient's ulcer
8.2 Teach proper use of appropriate pressure relief product
8.3 Teach management of contributing conditions (e.g., incontinence, nutrition, positioning)
8.4 Teach wound care management

ET, Enterostomal therapist; *NSS,* normal saline solution; *prn,* as needed; *q,* every.

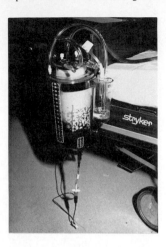

Fig. 13-1 Closed vacuum drainage system.

ployed at The Johns Hopkins Hospital uses the reservoir from cardiopulmonary bypass circuit (Fig. 13-1). This system allows for immediate postoperative autotransfusion of blood to the patient. These cardiotomy systems are placed on constant suction; suction is turned off only if ordered by the physician. If minimal drainage is anticipated or more precise measurement of drainage is required, a closed vacuum water suction system is used (Fig. 13-2). The usual level of water in the system is 20 cm.

Chest tubes and drains are usually removed on the first postoperative day if drainage is less than 50 ml for 4 consecutive hours.

The routine stripping of chest tubes has been found to be potentially hazardous, because stripping creates high negative pressures.[2] If there is a concern that clots are forming in the tubes, gentle milking is performed. Vigorous stripping of the tubes should be performed only if a sudden cessation of drainage from the tubes or large blood clots is observed in the tubing and at the connection site. Drainage canisters should be kept below the level of the patient to facilitate drainage.

Leg Drains

Areas of saphenous vein harvesting sites are sometimes drained to prevent hematoma formation. Small, self-contained suction

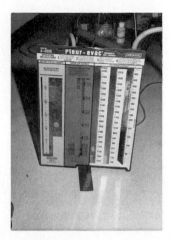

Fig. 13-2 Closed vacuum water suction.

drains are placed along the length of the wound (Fig. 13-3). If drainage is excessive, the physician should be notified, the wound inspected for specific bleeding sites, and corrective action taken. The small connecting tubes to the drain canister should be stripped frequently to assure patency. These drains are generally removed on the first postoperative day if drainage is minimal.

Psychosocial Considerations

With the ever-increasing advances being made in cardiac surgical procedures today and with an older, more complex population undergoing surgery, it becomes apparent that patient problems are increasing as well. It is vital for good patient care that a multi-disciplinary team approach be used in patient care. As a member of such a team, the social worker provides a unique perspective to both patients and families, resulting in a decreased length of stay and a increase in patient and family satisfaction with the health care process.

Given current guidelines on length of stay, patients and families should ideally be screened before admission for psychosocial problems. This allows for identification of issues related to emotional and physical response to surgery, the hospital stay, and discharge. Such issues include the following:

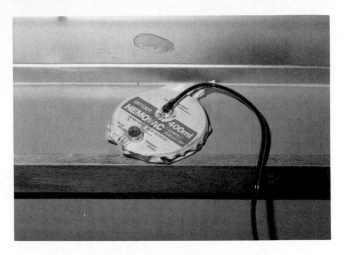

Fig. 13-3 Self-contained suction drain.

- Living alone; no caregiver available
- Immediate financial concerns
- Inadequate insurance coverage
- Lack of emotional support or coping mechanism
- Alcohol or drug dependency
- Patient who is a primary caregiver to an ill or disabled family member
- Inability to make decisions because of mental incapacity

With early problem identification the social worker can assist the patient and family in developing a plan to address these issues through interpersonal and community resources. Having some problem resolution preoperatively better enables the patient to cope with the rigors of surgery and hospitalization.

Some psychosocial problems may not be identified before admission but rather postoperatively. The members of the health care team quickly recognize indications such as:

- Aggression or agitation
- Alteration in mental status
- Repeated conferences with staff or family
- Self-reported inability to cope
- Inability to understand and make decisions

These are clues to the staff that the patient and family may have a need for immediate social work intervention. A complete assessment of patient and family needs enables formation of a plan to address current problems.

In the ICU the social worker's role is primarily that of a counselor, advocate, and resource person. With time constraints placed on the nursing staff caring for the critically ill patient, families may feel left out and confused. The worker can act as an liaison to help facilitate communication between staff and family, educate the family about the ICU experience, and assist with housing and financial needs. He or she can also assist the medical staff in understanding and accepting responses to crises that may be displayed by families; thus alleviating tension and possible conflict.

On occasion it is necessary to facilitate the transfer of a patient to another institution for either further acute care or long-term maintenance. The intubated critically ill patient has many medical and psychosocial problems requiring an understanding of possible transfer complications and the ability to organize a complex system. The social worker acts as coordinator and liaison between the medical staff and the receiving facility. A working knowledge of available air and ground transportation, equipment necessary for patient removal, and personnel necessary to provide care is essential. Careful consideration of associated costs and insurance must be considered before a move can be contemplated. Involvement of family and patients, if possible, extends to them some small degree of participation and control. Because of the anxiety such a move can evoke, close attention must be given to patients and families during this period to ensure that their emotional needs are met.

A standard of care for all patients undergoing cardiac surgery demands a complete analysis of the patients' discharge needs as they progress after surgery. The nursing staff, nutritionist, and physical and occupational therapists gain an understanding of the patient's needs and abilities. Multidisciplinary team conferences allow each group to provide this unique perspective on enhancing care and a successful transition to the community. Complete assessment of the patient's functional abilities allow the social worker to formulate a discharge plan that takes into consideration the patient's environment and available support. Issues such as respiratory needs, physical limitations, and knowledge about medications and dietary requirements can be successfully handled through family education and community agencies if identified early. The physical and occupational therapy teams often recommend environmental adaptations and equipment, enabling the patient to gain a higher degree of independence.

As the discharge planner, the social worker must consider all recommendations made by staff so a plan can be developed to address patient and family needs. With the process started early in the hospital stay, successful transition from hospital to community can be accomplished, resulting in an appropriate length of stay and decreased anxiety for patient and family. Given the frequent cutbacks, community resources may be limited. It is the charge of social work to keep abreast of changes in policy and service providers to ensure that the patient's needs are addressed in the community.

Unfortunately, occasional consequences from surgery result in an alteration in the normal pattern of recuperation. Wound infections and cardiovascular accidents can dramatically add days to the patient's hospital stay and further challenge the patient physically. Emotional responses to these sequelae such as anger and depression must be addressed while the patient's long-term physical needs are being planned. The social worker can be instrumental in providing support to the patient and family while also offering alternatives such as community support groups to help with adjustment.

Careful screening of patients' medical requirements results in the team's ability to plan for their successful return home. Home IV therapy, intravenous therapy, wound care, nursing, and physical and occupational therapy can be accomplished only after investigation of the community agencies' ability to handle such problems and the financial clearance of the patient's third-party payer. No discharge plan can be successful without interaction of all team members.

References

1. Allman R et al: Pressure sores among hospitalized patients, *Annals of Internal Medicine,* 105:337-342, 1986.
1a. Alterescu A, Cooper DM, Watt RC: *Guide to wound care,* 1983, Hollister.
2. Carroll P: The ins and outs of chest drainage systems, *Nursing '86* 16:26-33, 1986.

3. Culligan M et al: Preventing graft leg complications in CABG patients. *Nursing* '90 20:59-61, 1990.

4. David JA: *Wound care,* St Louis, 1986, Mosby.

5. Demmy TL et al: Recent experience with major sternal wound complications; *Ann Thorac Surg* 49:458-462, 1990.

6. Gallo J, Todd B: Mediastinitis after cardiac surgery, *Crit Care Nurs* 10:64-68, 1989.

7. Jeevanandam V et al: Single step management of sternal wound infections, *J Thorac Cardiovasc Surg*, 99(2):256-263, 1990.

8. Loop FD et al: Sternal wound complications after isolated coronary artery bypass grafting: early and late mortality, morbidity, and cost of care, *Ann Thorac Surg* 49:179-187, 1990.

9. Nahai F et al: Primary treatment of the infected sternotomy wound with muscle flaps: a review of 211 consecutive cases, 84(3):434-441, 1989.

10. Pairolero PC et al: Management of recalcitrant median sternotomy wounds, *J Thorac Cardiovasc Surg* Vol 88(3):357-363, 1984.

11. Phipps WJ et al: *Medical-surgical nursing: concepts and clinical practice,* St Louis, 1979, Mosby.

12. Pinchccofsky-Devin G: Why won't this wound heal? *Ostomy Wound Management* 42-51, 1989.

13. Rutledge R et al: Mediastinal infection after open heart surgery, *Surgery* 97(1):88-92, 1983.

14. Sarr MG et al: Mediastinal infection after cardiac surgery, *Ann Thorac Surg* 38(4):415-423, 1984.

15. Smith T et al: Hospital malnutrition, *Lancet* 1:689-693, 1977.

16. Stradtman JC: Nursing implications in sternal and mediastinal infections after open heart surgery, *Focus Crit Care* 16(3):178-183, 1989.

17. Voiriot P et al: *Staphylococcus aureus* mediastinitis: prognostic usefulness of an early medicosurgical therapy; *Infect Control* 8(8):325-328, 1987.

18. Westaby S: *Wound care,* St Louis, 1986, Mosby.

14

Care in the Intermediate Intensive Care Unit

Diane M. Burnett and Alfred S. Casale

Care of the patient undergoing cardiac surgery in the intermediate intensive care unit focuses on pulmonary and cardiovascular stability, neurologic assessment, maintenance of renal function, surveillance for infection, regulation of preexisting and current medications, and early physical rehabilitation. The patient's outcome depends on the ability of the physician and nurse to integrate pertinent preoperative data and routine postoperative care.

Pulmonary Function

The cause of respiratory insufficiency in patients who undergo surgery in which cardiopulmonary bypass is used may involve intracellular, extracellular, and mechanical aberrations. Most commonly, respiratory insufficiency in the intermediate intensive care unit is caused by interstitial edema and atelectasis. The practitioner must recognize preexisting lung disease (e.g., chronic obstructive pulmonary disease, tuberculosis, asbestos exposure, pulmonary resection) as well as obesity and cigarette smoking as important predictors of impaired postoperative pulmonary function. The following factors affect postoperative pulmonary function:

- Preexisting lung disease
- Obesity
- Cigarette smoking
- Decreased oncotic pressure
- Microemboli
- Paralysis of a hemidiaphragm

Other factors to be considered are decreased plasma oncotic pressure resulting from hemodilution, and microemboli from blood transfusions, which result in elevated pulmonary vascular resistance. In addition, paralysis of a hemidiaphragm because of phrenic nerve injury during topical cooling of the heart may alter chest wall dynamics, thus contributing to respiratory compromise.

Physical assessment of the patient's respiratory status includes auscultation and percussion. The most common findings from auscultation of the chest are decreased breath sounds (particularly the left lower lobe), the presence of rales, inspiratory and expiratory wheezes, and pleural friction rubs. Percussion can help determine the presence of atelectasis, consolidation, fluid (dullness), or a pneumothorax (hyperresonance).

The preoperative and postoperative chest x-ray films are compared. The most commonly noted abnormalities include lower lobe atelectasis, pleural effusion, elevated left hemidiaphragm, pneumothorax, and lobar infiltrate.

In addition, lateral decubitus films can help differentiate free-flowing pleural fluid from atelectasis or diaphragmatic elevation. Thoracentesis may be indicated even in asymptomatic patients because moderate to large fluid volumes impinge on the lung fields and thus promote atelectasis and consolidation. Symptomatic effusions should be evacuated.

Elevation of the left hemidiaphragm is usually related to phrenic nerve injury resulting from topical cold saline solution used to protect the heart during the operative period of ischemic arrest. On occasion the injury is a result of the electrocautery. The majority of patients with chest x-ray films showing an elevated hemidiaphragm have no symptoms. It generally resolves within 6 months.

Arterial blood gases are monitored as needed, but transcutaneous oxygen saturation monitoring is used for ongoing patient observation. Preoperative arterial blood gas determinations provide a baseline for interpretation of postoperative values. Usually the levels of arterial oxygen pressure (PaO_2) are maintained between 70 to 80 mm Hg with oxygen saturations ranging from 92% to 100% with oxygen delivered through nasal cannula (2 to 6 L/min) or through face mask (FiO_2 of 40% to 60%). Exceptions are commonly seen in chronic obstructive lung and congenital heart disease patients. Typically, the patient with chronic obstructive pulmonary disease has PaO_2 levels between 50 and 60 mm Hg with arterial carbon dioxide pressure occasionally observed in the 50 to 60 mm

Hg range. To maintain the respiratory drive that depends on hypoxemia, a lower PaO_2 is necessary in these patients. Similarly, the patient with congenital heart disease may have preexisting shunting, causing much lower PaO_2 and oxygen saturation values without signifying respiratory compromise.

Pulmonary embolism is an important cause of hypoxemia in cardiac surgical patients postoperatively. Findings include tachypnea and an acute decline in oxygenation with the presence of sharp inspiratory pain and restlessness. Cardiorespiratory arrest can develop quickly. Diagnostic maneuvers include arterial blood gas determinations demonstrating hypoxemia (po_2 <70 mm Hg) and hyperventilation, and a positive ventilation and perfusion scan or pulmonary arteriogram. Treatment consists of oxygen and ventilatory support, and heparinization with a bolus of 5000 U followed by 1000 U/hr, aiming for a doubling of the partial thromboplastin time. Administration of thrombolytic agents is generally contraindicated early after the operation.

Preventive therapy for respiratory compromise consists of incentive spirometry, achieving a minimum of 1000 cc for 10 breaths every 1 to 2 hours, and effective coughing to expectorate secretions. Chest percussion and postural drainage every 6 hours and nasotracheal suctioning with saline solution every 2 to 4 hours are prescribed for patients who have difficulty mobilizing secretions. Adequate analgesia should be provided with oral or parenteral agents. Early ambulation is initiated to promote deep breathing and lung expansion and prevent accumulation of secretions.

Medications in the treatment of respiratory compromise include bronchodilators, diuretics, and antiinflammatory drugs. The principal bronchodilators used are aminophylline (to maintain a theophylline level of 10 to 20 µg/ml) or inhalation treatments with β-agonists. These drugs directly relax the smooth muscle of the bronchial airways and pulmonary blood vessels. Because of the cardiac stimulant action of theophylline, the patient must be monitored for supraventricular and ventricular arrhythmias and treated by reduction of drug dose or initiation of antiarrhythmic drugs.

Diuresis is promoted (usually with oral furosemide 20-40 mg qd or bid) until the patient is within 2 kg of preoperative weight. Occasionally dopamine may be necessary to effect a diuresis by dilation of the renal vasculature. Potassium replacement is given concomitantly either intravenously or orally. Preferentially, potassium supplements are given through a central line (usually in place for approximately 48 hours after the operation) to prevent nausea associated with oral administration. A total fluid restriction of 1200 ml/day of both intravenous and oral liquids is maintained until the patient has reached the desired goals as noted above.

Lastly, antiinflammatory drugs may be prescribed to treat the pain associated with pleuritic irritation. This pain can prevent the patient from performing the necessary deep-breathing and coughing and thus compromise pulmonary function. A nonsteroidal antiinflammatory agent (indomethacin, 25 mg orally three times daily; ibuprofen, 600 mg orally four times daily) is prescribed to provide both analgesic and antiinflammatory effects.

Cardiovascular Function

The cardiovascular assessment includes auscultation of heart sounds, interpretation of the electrocardiogram (ECG), management of arrhythmias, blood pressure control, and evaluation of peripheral circulation.

Auscultation

Auscultation of the heart in the postoperative cardiovascular surgical patient in the intermediate care unit focuses on murmurs, prosthetic valve sounds, the presence of a pathologic S_3, and pericardial friction rubs.

Particular attention is given to the presence of systolic and diastolic murmurs, especially in patients who have undergone valvular surgery. The development of a new murmur may indicate dehiscence of a prosthetic valve or ring. A Doppler echocardiogram is performed to measure the amount of regurgitation. The results are correlated with the patient's clinical course to denote the necessity and timing of intervention.

The presence of an S_3, which signifies rapid filling of the ventricle during early diastole, may denote myocardial failure or incompetence of the mitral or tricuspid valve. The practitioner must correlate this finding with the presence of a new murmur in the valvular heart patient or with ECG evidence of myocardial damage in the patient undergoing coronary artery bypass.

The detection of a pericardial friction rub indicates pericardial inflammation. Postpericardiotomy syndrome develops in approximately 30% to 40% of all patients undergoing surgery that requires opening of the pericardium.[1] This syndrome consists of a pericardial friction rub that can be heard best on end-expiration and is accompanied by chest pain radiating to the scapular area, low-grade fever, and/or diffuse ST elevation on the 12-lead ECG. The pain associated with this syndrome can be similar to angina and requires these other components to make the differentiation.

ECG Interpretation

Frequently seen in this patient population are ST-T wave changes of pericarditis, myocardial ischemia and infarction, digitalis effect, and QRS aberrations noted in bundle branch block and intraventricular conduction delay. The 12-lead ECG changes typical of pericarditis or epicarditis are global J-point elevation or inverted T waves. On occasion these changes may be localized to various regions of the heart as signified by ECG changes. Usually these changes are noted between 6 to 48 hours postoperatively.

Nonspecific ST-T wave elevation or depression of 0.5 to 1 mm is common. However, symptomatic regional ST-T elevation or depression of more than 1 mm with or without reciprocal changes may be indicative of myocardial ischemia. Interpretation of the ECG is difficult in patients receiving digoxin because ST sloping may be present from the drug's effect.

With the suspicion of myocardial ischemia, sublingual nitrates are prescribed to promote coronary vasodilation. Topical nitrates and nifedipine (10 mg 96° SL) are added to the patient's medical regimen. Depending on the degree or persistence of symptoms, an echocardiogram is ordered, to determine regional wall abnormalities. Recurrence of myocardial ischemia or typical anginal symptoms during the postoperative period prompts a low-level stress test and cardiac catheterization, alone or in combination, to determine the patency of the bypass grafts.

Another commonly seen ECG aberration is the development of a bundle branch block or intraventricular conduction delay. In the absence of other ECG changes, such as ischemic ST-T wave changes or bifascicular block, which may be predictive of high degrees of block, continued observation is sufficient.

Arrhythmias

Approximately 30% of all patients who undergo procedures requiring cardiopulmonary bypass are prone to supraventricular and/or ventricular arrhythmias. Diagnosis of the arrhythmia can be made with the use of atrial pacing wires inserted at the time of operation. Together with the use of antiarrhythmic drugs, metabolic abnormalities such as low potassium, magnesium, and calcium levels should be corrected to normal to high-normal range and hypoxemia corrected to normal values for the individual patient.[3]

Atrial fibrillation and flutter with rapid ventricular response are the most common arrhythmias noted within the early postoperative period. Atrial flutter should be overdriven with atrial wires as described in Chapter 10. Digoxin is given to control the ventricular response by blocking impulses at the atrioventricular node. If the patient's ventricular response remains greater than 120 beats/min after the initial 0.5 mg of digoxin is given, verapamil is administered to slow the heart rate (see Chapter 10). Prior to administering verapamil, a backup ventricular demand pacemaker is attached to the patient.

Beta blockade can be instituted in patients with ejection fractions >40% to control heart rate. Low dose propanolol post-operatively in patients who received pre-operative beta blockers has been shown to be effective in reducing clinically important arrhythmias after coronary artery bypass grafting.[2,6]

If conversion to normal sinus rhythm does not occur within 24 to 36 hours, a type I agent such as procainamide or quinidine is instituted to promote chemical conversion. Electrical cardioversion is performed for patients who are hemodynamically unstable or who remain in atrial fibrillation or flutter despite therapeutic levels of type I agents. Patients whose blood is anticoagulated because of valvular replacement or repair are discharged, and elective cardioversion is performed approximately 8-12 weeks postoperatively.

The incidence of all types of ventricular arrhythmias in patients undergoing coronary artery bypass and valvular heart surgery can be as high as 36% to 50%.[4,5] Typically, ventricular arrhythmias are potentiated by hypoxemia, electrolyte imbalance, myocardial ischemia, or direct myocardial irritation by devices. Greater than 12 unifocal premature ventricular contractions (PVC)/min, multifocal ectopy, or frequent couplets or triplets within the first 24 hours after the operation should be investigated with an arterial blood gas and electrolyte determination, and a 12-lead ECG. Any deficits should be corrected and drug therapy started if arrhythmias persist. A lidocaine bolus of 1 mg/kg is administered, followed by a continuous infusion of 20 to 40 µg/kg/min.

For long-term arrhythmia management, an oral type I agent such as procainamide or quinidine is added for patients with impaired left ventricular function. Lidocaine is discontinued after the third oral dose of drug, and Holter monitoring is used to confirm the efficacy of the therapy when the patient has attained a therapeutic level of the drug. Procainamide is well tolerated by most patients; however, the side effects of nausea and lupus may occur, necessitating discontinuation of the drug. Quinidine's predominant side effects are diarrhea, drug fever, and thrombocytopenia which resolve with withdrawal of the drug. Both drugs have the potential for proarrhythmic effects and the idiosyncratic reaction of torsades des pointes, which is treated by conventional methods, overdrive pacing, and discontinuance of the drug.

The use of overdrive suppression may also be employed short-term for ablation of nonsustained ventricular ectopy. Increasing the heart rate decreases the QT interval and suppresses ectopic impulses.

When arrhythmias are not successfully controlled by the traditional drugs, type Ic drugs such as mexiletine or amiodarone may be necessary. When the presenting arrhythmia is sustained ventricular tachycardia or fibrillation requiring direct-current cardioversion, the arrhythmia must be treated more aggressively. The cause of the arrhythmia must be discerned and corrected whether it is due to metabolic abnormalities, hypoxemia, or myocardial ischemia secondary to graft thrombosis or spasm.

Atrioventricular Blocks

Temporary or permanent atrioventricular (A-V) block may develop in the postoperative valvular cardiac patient. In particular, patients undergoing aortic valve surgery may have A-V conduction disturbances ranging from first-degree heart block to complete heart block because of swelling around the nodal pathways or disruption of the pathways by suture material. A temporary ventricular demand pacemaker is necessary to avoid bradycardic episodes in patients with low degrees of block. In patients with high degrees of A-V block and compromised function, an A-V sequential pacemaker is necessary to synchronize the atrial and ventricular activity to maximize cardiac output. A decision to place a permanent pacemaker is made after approximately 10 days to allow edema to resolve. The threshold required to capture the ventricle in a pacemaker-dependent patient must be checked daily because increasing energy requirements may necessitate earlier permanent pacemaker insertion.

Hemodynamic Factors

Hypertension is noted for approximately 24 to 48 hours in many postoperative cardiac surgical patients. At this stage of recovery most patients respond well to diuretics, topical nitrates, and nifedipine. Patients who required antihypertensive medications before the operation often do not require reinstitution until 2 to 3 weeks after the operation. If indicated in the early postoperative period, the drug is usually administered at half doses, with appropriate changes as needed.

Patients who have increased systemic vascular resistance and poor left ventricular function may benefit from an angiotensin converting enzyme inhibitor such as captopril or enalapril.

Peripheral Circulation

Routine pulse checks are monitored every 8 hours on all patients, and special notation is made of intraaortic balloon pulsation (IABP) or femoral cannulation sites. Occasionally a pseudoaneurysm may develop or pulses may be decreased or absent distally in the affected extremity. These findings require urgent vascular surgical evaluation.

Venous circulation is altered because of the removal of the greater saphenous vein. Patients are instructed to elevate their legs when sitting, to reduce edema formation. Thigh-length thromboembolic stockings may be ordered for patients with excessive edema.

Neurologic Assessment

The patient's neurologic status is assessed every 8 hours and as needed to discern subtle or profound deficits. Subtle changes are often noted by family members and brought to the attention of the medical and nursing staff. Commonly patients or family members note the patient's memory loss, visual changes such as flashing lights, and inability to focus while reading. Visual changes may necessitate an ophthalmologic consultation. Another common neurologic abnormality noted is numbness in the last two or three digits of either hand. This usually indicates a brachial plexus injury from stretching or compression of the nerves during retraction of the sternum. Typically sensation returns without intervention within 1 to 3 months.

Profound neurologic deficits indicative of a cerebrovascular event prompt a neurologic consultation for diagnosis and prognosis. The majority of cerebrovascular accidents occur intraoperatively or within the first 24 hours thereafter and are usually discovered in the intensive care unit. Rehabilitative needs are identified, and supportive services such as physical, occupational, speech, and swallowing therapy are arranged on the basis of the individual patient's needs.

Another central nervous system disorder noted in this patient population is intensive care unit psychosis. Predisposing factors such as stress, substance abuse, alteration of sleep patterns, history of psychiatric illness, and thromboemboli from cardiopulmonary bypass have been identified.[1] The patient may have disorientation, paranoid delusions, and auditory or visual hallucinations.[7] Reorientation of the patient to date, time, and place with visual aids such as a calendar and clock is helpful. If the patient is combative or extremely agitated, a sedative such as haloperidol should be administered to calm the patient.

Renal Impairment

Increases in total body water and interstitial edema occur in patients who have undergone cardiopulmonary bypass, because of increased secretion of antidiuretic hormone and aldosterone, activation of serum complement (increasing vascular permeability), and the use of crystalloid prime. Intravenous and oral fluid restrictions of 1200 ml/day remain in effect until the optimum weight has been achieved.

Renal doses of dopamine promote perfusion of the kidneys and is added to the diuretic regimen described earlier in this chapter for patients who are excessively overloaded with fluid or who demonstrate a poor response to diuretics. Electrolyte levels are checked at least daily in these patients.

Infection Control

Prevention, recognition, and prompt treatment of infection is important in the cardiac surgical patient postoperatively. The primary infections noted in this patient population are pulmonary, wound, and urinary infections, with or without resultant bacteremia and septicemia.

To prevent and treat pulmonary infections, chest physiotherapy is initiated as outlined earlier in this chapter. All surgical wounds are covered with an occlusive dressing for 48 hours postoperatively and are cleansed daily with hydrogen peroxide thereafter until discharge. Mediastinal wounds that appear erythematous or culture positive are treated with broad-spectrum antibiotics until a specific pathogen is identified. Particular attention is given to those patients at high risk for mediastinitis. They include elderly, obese, immunosuppressed, and diabetic patients, and patients undergoing internal mammary artery grafts.

All central intravenous lines and urinary catheters are removed within 24 to 48 hours of the operation in patients without complications. Typically fevers in the first 48 hours after surgery are due to atelectasis and signal the need for aggressive chest physiotherapy. Fevers of more than 38.5° C after the second postoperative day should lead to blood, sputum, and urine cultures, and a careful physical examination.

Medications

Patients undergoing coronary artery bypass receive aspirin postoperatively (325 mg/day) to maintain the patency of the grafts.[8] The patients are then discharged with instructions to take one aspirin a day.

Warfarin (Coumadin) is initiated in the valvular heart surgery patient after removal of the mediastinal tubes. The aim of therapy is to maintain a prothrombin time of 1.5 to 2.0 times control values. To achieve this goal, patients who have undergone aortic valve replacement initially receive 5 mg/day and doses are increased appropriately, whereas mitral valve patients receive smaller doses of 2.5 mg because of the likelihood of preexisting passive liver congestion. The practitioner must also take into account the interaction of warfarin with numerous drugs. The most prevalent interaction seen is that of warfarin with antibiotics (particularly the cephalosporins). The prothrombin time is elevated because of interaction of antibiotics and vitamin K synthesis.

Most *noncardiac medications* taken preoperatively, such as anticonvulsants, glaucoma medicines, hypoglycemic agents, steroids, and thyroid supplements, are resumed at this time. Anticonvulsants, glaucoma medications, and thyroid supplements can be resumed at their preoperative doses. However, steroid replacement is tapered from perioperative doses initiated in the intensive care unit to the patient's preoperative dose. Glucose level is controlled by the administration of regular insulin by sliding scale for the first 24 to 48 hours postoperatively. Oral hypoglycemics and long-acting preparations of insulin are ordered when the patient is receiving a substantial amount of calories and requires periodic coverage with sliding-scale insulin administration. Generally, long-acting insulin preparations are begun at one third the amount of regular insulin coverage required by the patient and are increased depending on patient need during the ensuing days of hospitalization.

Physical Activity

The patient begins a cardiac rehabilitation program to promote lung expansion, venous circulation, and endurance. A physical therapist examines the patient for preexisting and current mobility deficits caused by a stroke, accident, or prolonged bed rest or limited preoperative activity. Working with each individual patient's need, the therapist begins low-level arm and leg stretching exercises. The patient is helped to a chair three times a day and takes short walks of approximately 20 to 50 feet one or two times a day. The patient's vital signs are monitored before, during, and after activity. A progressive structured exercise program is designed for the patient and guides him or her through recovery on the general nursing floor and at home.

References

1. Bartle SH: Psychiatric complications of cardiac surgery. In Litwak RS, Jurado RA, eds: *Care of the cardiac surgical patient,* Norwalk, Conn, 1982, Appleton-Century-Crofts.
2. Matangi MF: Arrhythmia prophylaxis after coronary artery bypass: The effect of minidose propranolol, *J Thorac Cardiovasc Surg,* 89:439-443, 1985.
3. Parikka H, et al: The influence of intravenous magnesium sulphate on the occurrence of atrial fibrillation after coronary artery bypass operation, *Eur Heart J,* 14:251-258, 1993.
4. Rubin DA, et al: Ventricular arrhythmia after coronary artery bypass graft surgery: Incidence, risk factors and long-term prognosis, *J Am Coll Cardiol* 6:307-310, 1985.
5. Smith RC, et al: Ventricular dysrhythmias in patients undergoing cor-

onary artery bypass graft surgery: Incidence, characteristics and prognostic importance, *Am Heart J* 123(1):73-81, 1992.

6. Stephenson LW, et al: Propranolol for prevention of postoperative cardiac arrhythmias: A randomized study, *Ann Thorac Surg* 29(2)113-116, 1980.

7. Utley JR: Postperfusion syndrome, visual syndromes, and bacterial infection after cardiopulmonary bypass. In Utley JR, ed: *Pathophysiology and techniques of cardiopulmonary bypass,* Vol 3, *Cardiothoracic Surgery series,* Baltimore, 1983, Williams and Wilkins.

8. van der Meer J, et al: Prevention of one-year vein-graft occlusion after aortocoronary-bypass surgery: A comparison of low-dose aspirin, low-dose aspirin plus dipyridamole, and oral anticoagulants, *Lancet* 342:257-264, 1993.

Convalescence Before Discharge

15

Cathy Custer and Alfred S. Casale

On transfer to the regular cardiac surgical floor the nursing staff performs an admission assessment and initiates an appropriate nursing care plan. Standardized care plans form the groundwork from which care is individualized. A problem list identifies common areas for assessment: circulatory function, respiratory function, nutrition, neurocerebral function, structural integrity, emotional response, social system, cognitive response, health management patterns, sensory function, sexual function, and sleep patterns. Once problems are identified, appropriate interventions are implemented and the outcomes evaluated every 24 hours.

The prevention and early detection of postoperative complications are goals shared by medical and nursing staff. Infection, arrhythmias, postpericardiotomy syndrome, and late cardiac tamponade may occur during this period and are discussed in Chapter 14. Priorities in this phase of convalescence include physical rehabilitation, nutrition, risk factor modification, and discharge planning and anticoagulation.

Physical Rehabilitation

Early mobilization of patients after cardiac surgery has been shown to be both safe and beneficial.[3,8] Phase I, or acute, in-hospital rehabilitation programs, can decrease the detrimental effects of prolonged bed rest, increase patient self-confidence, and decrease the cost and length of the hospital stay.[11]

The inpatient cardiac rehabilitation program at The Johns Hopkins Hospital consists of a supervised progression of low-level activity together with a patient-family education component. The goals of the program are to:

- Decrease the total recovery period
- Provide the patient with a progressive, structured exercise program
- Initiate the return to previous activity levels
- Develop and maintain cardiovascular fitness

The benefits of the program to the patient include the following:

- Increased strength and endurance
- Decreased lung congestion
- Increased energy
- Toning and stretching of chest wall and leg muscles
- Increased activity levels according to tolerance
- Increased confidence
- Increased readiness for discharge home

Assessment

Physical therapists from the cardiac rehabilitation division of the department of rehabilitation medicine examine each cardiac surgical patient within 48 to 72 hours of the operation for ability to begin the inpatient program. A written evaluation notes the following information:

- Patient's mental status
- Inspection of sternal and leg incisions
- Stability of the sternum
- Auscultation of the lungs
- Cough effort and productivity
- Incentive spirometry effort
- Presence of supplemental oxygen
- General muscle strength
- Mobility
- Resting cardiovascular parameters (heart rate, respiratory rate, and blood pressure)

Special attention is paid to preexisting medical conditions such as obesity, orthopedic limitations, and pulmonary or peripheral vascular disease because their presence often requires modification of the exercise program. Postoperative complications such as myocardial infarction, cerebrovascular accident, pneumonia, and arrhythmias are noted, and the rehabilitation program is appropriately modified. Also assessed are psychosocial factors including patient support systems, preoperative and current emotional status, and compliance with the medical regimen.

Intervention

Once the evaluation is completed, an individualized exercise program is initiated. The general exercise protocol developed for the cardiac surgical population includes three components: warm-up exercises, endurance activity, and cool-down exercises.

Warm-up exercises are an integral component of any exercise program. They allow for the gradual circulatory adjustments necessary to meet increased metabolic demands.[4] The inclusion of warm-up exercises in the postoperative cardiac surgical population is particularly important. Warm-up exercises decrease the potential for injury, ischemic electrocardiographic changes, and arrhythmias associated with sudden exertion.[4]

The warm-up exercises involve both musculoskeletal exercises (static stretching, flexibility, and muscle-strengthening exercises) and cardiovascular exercises (total body movement at slightly lower than endurance level). Examples of warm-up exercises are listed in Table 15-1. The purpose of the endurance phase of the exercise program is to stimulate directly the oxygen transport system.[4] Walking is the most common form of endurance activity in inpatient settings. Cycling may be added where appropriate.

The walking or endurance phase of the rehabilitation program is tailored to each patient. Intensity, duration, and frequency of the endurance activity is modified to ensure that patients exercise safely within their limits.

Cool-down exercises follow the endurance component of the program. Cool-down exercises are necessary to prevent light-head-

Table **15-1**   Warm-up Exercises

Sitting	Standing
Knee extension	Toe rises
Hip flexion	Shoulder shrug
Shoulder abduction	Side leg lifts
Shoulder flexion	Knee touches
	Arm circles
	Side bends

edness, syncope, and arrhythmias associated with the abrupt cessation of exercise. During the endurance phase of exercise, vasodilation occurs to accommodate the increased volume of blood required to meet metabolic demands. Venous return increases, resulting in an increased stroke volume. Sudden cessation of exercise creates a rapid fall in cardiac output without allowing time for appropriate compensatory changes to occur in peripheral vascular resistance. Blood therefore pools in the extremities, further decreasing venous return and often leading to cardiovascular compromise. The best way to prevent pooling of blood after endurance activity is to maintain the massaging action of muscles through continued movement.[4] To cool down, patients walk at a slower pace for approximately 10 minutes. This allows for the return of heart rate and blood pressure to near preexercise levels, and for the dissipation of heat accumulated during the endurance phase.

The cardiac surgical patient is closely monitored through each phase of the program by the physical therapist. Vital signs are measured and recorded before, during, and after exercise. The following changes exceed expected responses:

- Heart rate 20% greater than resting heart rate
- Fall in systolic blood pressure of more than 10 mm Hg
- Rise in systolic blood pressure of more than 30 mm Hg
- Increase in respiratory rate of more than 15 breaths/min

These are noted and reported to the patient's physician. The occurrence of dyspnea, dizziness, or chest pain during exercise leads to termination of the exercise and investigation of the symptoms.

The physical therapist sees each cardiac surgical patient daily to review, monitor, and assist the patient through the cardiac rehabilitation program. Exercise intensity, duration, and frequency gradually increase as the patient progresses toward discharge.

Patient Education

Patients are given a written booklet with diagrams and instructions for each exercise they are to perform. The patient is instructed to perform the prescribed exercises three times a day; once with the therapist and twice on his or her own or with assistance when necessary. A patient log is provided for the patient to record the performance of the prescribed activity. In addition to recording exercise, the patient is asked to rate the perceived level of exertion during exercise according to a scale. This log provides the patient with objective and subjective feedback as to his or her progress.

Patients and their families are taught the purposes, goals, and benefits of the inpatient cardiac rehabilitation program. In addition, preoperative physical inactivity as a risk factor of coronary artery disease is identified in appropriate patients. Counseling in this area of risk factor modification is provided by the physical therapist.

Discharge Planning

Before discharge the patient's overall progress, home environment, resources, and support systems are evaluated to determine whether a need exists for further inpatient, outpatient, or home physical therapy. Routinely, cardiac surgical patients are discharged with a 6-week home exercise program incorporating the basic three components of the inpatient rehabilitation program. The home program increases the intensity, duration, and frequency of exercise weekly. Individualized realistic goals are set for each patient.

For those patients who may require additional physical therapy, appropriate referrals are made. Arrangements for delivery of equipment required at home, such as walkers, canes, or bedside commodes, are made by the physical therapist or the social worker. Patients whose mobility has been compromised by perioperative cerebrovascular accidents may be referred to an inpatient rehabilitation facility for further intensive physical therapy.

The physical therapist reviews guidelines for home activity and specific activity restrictions with the patient and family before discharge. Activities such as driving, returning to work, sports, and hobbies; and resuming sexual activity are discussed. Restrictions on lifting more than 10 to 15 lb, straining, twisting, pushing, pulling, and avoidance of extreme weather are reviewed. Returning to a normal lifestyle is stressed.

Cardiac surgical patients return for a postoperative visit approximately 4 weeks after surgery. At this time a person is occasionally referred to a phase III program, a community-based supervised conditioning and maintenance exercise program.

Nutrition

Studies indicate that malnutrition increases morbidity and mortality rates in surgical patients postoperatively.[5] These studies recognize that inadequate nutrition impairs wound healing and may predispose to septic complications. It is therefore imperative that the nutritional status of patients undergoing cardiac surgery be carefully considered.

Assessment

Evaluation of the cardiac surgical patient's nutritional status is performed by a registered dietitian early after the operation. The initial assessment involves a dietary history documenting preoperative dietary habits, difficulties with chewing or swallowing, the presence of dentures, food intolerances or allergies, and food preferences. Medical conditions such as diabetes, renal insufficiency, and colitis are noted. Usual and current weights are recorded. Ideal body weight is determined, and current percentage of ideal body weight is calculated.

Laboratory values are documented. Preoperative serum lipid profiles (including cholesterol, high-density lipoprotein, low-density lipoprotein, and triglyceride levels) identify patients with hypercholesterolemia and hypertriglyceridemia who may require more intense nutritional instruction. Baseline serum albumin level is also noted. The dietitian records medications currently prescribed for the patient.

Intervention

Most patients undergoing cardiac surgery follow a standardized progression of diet. Clear liquids are allowed within 24 hours of the operation if the patient is extubated and demonstrates evidence of bowel function (flatus, bowel sounds). If clear liquids are tolerated well, the diet is advanced rapidly to a full liquid diet and then a no-added-salt (sodium intake restricted to 4 g/day) diet within the next 24 hours. Modifications are made for patients with coexisting medical disorders (i.e., diabetes), food intolerances (i.e., lactose intolerance), or food preferences (i.e., kosher diet).

After the initial nutritional evaluation the dietitian visits each cardiac surgical patient at mealtime to assess the patient's tolerance of the current diet and ability to meet nutritional demands. Nausea and anorexia are frequent complaints in the postoperative period. Recommendations for small frequent feedings, specific food preferences, liberalization of dietary restrictions where possible, and alteration of medication schedules may decrease some of these complaints.

In situations where the patient consistently fails to meet nutritional needs, vitamins and high-calorie, high-protein supplements may be recommended. In extreme cases where the patient is unable to meet nutritional needs orally because of an altered level of consciousness or because of inadequate airway protecting reflexes, enteral or parenteral nutrition is initiated (see Chapter 11).

The effectiveness of these dietary interventions can be evaluated with daily calorie counts, weekly serum albumin determinations, measurement of transferrin and iron levels, and nitrogen balance studies. In patients with normal hepatic function, nutritional status correlates well with serum albumin levels. A serum albumin level of less than 2.5 g/dl has been shown to correlate with increased rates of surgical complications and mortality. However, serum transferrin may be a more reliable indicator of nutritional status because it has a shorter biologic half-life than albumin (8 days compared with 17 days). Serum iron levels should also be determined in cases of suspected iron deficiency anemia because serum transferrin may be falsely elevated in this situation.

Patient Education

Before discharge the dietitian meets with the patient and family to provide individualized dietary instructions. The basic diet is modified for patients with coexisting medical disorders (i.e., diabetes, renal disease).

The current recommended diet is similar to phase I of the unified diet developed by the American Heart Association.[6] The diet follows five basic principles:

- Reduction of total fat intake, particularly saturated fat (total fat should not exceed 30% of total daily caloric intake)
- Replacement of some (10%) of the saturated fat with polyunsaturated fat
- Reduction of cholesterol intake to less than 300 mg/day
- Achievement and maintenance of appropriate body weight
- Increased intake of soluble fiber

Practical ways to implement these recommendations are provided by the dietitian.

Reduction in caloric intake is discouraged in the immediate recovery period; rather, changes in eating habits are stressed. Patients with newly diagnosed hypercholesterolemia or hypertriglyceridemia are referred to the Preventive Cardiology Clinic for outpatient follow-up and counseling.

Risk Factor Modification

It is widely accepted that there are certain risk factors associated with the incidence of coronary artery disease. Major risk factors identified by the Framingham Heart Study include hypertension, hypercholesterolemia, and cigarette smoking. Other contributory risk factors include age, sex, obesity, inactivity, glucose intolerance, genetic predisposition, race, and stress. Of these risk factors only diet (hyperlipidemia, obesity, glucose intolerance), inactivity, cigarette smoking, hypertension and stress can be altered.

Identification of risk factors is made on admission during the history and physical examination. Modifiable risk factors are addressed by a multidisciplinary team in the postoperative period.

Diet

As discussed earlier, the dietitian provides verbal and written information regarding the reduction of dietary risk factors, specifically the lowering of cholesterol and triglyceride levels, maintenance of ideal body weight, and importance of adequate glucose control.

Inactivity

In addition to the discharge exercise program, physical therapists educate patients as to the importance of regular physical activity. Recommendations are made for exercise programs beyond the recovery period. Community resources and programs are identified.

Cigarette Smoking

For those patients who smoked cigarettes before cardiac surgery, smoking cessation begins with the admission to the hospital. Currently a no-smoking policy is in effect for all patients and employees of the hospital. Patient charts are screened by counselors of the Smoking Cessation Service and appropriate persons are interviewed. The counselors provide the patient and family with information regarding smoking cessation. If the person is receptive, the counselor devises an individual plan for the patient or family member desiring to quit smoking. Follow-up is made on an outpatient basis.

Hypertension

Fluctuations in blood pressure associated with physiologic changes at the time of cardiac surgery influence the care of the patient with hypertension. Antihypertensive medications may be increased, decreased, or even temporarily discontinued during the postoperative period. Patients are educated as to the rationale for these changes and are instructed to resume routine visits to their referring physicians for further treatment.

Newly diagnosed hypertension is noted and appropriately treated during the hospital admission. A letter to the patient's referring physician at the time of discharge describes the patient's antihypertensive regimen and the need for follow-up.

Stress

After the operation cardiac surgical patients may exhibit a wide variety of emotional and behavioral changes.[7] These include confusion; paranoia; depression; exhilaration; annoyance; guilt; attention-seeking behaviors; fatigue; anxiety; and decreased ability to reason, write, or think clearly. The cause of these changes is often multifactorial (metabolic, psychological, drug- or environment-related) and are usually temporary. During the hospital stay patients manifesting these changes are seen by a psychiatric occupational therapist. This therapist discusses the patient's current emotional status and identifies coping strategies for individual patients and their families. Diversional activities (crafts) and opportunities to socialize with other cardiac surgical patients and their families (weekly "heart to heart" lunches) are organized by the psychiatric occupational therapist.

Patients identifying high levels of stress in their life, whether job, family, or personal stress, are counseled as to alternative coping strategies and ways of dealing with stress. In extreme cases a psychiatric consultation may be indicated and initiated.

Discharge Planning

Potential discharge problems or special discharge needs are initially identified by the nurse the day the patient is admitted to the hospital. The nurse records information on the admission data base that ultimately affects the patient's discharge. This includes information about the patient's living environment (e.g., number of stairs, bathroom facilities, etc); support systems and their availability to assist the patient at home; health insurance and coverage for home visiting nurse services if necessary; and local residence, including whether the patient is from another state or country. This information provides the groundwork for discharge planning.

Reassessment of discharge needs occurs early in the postoperative course. Postoperative complications such as cerebrovascular accident and infection can significantly alter the person's discharge needs. Discharge planning is a multidisciplinary effort, involving the dietitian, physical and occupational therapists, nursing staff, physician, and social worker.

Routinely, patients undergoing cardiac surgery receive discharge information through both verbal and written instructions. It is well recognized that the postoperative period is suboptimal for learning.[2] Anxiety, depression, and physical discomfort affect the patient's ability to learn. Narcotics, given frequently for analgesia, impair memory and attention span. For these reasons it is crucial that family members be included in the discharge planning process. When involved they are able to facilitate patient understanding of content and improve patient compliance with discharge instructions.

Discharge classes are held five times a week and cover topics such as activity restrictions, wound care, and signs and symptoms of infection. Classes allow patients and family members the opportunity to ask questions that others may not have addressed. Supplemental written materials are given to the patient and family covering topics discussed in class. Patients and family members are given phone numbers of persons to contact after discharge if questions or concerns arise.

Medications are reviewed by the nurse with the patient and family before discharge. Rationale, method of actions, dose, frequency, and side effects are discussed. Preoperative medications are reviewed and unnecessary medications discontinued. Special attention is paid to those patients requiring anticoagulation therapy.

Anticoagulation

Thromboembolism can be a major complication that limits the success of prosthetic valve replacement and is influenced primarily by valve design and site of implantation.[9] Three general types of prosthetic valves are available: mechanical prostheses and porcine and pericardial bioprostheses. Mechanical prostheses are durable but are prone to thrombogenic complications and require lifelong anticoagulation therapy. Porcine and pericardial bioprostheses are less thrombogenic but have limited durability and can fail, necessitating a second operation for replacement within the patient's life span.

In general, thromboembolic complications are seen more frequently with mechanical prostheses and more often in the mitral position. Standard practice at The Johns Hopkins Hospital is to use the St. Jude bileaflet mechanical prosthesis or the Carpentier-Edwards porcine or pericardial bioprosthesis. (For more specific information see Chapter 16.)

Thrombosis of the valve may cause obstruction of the valve orifice, interference with valve closing, or pulmonary or systemic embolization. Thromboemboli from prosthetic valves frequently travel to cerebral vessels, with variable neurologic sequelae.

Although it is widely accepted that prosthetic valves require anticoagulation therapy, different medical centers vary widely on the type, dose, and duration of anticoagulation therapy. Heparin and warfarin (Coumadin) are the two most common anticoagulants used at The Johns Hopkins Hospital. The goals of anticoagulant therapy include effective anticoagulation, convenient administration, and minimal incidence of side effects.

Heparin is not absorbed from the gastrointestinal tract and therefore must be given parenterally (see Chapter 9 for mechanisms of action). When heparin is given by continuous intravenous infusion, constant levels of anticoagulation are achievable with resumption of normal hemostasis within 1 to 2 hours of discontinuing the infusion. Serial serum activated partial thromboplastin times are measured while the patient is receiving heparin therapy to monitor the efficacy of treatment and to decrease the incidence of complications. Activated partial thromboplastin times are kept at approximately 1.5 to 2.0 times laboratory control values. The temporary use of heparin is indicated when anticoagulation therapy with warfarin alone is inadequate.

Warfarin acts by interfering with the action of vitamin K, thereby preventing the synthesis of clotting factors in the intrinsic pathway (factor IX), extrinsic pathway (factor VII), and common pathway (factors X and II). Vitamin K is a part of the normal diet and is synthesized by bacteria in the small intestine.

Warfarin may be given intramuscularly but is more commonly administered orally. Peak effect occurs 36 hours after ingestion.

The prothrombin time (PT) is the laboratory test used to monitor warfarin activity. The PT often rises to a therapeutic range within 1 to 2 days but can be misleading. The rise reflects a decrease in factor VII, which has a very short half-life. Suppression of factors IX, X, and II requires 3 to 6 days and argues against the practice of high loading doses of warfarin. This practice may lead to a higher incidence of complication and does not adequately protect against thrombus formation.

Platelet activity is of prime importance in maintaining hemostasis in the patient receiving anticoagulant therapy. For this reason patients with decreased platelet counts after cardiopulmonary bypass begin receiving modest doses of warfarin (2.5 to 5 mg) on a daily basis. Daily PTs are taken to monitor and guide therapy. Drugs that affect platelet activity, specifically aspirin and indomethacin, are used rarely with concomitant anticoagulation therapy.

PTs are maintained approximately 1.5 times control values. The patient who is initially resistant to modest doses of warfarin may temporarily require a continuous infusion of heparin to decrease incidence of early thromboembolic complications. However, when heparin and warfarin are given simultaneously, the PT may be affected. At low doses of heparin the effect is minimal, but at high doses the PT may be artificially prolonged by several seconds.

In emergency situations heparin may be reversed by giving intravenous protamine sulfate, 1 mg/100 U heparin. Vitamin K restores normal clotting factor synthesis in the liver in cases of hypoprothrombinemia. When given intramuscularly or intravenously, vitamin K restores normal hemostasis within approximately 6 to 12 hours. However, vitamin K should be used judiciously because it makes patients refractory to warfarin for 1 to 2 weeks. Daily vitamin supplements containing vitamin K should be avoided.

Before discharge patients receiving warfarin therapy are taught the purpose of anticoagulation; its side effects, precautions, and drug interactions; and duration of therapy. Patients who receive a St. Jude prosthesis require lifelong anticoagulation. Anticoagulation therapy for the Carpentier-Edwards bioprosthesis ranges from 1 to 3 months.

Cerebrovascular hemorrhage is the most serious risk associated with anticoagulation therapy but occurs infrequently.[10] It is therefore imperative that monitoring of PT continues after discharge from the hospital. Referring physicians are contacted before patient discharge and are alerted to the current warfarin dose and recent PT values. Any difficulties the patient encountered with anticoagulation are also discussed. The patient is instructed to contact the referring physician to arrange to have a PT drawn within 3 days of discharge. It is recommended that weekly PTs be drawn until a series of stable results are obtained. Some institutions, such as The Johns Hopkins Hospital, have a Coumadin Clinic where anticoagulation therapy can be monitored and inpatient education reinforced. A recent development, the Coumatrak, allows PTs to be calculated from finger stick sample and avoids venipuncture. This allows for immediate PT results, which can be interpreted in the patient's presence, thereby allowing warfarin doses to be adjusted appropriately.

In addition to anticoagulation education, persons with prosthetic valves receive information pertaining to infection prophylaxis. Patients are given the current guidelines of the American Heart Association for antibiotic prophylaxis of invasive dental and surgical procedures. The role of prophylaxis in the prevention of endocarditis is explained.[1]

References

1. American Heart Association: Prevention of bacterial endocarditis: recommendations by the American Heart Association, *JAMA* 264:2919-2922, 1991.
2. Argondizzo NT: Education of the patient and family. In Wenger NK, Hellerstein HK, eds: *Rehabilitation of the coronary patient,* New York, 1984, Wiley.
3. Dion WF et al: Medical problems and physiological responses during supervised inpatient cardiac rehabilitation: the patient after coronary artery bypass grafting, *Heart Lung* 11:248, 1982.
4. Hellerstein HK, Franklin BA: Exercise testing and prescription. In Wenger NK, Hellerstein HK, eds: *Rehabilitation of the coronary patient,* New York, 1984, Wiley.
5. Imbembo AL, Walser M: Nutritional assessment. In Walser M et al: eds: *Nutritional management: the Johns Hopkins handbook,* Philadelphia, 1984, Saunders.
6. Margolis S, Elfert G: Dietary modification of plasma lipid and lipoprotein levels. In Walser M et al, eds: *Nutritional management: the Johns Hopkins handbook,* Philadelphia, 1984, Saunders.

7. McElligott MT: The person undergoing cardiac surgery. In Guzzetta CE, Dossey BM, eds: *Cardiovascular nursing: bodymind tapestry,* St Louis, 1984, Mosby.

8. Robinson G, Froelicher VF, Utley JR: Rehabilitation of the coronary artery bypass graft surgery patient, *J Cardiac Rehabil* 4:74, 1984.

9. Seth JC: The person with coronary artery disease and risk factors. In Guzzetta CE, Dossey BM, eds: *Cardiovascular nursing: bodymind tapestry,* St Louis, 1984, Mosby.

10. Shapiro RM: Anticoagulant therapy. In O'Connor AB, ed: *Advances in cardiovascular nursing,* New York, 1975, American Journal of Nursing.

11. Wenger N: Early ambulation physical activity: myocardial infarction and coronary artery bypass surgery, *Heart Lung* 13:14, 1984.

Ischemic Heart Disease and Its Complications

16

Peter W. Cho, R.C. Stewart Finney, Jr. and Timothy J. Gardner

Ischemic heart disease is a major cause of morbidity and mortality in the United States. Each year about 1.5 million Americans have myocardial infarctions, and more than 500,000 die of complications of ischemic heart disease. Some of the most spectacular advances in modern medicine, including catheter-based angioplasty and heart surgery with cardiopulmonary bypass, have been devised to treat this disease and its complications.

Normal Anatomy and Physiology

The left main and right coronary arteries branch from the ascending aorta at the level of the aortic valve leaflets (Fig. 16-1). The right coronary artery originates from the aorta anterolaterally, courses deep in the atrioventricular groove around the acute margin of the heart, and terminates in the posterior descending artery, which runs toward the apex in the posterior interventricular groove. Branches of the right coronary artery supply the anterior and posterior right ventricle, the sinus node, and often the adjacent half of the posterior left ventricle and the posterior third of the interventricular septum. The left main coronary artery branches into the left anterior descending (LAD) and the circumflex arteries. The LAD artery courses in the anterior interventricular groove and terminates near the apex of the heart, often anastomosing with the posterior descending artery. Diagonal branches from the LAD artery supply the proximal half of the anterior left ventricular surface and medial third of the anterior right ventricle, and the anterior

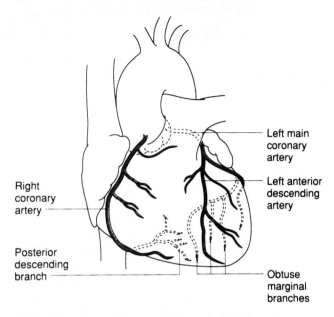

Fig. 16-1 Coronary arteries and their major branches.

two thirds of the interventricular septum. The circumflex branch of the left coronary artery courses laterally in the left atrioventricular groove and eventually communicates with the posterior descending artery. The circumflex artery and its marginal branches supply the lateral aspect of the left ventricle.

Most of the myocardial venous blood returns through the superficial epicardial veins to the coronary sinus, and from there to the right atrium. Deep intramyocardial thebesian veins carry the balance of the coronary venous blood directly into the four cardiac chambers.

In normal hearts there is little blood flow through the numerous intercoronary collateral vessels because there are no significant pressure gradients between regional arterial beds. However, these collaterals can become a source of blood flow to an ischemic region of the myocardium when a significant coronary artery obstruction alters local flow dynamics. Although the collateral channels are generally inadequate to compensate for an acute coronary artery occlusion, they can enlarge over time in response to progressive coronary obstruction.

Unlike blood flow to other tissues, flow to the heart decreases during systole because of partial obstruction of the coronary ostia by the opened aortic valve leaflets and to compression of blood vessels by contracting myocardium. Flow increases during diastole as aortic valve leaflets close and the myocardium relaxes. Furthermore, there may be blood flow gradients across the ventricular wall due to relatively higher wall tension toward the endocardium. During ventricular systole, subendocardial blood flow ceases whereas subepicardial blood flow is markedly reduced. During diastole, blood flow is greater to the subendocardium. The net result is uniform perfusion to all regions of the normal myocardium.[7]

The metabolic needs of the myocardium are the primary regulators of coronary blood flow. Cardiac muscle requires relatively large amounts of energy because it is constantly contracting. The major source of energy is adenosine triphosphate (ATP) generated by oxidative metabolism in mitochondria, which constitute one third of myocyte mass. During periods of ischemia, ATP can be produced anaerobically by glycolysis, but this inefficient process cannot sustain the heart for an extended period of time.

The heart requires large quantities of oxygen. It is estimated that the heart, which comprises only 0.2% of the body by weight, accounts for approximately 4% of the total body oxygen consumption. Even the resting heart extracts much of the available oxygen delivered by coronary blood flow. Compared with most other organ systems, which extract less than 50% of the oxygen in arterial blood, myocardial oxygen extraction often exceeds 70% and may increase to 80% during exercise. Given this high baseline oxygen extraction, any inotropic or chronotropic stimulus that increases myocardial metabolic activity and oxygen consumption soon forces the heart to rely on coronary vasodilatation and increased myocardial blood flow to ensure adequate oxygen delivery. Hence the heart is particularly vulnerable to occlusive arterial disease.

Many factors can induce regional or global coronary vasodilation. Among the most potent stimuli are myocardial ischemia and hypoxia, which cause increases in hydrogen and potassium ions, carbon dioxide, and adenosine levels. Myocardial hypoxia also leads to the local release of vasodilators such as bradykinins and prostaglandins. Endogenous neurotransmitter substances such as acetylcholine, epinephrine, and norepinephrine all result in complex fluctuations of coronary vasoconstriction and dilatation, as determined by overall physiologic activity and metabolic demand.

Pathogenesis of Ischemic Heart Disease

Ischemic heart disease is a result of inadequate coronary artery blood flow. The underlying pathologic mechanism in virtually all cases is fixed atherosclerotic narrowing of the coronary arteries. Intermittent coronary arterial vasospasm may play a role in acute myocardial infarctions by further reducing regional coronary flow and predisposing to thrombosis. The obstructing lesion, the atheromatous plaque, is a subintimal collection of cholesterol and its esters (atheroma) with a fibrous cap of collagen fibers intermixed with smooth muscle fibers. Extracellular material such as collagen, proteoglycans, elastic fibers, calcium or calcium crystals, and inflammatory cells may also be present in the plaque.

The cause of plaque formation is not completely understood. The most widely accepted theory proposes that factors such as turbulent blood flow and immunologic or infectious processes cause injury to the endothelial surface, where platelets aggregate and release platelet-derived growth factor and other substances that stimulate the migration and proliferation of smooth muscle cells, which in turn result in the deposition of collagen, elastic fibers, and proteoglycans. The altered intima is more permeable to lipoproteins, which accumulate in the subintimal area. Eventually, with repeated endothelial surface injury, a fibrous plaque forms. Diets high in cholesterol may accelerate the progression to atherosclerotic plaque formation.

Atherosclerotic lesions typically form in the proximal third to half of large coronary arteries, often at or just beyond branching points. These lesions are most common in the main trunks of the LAD and the right and circumflex arteries and their main branches. Disease of the distal vessels and intramyocardial arterioles is less common. This proximal pattern of coronary arterial involvement in atherosclerosis makes bypass grafting of obstructed coronary arteries efficacious in most instances.

Table 16-1   Risk Factors for Coronary Artery Disease

Family history
Hyperlipidemia
Hypertension
Cigarette smoking
Male gender
Menopause/oral contraceptive agents
Diabetes mellitus
Obesity
Personality type/behavior pattern
Sedentary lifestyle
Excessive alcohol intake

Hypercholesterolemia, whether caused by a genetic predisposition or by excessive intake, is strongly associated with coronary artery disease, as are elevated levels of low-density lipoproteins and decreased levels of high-density lipoproteins[2] (Table 16-1). Other risk factors include untreated hypertension, cigarette smoking, diabetes mellitus, a positive family history, peripheral vascular disease, and obesity. Although male gender is associated with a much higher risk up to late middle age, thereafter the difference between genders quickly disappears.

Clinical Syndromes

Angina Pectoris

Angina pectoris is the pain caused by myocardial ischemia and is classically described as a heavy, often crushing substernal chest pain that is precipitated by physical exertion and relieved promptly by rest. The pain often radiates to the left shoulder, arm, or side of the neck or face. By definition, the ischemia that causes angina pectoris is reversible and results in no myocardial cell necrosis.

There are two broad clinical types of angina with variable causes. Stable angina pectoris consistently occurs with exertion and is relieved quickly by rest and/or nitroglycerin; it is generally due to fixed atherosclerotic narrowing of coronary arteries. Unstable angina, also referred to as Prinzmetal's, variant, or atypical angina, often occurs spontaneously, even when the patient is at rest. It is thought to result from coronary arterial spasm in association with a fixed intraluminal lesion. Such spasm may be mediated by the autonomic nervous system, by local platelet-derived vasoconstrictive agents such as serotonin or thromboxane, or by smooth muscle irritation caused by material in adjacent plaques. Symptomatic coronary artery spasm without demonstrable atherosclerotic disease is relatively rare.

The clinical presentation of patients with angina pectoris varies considerably. The diagnosis of myocardial ischemia may be suggested by typical symptoms of angina pectoris, but it must be confirmed by documentation of electrocardiographic changes of ischemia during chest pain or exercise testing, with further confirmation of coronary obstructive disease provided by radionuclide scanning of the heart or by coronary angiography (Fig. 16-2). The differential diagnosis includes esophagitis secondary to gastrointestinal reflux, peptic ulcer disease, biliary colic, visceral artery ischemia, pericarditis, pleurisy, thoracic aortic dissection, and a variety of musculoskeletal disorders. In some persons so-called angina equivalents develop with the onset of myocardial ischemia such as shortness of breath caused by a sudden reduction in ventricular contractility, whereas others have episodes of "silent" or asymptomatic myocardial ischemia, which can be documented only by continuous electrocardiogram (ECG) monitoring.

Myocardial Infarction

Prolonged myocardial ischemia eventually leads to irreversible injury and cell death. The myocardium ceases to contract as early as 10 or 15 seconds after the onset of ischemia as a result of depletion of high-energy phosphate compounds and oxidative metabolism shifts to less efficient anaerobic glycolysis within 15 to 30 seconds after the onset of ischemia. The absence of tissue washout during ischemia causes accumulation of glycolytic end products (including carbon dioxide, hydrogen ions, and lactate) and falling intracellular pH, which eventually inhibit even glycolysis. Accumulating products of high-energy phosphate metabolism and of glycolysis increase the intracellular osmotic load and lead to cell swelling, which together with elevated intracellular calcium, decreased protein synthesis, and activation of lytic enzymes damage cell membranes, with eventual rupture and cell death.

Diagnosis of acute myocardial infarction is based on the clinical history of the patient, the presence of ECG changes, and elevation

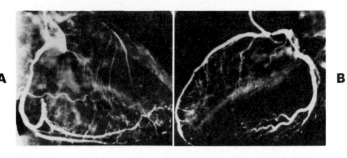

Fig. 16-2 Right and left coronary angiograms. *(A),* Right coronary injection faintly fills LAD coronary artery system through septal collateral channels, suggesting major obstruction of LAD. *(B),* Left coronary artery injection in left lateral projection demonstrates very tight obstructing lesion in proximal part of LAD coronary artery.

of specific serum enzyme levels. Typically the patient has severe crushing chest pain, which may radiate to the left shoulder, arm, or face and which is often accompanied by nausea, diaphoresis, and/or shortness of breath. Transmural infarction produces acute ST segment elevations on ECG. Later the ST segments return to baseline levels and T wave inversions may appear; finally new Q waves appear. ECG changes of a subendocardial infarction usually include ST wave depression and T wave inversions acutely; Q waves do not develop. The myocardial creatine kinase isoenzyme CK-MB, the most specific serum marker of myocardial cell injury, appears in the blood a few hours after infarction and peaks at 8 to 24 hours after infarction.

Acute complications of myocardial infarction

Arrhythmias and cardiogenic shock

Within hours of an acute myocardial infarction 20% of patients have sudden cardiac death, presumably from ventricular fibrillation. In the majority of survivors some form of arrhythmia or conduction defect develops. There is little clinical evidence to demonstrate that emergency coronary artery bypass grafting effectively reverses the patient's arrhythmic tendency.

When 40% or more of the left ventricle infarcts acutely, cardiogenic shock usually ensues. The mortality rate associated with postinfarction cardiogenic shock is high, but again the effectiveness of surgical revascularization for cardiogenic shock has not been demonstrated.[11]

Free wall or ventricular septal rupture

The greatest risk of free wall or septal rupture occurs within the first 10 days after acute myocardial infarction, when maximal necrosis of the infarcted myocardium causes the infarcted ventricular wall or septum to become thin. Any factor that increases ventricular wall tension, such as abrupt rises in preload or afterload, predisposes to ventricular rupture. Ventricular free wall rupture almost invariably results in a massive hemopericardium, severe tamponade, and sudden death. Rupture of the interventricular septum, which occurs in approximately 1% of patients after infarction, usually causes a sudden hemodynamic decompensation but is rarely the cause of sudden death; an unrepaired defect is, however, associated with high mortality rates of about 50% at 1 week and more than 80% at 2 months.

Clinically the patient with a postinfarct ventricular septal defect manifests the immediate onset of congestive heart failure and often cardiogenic shock. Right-sided heart catheterization demonstrates right ventricular and pulmonary artery pressure elevations caused by left-to-right shunting, with abnormally high oxygen tension and saturation in the pulmonary artery or mixed venous blood. Diagnosis is facilitated with transesophageal echocardiography (TEE). Surgical intervention is nearly always necessary because these patients do not stabilize with medical treatment alone.[6] Early repair of a necrotic ventricular septal defect, however, can be difficult technically, with surgical failure caused by disruption of the repair or by extension of the defect fairly common.

Mitral regurgitation

Acute mitral valve incompetence may develop as a result of papillary muscle dysfunction or rupture; the majority of cases involve a posteroinferior myocardial infarction resulting in necrosis of the posterior papillary muscle. The mortality rate in this group is high, with 70% of patients dying within 24 hours after the onset of mitral regurgitation and a 90% mortality rate without surgery within 2 weeks. The clinical presentations of such patients are similar to those of patients with acute septal rupture. Rapid hemodynamic deterioration, acute left ventricular failure, pulmonary edema, and cardiogenic shock are present. Right heart catheterization in these patients, however, although frequently demon-strating elevated right ventricular and pulmonary artery pressures, does not show an increase in oxygen saturation in the right ventricle or pulmonary arteries. There is usually marked elevation of the pulmonary capillary wedge pressure with prominent V waves. TEE obviates the need for left-sided ventriculography. Although the patient's condition occasionally can be improved or even stabilized with medical management, including the use of the intraaortic balloon pump, surgical repair or replacement of the valve is almost always required and is the definitive treatment of this condition.

Chronic complications of myocardial infarction

Left ventricular aneurysm

In up to 10% of patients after major acute myocardial infarctions the infarcted area of ventricular wall develops a localized aneu-rysm. More than 80% of these aneurysms result from anterolateral transmural infarctions caused by a proximal LAD coronary artery occlusion. Small aneurysms measuring less than 5 cm in diameter generally are of no functional significance, but larger aneurysms can exhibit dyskinetic ventricular wall motion, which increases wall stress in adjacent regions and dissipates the work of ventricular contractions.

In patients with evolving left ventricular aneurysms progres-sively worsening left ventricular failure often develops and conges-tive heart failure or angina secondary to the increased work demand in the uninvolved area of the heart may be present. Other com-plications include systemic emboli and recurrent ventricular ar-rhythmias.

A left-sided ventriculogram can demonstrate the dyskinetic movement of the aneurysmal portion of the ventricular wall and the presence of mural thrombus. Surgical resection of the aneurysm is mandated most often by intractable congestive heart failure, and by recurrent ventricular arrhythmias or systemic emboli. Surgical resection is optimally performed 2 months or later after infarction to allow for scar maturation and better delineation of the true margins of the aneurysm.

Chronic Ischemic Cardiomyopathy and Congestive Heart Failure

Many patients have during the course of years a series of smaller, individually less debilitating infarctions that lead to chronic heart failure. A gradual increase in left ventricular end-diastolic pressure increases subendocardial wall tension, further compromising coronary perfusion in that area. With progressively worsening coronary obstructive disease, the patient often manifests episodic ventricular failure associated with recurrent episodes of myocardial ischemia.

Although these patients frequently have impaired left ventricular function, surgical revascularization is often indicated to avoid recurrent episodes of heart failure associated with ischemia in still-viable portions of the heart. In patients with so-called hibernating myocardium, that is, viable portions of the heart that contract poorly because of insufficient blood flow,[15] ventricular failure often improves dramatically with surgical reperfusion. Preoperative prediction of improvement may be difficult, but in general those with recurring heart failure and reversible ischemic episodes benefit from coronary artery bypass surgery.

In another subgroup of patients the syndrome of ischemic cardiomyopathy develops. Such patients often have diffuse ventricular wall scarring and fibrosis, the result of slow but progressive limitation of coronary blood flow to the myocardium. These patients have worsening cardiomegaly and chronic congestive heart failure, and may or may not have angina pectoris. This condition may be more common in patients with diffuse distal coronary arterial disease or in those with small-vessel disease, as occurs in many patients with severe diabetes mellitus. These patients generally do not benefit from coronary revascularization because of the extensive myocardial dysfunction or because of diffuse small-vessel coronary artery disease.

In surgical candidates it is important to demonstrate the reversibility of myocardial perfusion defects. A "stress" thallium study is a sensitive method of identifying reversibly ischemic myocardial tissue. This study uses thallium 201, a radioactive potassium analogue, which is taken up by normal myocytes in proportion to the regional flow and metabolic activity.[10] Relatively decreased perfusion with exercise, correlated with angina or reduced ventricular wall contractility, suggests good potential for improvement with surgical revascularization.

Estimates of left ventricular function can be obtained with multiple-uptake gated acquisition scanning (MUGA)[13] or echocardiography. MUGA scans together with exercise stress testing can demonstrate regional and global left ventricular dysfunction, and

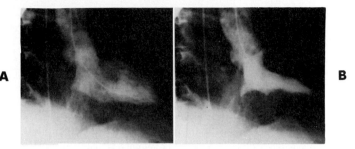

A

B

Fig. 16-3 Left ventriculograms in right anterior-oblique view at end-diastole *(A)* and end-systole *(B)*.

decreases in ejection fraction accompanying exercise-induced ischemia. Echocardiography is a commonly used alternative, although it is not as quantitatively accurate as MUGA scanning techniques to evaluate left ventricular function, ejection fraction, and abnormal wall motion noninvasively.

Cardiac catheterization is usually necessary to define coronary anatomy and the extent of atherosclerosis, and to define further left ventricular function and contractility. The degree of coronary stenosis is conventionally estimated as a percent reduction in luminal diameter compared with the diameter of normal adjacent segments of artery. A left-sided ventriculogram provides an estimate of ejection fraction by comparing end-systolic and end-diastolic volumes (Fig. 16-3).

Medical Treatment of Ischemic Heart Disease

The rationale for pharmacologic intervention in coronary artery disease is to improve coronary blood flow and/or decrease myocardial oxygen demands. Three classes of drugs are commonly used to treat coronary artery disease: nitrates, β-adrenergic blockers, and calcium channel blockers.

Nitrates cause vasodilatation of vascular smooth muscle, primarily in venous capacitance vessels, but at higher doses also in systemic arterioles. Nitrates may result in some dilatation of the coronary arterioles and improvement in collateral blood flow in patients with extensive atherosclerotic disease. However, the primary benefit of nitrates appears to be the reduction of myocardial oxygen demand by reducing ventricular work. Dilatation of venous capacitance vessels and systemic arterioles lowers ventricular filling pressures, wall stress, and afterload. Similarly, the primary benefit of β-*adrenergic* blockers is also a reduction in myocardial oxygen demand by decreasing both cardiac contractility and heart rate. Adrenergic blockers may also reduce blood pressure and systemic vascular resistance, further reducing the work of the heart. *Calcium channel blockers* have more complex cardiac and vascular effects, including reduction in ventricular contractility, variable degrees of vasodilatation, and possibly some direct protection of hypoxic myocytes. Calcium channel blockers may be particularly effective in those patients with a component of coronary vasospastic disease. It is unclear whether the use of these drugs affects the progression of atherosclerotic disease.

Management of acute myocardial infarction now also includes the use of newly developed *thrombolytic agents* to lyse the occluding arterial blood clot. Streptokinase, urokinase, or recombinant tissue plasminogen activator is administered intravenously or directly into the involved coronary artery as soon as possible after diagnosis of acute myocardial infarction. If administered early enough in the course of infarct evolution, such agents can result in recanalization of the occluded artery with salvage of ischemic myocardium at risk of infarction. Clinical trials of thrombolytic agents have demonstrated improved survival rates after an acute myocardial infarction.[5] The use of thrombolytic therapy may result in bleeding complications if the patient requires surgical intervention within hours after administration of these agents.

Percutaneous Transluminal Coronary Angioplasty

Since the 1970s balloon dilatation catheters have been used to dilate discrete coronary arterial stenotic lesions. With increasing experience the presence of multivessel coronary artery disease or even complex coronary arterial obstructive lesions is no longer an absolute contraindication for percutaneous transluminal coronary angioplasty (PTCA). It is generally accepted that PTCA should be considered for medically intractable angina pectoris caused by a significant stenosis of one major coronary artery or for patients with a favorable pattern of coronary occlusive disease involving more than one coronary artery. Whether PTCA is superior to coronary artery bypass grafting (CABG) in patients with more complicated multivessel coronary artery disease remains controversial. In general, PTCA is contraindicated if significant disease is in the left main coronary artery, if the target coronary artery is less than 2 mm in luminal diameter, if multiple significant obstructive lesions are in the same artery, or if there are complex obstructive lesions such as those involving or straddling arterial bifurcations.

Initial success rates of angioplasty in large series exceeds 90%. About 2% to 4% of patients require emergency or urgent CABG for acute ischemic problems, an equal number of patients have myocardial infarction, and in about 5% of patients some arrhythmia develops during or immediately after dilatation, thereby requiring electrical cardioversion.

The most significant problem with PTCA to date is the relatively high incidence of restenosis, which has been defined as a 50% or greater reduction of the initial dilatation. Restenosis is likely the result of postdilatation proliferation of intimal and smooth muscle cells in response to the angioplasty. Restenosis rates of between 30% and 40% within the first 4 to 6 months after PTCA have been reported in patients with initially successful dilatation for simple lesions and has been reported to be as high as 60% for patients with complex lesions that have required multiple dilatations. Although redilatation or recurrent stenotic lesions can be carried out successfully, many of these patients ultimately require CABG.

The 5-year survival rate in one large series was 96%; patients with single vessel disease had generally better results than those with complex multivessel disease. The repeated angioplasty rate was 19% within 5 years, with 15% of patients having coronary bypass surgery.[12]

Surgical Treatment of Coronary Artery Disease

Indications

Atherosclerotic lesions that narrow the lumen of an artery by at least 40% to 50% are generally considered significant. Obstructions of greater than 70% do not permit increases in blood flow distally despite maximal coronary vasodilatation. Patients are referred to as having single-, double-, or triple-vessel disease according to the number of major coronary arteries (LAD, circumflex, and right coronary arteries) involved. Data from clinical trials and retrospective studies suggest that as the number of diseased major coronary arteries increases, the greater the survival benefit of surgical therapy over medical therapy alone.[4,9,16] For example, the presence of severe proximal triple-vessel coronary artery disease, especially in patients with impaired left ventricular function, is an indication for surgical revascularization.

A well-accepted indication for CABG is significant stenosis of the left main coronary artery. Two major studies provide evidence for improved survival with surgical treatment of left main disease.[4,9] Similarly, stenosis of the proximal LAD artery is a relative indication for surgical treatment.[16] The need for surgery in patients with single- or double-vessel disease and adequate left ventricular function has not been clearly established. Patients with mild angina and single-vessel disease benefit no more in terms of survival than medical versus surgical treatment.

Unstable angina

Patients with unstable angina, defined as severe angina at rest accompanied by ischemic ECG changes that last for more than 15 minutes, have variable onset and progression of symptoms. In general, the occurrence of unstable or crescendo angina suggests that the patient is at risk for myocardial infarction and death. These patients may require aggressive medical treatment including ECG monitoring, effective vasodilator and β-adrenergic blocker therapy, and heparin anticoagulation to forestall coronary arterial thrombosis. If the patient continues to have unstable or rest angina despite such medical treatment, urgent coronary angiography is indicated and the patient often will require PTCA or surgery. The collective outcome data from several series of patients with unstable angina who underwent surgical revascularization demonstrated increased rates of perioperative myocardial infarction, postoperative low cardiac output, and death compared with patients having CABG for chronic stable angina. However, for patients with unstable angina late outcome after CABG was similar to that in patients with chronic stable angina in that relief of angina was excellent, the late myocardial infarction rate was low, and, most important, short- and long-term survival rates were similar. In general, CABG in patients with unstable angina remains a relatively safe procedure, even in this higher-risk patient group and is certainly indicated when medical therapy fails to alleviate worsening myocardial ischemia.

Acute myocardial ischemia or infarction

Coronary artery surgery for salvage of infarcting myocardium has been largely abandoned because of a high operative mortality rate in patients with evolving myocardial infarction and cardiogenic shock. There is little evidence of benefit with surgical therapy in this situation. Recently, thrombolytic agents have been used successfully to provide rapid reperfusion of ischemic myocardium. Clinical use has clearly demonstrated that thrombolytic therapy can salvage myocardium at risk, improve ventricular function, and increase early survival rate.

Although the role for CABG in the setting of acute myocardial infarction does not appear to be clear, the development of recurrent angina early after infarction has become an accepted indication for PTCA or surgical revascularization. A significant number of patients who have an acute myocardial infarction have postinfarction angina, either because of recurrent ischemia in the infarct region or because of ischemia in other areas of the heart. These patients are at risk for infarct extension or for a second infarction. Patients who have postinfarction angina and do not undergo revascularization have a 1-year mortality rate of 17% to 50%. CABG is clearly indicated in this group because of the presence of multivessel disease.

Left ventricular dysfunction

Myocardial revascularization can markedly improve ventricular function, and occasionally patients with very poor preoperative heart function derive the most benefit from bypass surgery. Severe ventricular dysfunction with ejection fraction as low as 15% to 20% is no longer an absolute contraindication to bypass surgery. It can be difficult to predict, however, which patients with poor left ventricular function clearly benefit from surgery, because it is often difficult to distinguish fixed from reversible left ventricular dysfunction.

The concept of stunned myocardium has been developed to explain reversible left ventricular dysfunction that accompanies acute myocardial ischemia or infarction.[14] In addition, the term *hibernating myocardium* has been used recently to describe ventricular dysfunction secondary to inadequate coronary flow even in the absence of ECG changes or anginal symptoms.[1] In patients with hibernating myocardium atherosclerotic obstructive lesions appear to limit coronary blood flow into the ischemic regions during exercise and cause a reduction in regional or even global left ventricular function. Radionuclide scanning during exercise is a useful method of evaluating the potential for improved ventricular function after revascularization. Exercise stress thallium testing identifies poorly functioning ischemic areas as exercise-induced perfusion defects. Surgical revascularization improves the contractile function of hibernating and stunned myocardium, whereas little functional benefit is derived from revascularization of extensively scarred or infarcted myocardium.

Another technique for the identification of reversible ventricular dysfunction is the assessment of postextrasystolic potentiation of contractility. The degree of augmentation in regional function that occurs after a premature ventricular contraction can be used as a predictor of the reversibility of wall motion abnormalities after coronary revascularization.

Although most patients with chronic congestive heart failure resulting from long-standing ischemic heart disease may not derive functional benefit from revascularization, that subset of patients in which intermittent congestive failure associated with myocardial ischemia develops is often improved by revascularization. Like patients with hibernating myocardium, these patients with intermittent ventricular dysfunction are appropriate candidates for CABG. In more advanced cases of chronic congestive heart failure, however, surgery is rarely effective in improving ventricular function.

Indications for Emergency Coronary Artery Bypass Surgery

Angina at rest, unstable angina progressively worsening despite medical therapy, and postinfarct angina likewise all require urgent surgical intervention. In patients with completed acute myocardial infarction, emergency surgery may be indicated for acute mechanical complications such as ruptured ventricular septum or papillary muscle but is rarely effective as a primary treatment of cardiogenic shock associated with massive infarction.

Emergency CABG is necessary in most patients in whom coronary occlusive complications develop during PTCA. The majority of these occlusions result from coronary artery dissections proximal or distal to the site of dilatation starting at an intimal defect caused by the guide wire or by balloon dilatation. Ischemic injury can be attenuated and greater hemodynamic stability provided as needed by intraaortic balloon counterpulsation established promptly in the catheterization laboratory before transport to the operating room. Severe instability despite balloon pump support may require portable cardiopulmonary bypass support with peripheral cannulation for transport to the operating room and subsequent initiation of full cardiopulmonary bypass support with central cannulation. In general, one should attempt to give these patients cardiopulmonary bypass support as quickly as possible and to initiate cardioplegic arrest and myocardial cooling to reduce further extension of the infarction.

The condition of some patients who sustain PTCA complications can be stabilized by repeated dilatation of the coronary occlusion or by placement of a so-called bailout catheter across the site of complete obstruction and/or dissection. Although these maneuvers may abort the myocardial infarction that begins at the time of initial artery occlusion, the patient remains in a precarious situation and generally requires urgent or emergent CABG to avoid reinitiation of the infarction process.

The operative mortality rate associated with emergency revascularization in the PTCA failure group has been greater than the operative mortality rate even in urgently operated patients, emphasizing the fact that despite surgery undertaken early in the course of infarct evolution, the presence of an infarction increases operative risk. Likewise, the operative mortality rate associated with repair of mechanical defects in patients after acute myocardial infarction with or without CABG is substantial, reflecting both the complexity of the surgical repair and the patient's poor status preoperatively.

Operative Techniques

The standard operative technique for most open heart procedures is discussed in Chapter 4. The sequence of coronary arterial grafting varies considerably and is dictated by several considerations. These include the individual surgeon's myocardial protection strategy, the grafts to be implanted, the types of conduits to be used, and whether additional procedures are to be performed. If the surgeon relies on reinfusion cardioplegia during distal artery grafting, the most critically obstructed coronary artery will likely be grafted first to allow for early, direct cardioplegic solution administration into this distal arterial bed. The surgeon who relies on topical myocardial cooling with continuous cold saline solution infusion is likely to perform anastomoses to circumflex branches later in the cross-clamp period because these distal anastomoses necessitate elevation of the heart out of the pericardium and less efficient contact between the heart and the pericardial saline bath. Mammary artery anastomoses are generally performed late in the cross-clamp period because an attached mammary pedicle to either the right or left coronary artery limits manipulation of the heart.

Anastomotic techniques vary considerably. Most surgeons perform coronary artery grafting with $2.5\times$ to $4.5\times$ magnification, generally with loupes. Monofilament sutures are used by most surgeons, with continuous or interrupted anastomosis. In addition to individual vein or mammary artery graft anastomoses to specific arterial branches (Fig. 16-4), two or more distal anastomoses can be constructed from a single graft. These "in-continuity" or "skip" grafts are especially favored in situations where multiple distal sites require grafting or when there is a shortage of suitable conduit material. In addition, the construction of multiple distal anastomoses with mammary artery grafts, although limited somewhat by the length of the artery pedicle, can be performed when there is severe disease of the ascending aorta, which precludes safe placement of aortosaphenous vein anastomoses.

After the distal anastomoses are completed, the aortic and/or mammary artery clamp is released and coronary flow reestablished. A fibrillating heart can be cardioverted with a single direct-current electrical shock. The proximal aortosaphenous vein graft anastomoses can then be constructed as myocardial perfusion is maintained, by placement of a partially occluding clamp on the left or right lateral aspect of the ascending aorta, around the anastomotic site. Small aortotomies 4 to 5 mm in diameter are constructed, and after the lengths of the individual vein grafts are appropriately sized, the proximal anastomoses are constructed with monofilament suture. Blood flow is then established through the grafts into the distal coronary arteries and the patient is subsequently prepared

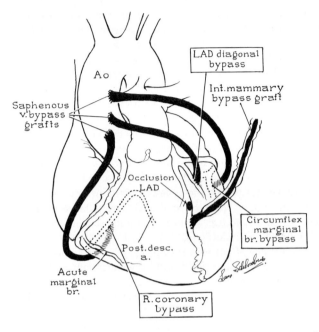

Fig. 16-4 Saphenous vein and IMA bypass grafts to coronary arteries.

for separation from bypass. Final stages of the operative procedure include removal of the cardiopulmonary bypass perfusion cannulas, reversal of the systemic heparinization with protamine, surgical hemostasis, and wound closure.

Most patients requiring multiple CABG have 30 minutes or more of complete myocardial ischemia and require at least an hour of cardiopulmonary bypass. For complex operations, especially those involving an additional procedure, such as repair of ventricular aneurysm, cardiac ischemia time can exceed 2 hours and cardiopulmonary bypass time can exceed 3 hours.

Selection of conduits for grafting

Clinical follow-up series compellingly demonstrate improved long-term patency and survival times for patients receiving internal mammary artery (IMA) grafts compared with saphenous vein grafts. It is increasingly clear from late follow-up studies that late vein graft occlusions develop at a predictable rate in many patients. On the basis of these data, the IMA is being used increasingly as the conduit of choice. Extended use of the mammary arteries, either as pedicle grafts or free grafts, or for multiple distal anastomoses, has been advocated by many experienced surgical groups, although convincing evidence to support such use is not available.

The preferred use of the mammary artery is as a pedicle graft, but either mammary artery can be used as a free graft to compensate for subclavian artery obstruction or insufficient graft length. In the latter case the free mammary artery can be anastomosed directly to the ascending aorta or to the proximal portion of a saphenous vein graft. Other arterial conduits include free radial artery, free or pedicled gastroepiploic artery, and free inferior epigastric artery grafts. Late patency of free radial artery grafts has been disappointing, and it is unclear whether other arterial segments used as free grafts will fail as quickly.

The poor rate of late vein graft patency is difficult to explain. Severe atherosclerotic changes, with or without native artery disease progression typically develops in the vein graft. This occurs with greater frequency and severity in patients poorly compliant with coronary risk factor reduction. The use of preoperative dipyridamole and postoperative aspirin has been demonstrated to reduce postoperative saphenous vein graft occlusion.

Other coronary graft conduits have included cryopreserved saphenous veins from cadaver donors and small-caliber synthetic grafts such as expanded polytetrafluorethylene. Cryopreserved vein grafts harvested from cadavers have not been used widely but appear to have high early and midterm occlusion rates. Likewise, synthetic grafts appear to be very susceptible to thrombosis.

Coronary endarterectomy

An important factor affecting late graft patency appears to be the rate of blood flow through the graft. Assuming no technical problems with the proximal aortic and distal coronary artery anastomoses and no obstruction caused by twisting or conduit injury during harvest, graft blood flow is determined by the size and quality of the distal artery bed. Extensive atherosclerotic disease of the distal coronary artery may dictate endarterectomy to allow more reliable graft-artery anastomosis and to improve blood flow into the distal arterial bed. The atherosclerotic core with arterial intima and media can be separated from the surrounding outer

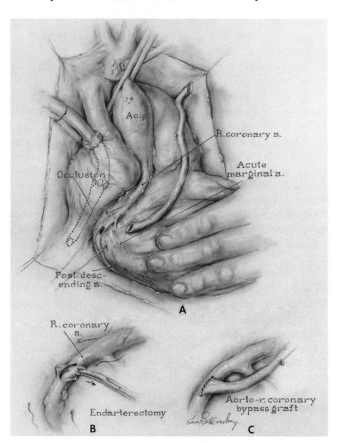

Fig. 16-5 Endarterectomy and coronary bypass. Obstruction of right coronary artery *(A)* is partially removed by endarterectomy *(B)* and vessel bypassed with saphenous vein graft *(C)*.

muscular wall and adventitia. The surgeon can choose direct dissection of the atherosclerotic plaque through a long longitudinal-arteriotomy or extraction in one piece of a long segment of the plaque through a short arteriotomy (Fig. 16-5). The former technique is favored for the LAD coronary artery, whereas the latter is most useful in larger, severely diseased right coronary arteries.

Data are conflicting regarding the safety and efficacy of coronary endarterectomy. Endarterectomy of the distal right coronary artery, which is the most common site of endarterectomy, appears to be relatively safe and well tolerated, presumably in part because the right coronary artery is very often nearly totally occluded when an endarterectomy is carried out. Collateralization is often present. Endarterectomy sites are widely believed to be more prone to early thrombosis and reocclusion, hence most of these patients are prescribed low doses of aspirin or other antiplatelet medication. Data regarding the long-term comparative value of endarterectomy on the LAD coronary artery versus grafting alone are not available. Endarterectomy is reserved for patients with such severe distal disease that it is necessary to open and decorticate long segments of the LAD to have any expectation of distal flow. Because patients with diffuse distal disease are already prone to poor outcome, it may prove difficult to demonstrate a beneficial effect with coronary endarterectomy, either in the short or the long term.

Ventricular aneurysm

An aneurysm of the ventricular wall is invariably a result of a major transmural myocardial infarction with progressive aneurysmal ballooning of the infarct scar. Scar maturation occurs over weeks to months, and at the end of this period a ventricular aneurysm has easily identifiable margins of scar-myocardial interface. However, before full scar maturation, especially early after acute myocardial infarction, it can be difficult to determine the precise margins for ventricular wall resection and it may prove to be troublesome to close the ventriculotomy securely.

Before cardiopulmonary bypass the heart is minimally manipulated to prevent embolization of any mural thrombus. Any pericardial adhesions are dissected after cardiopulmonary bypass is begun, and the heart is inspected before aortic cross-clamping. Once the margins of the aneurysm have been identified, the scarred area is opened near its center and the intracavity thrombus removed. Generally, the aneurysm is excised, leaving about a 2-cm rim of fibrous scar tissue (Fig. 16-6). Secure ventriculotomy closure may require felt strips or pledgets to reinforce the suture line. Occasionally, direct closure of the ventriculotomy distorts the ventricular geometry or reduces residual ventricular volume so much that it is necessary to incorporate a synthetic prosthetic patch in the ventricular closure. The left ventricle requires careful deairing before weaning from cardiopulmonary bypass.

If a ventricular septal defect is present in conjunction with an aneurysm, a synthetic prosthetic patch, usually a polyester or Teflon patch, can be used to close the defect. If the infarct scar is mature, the septal or free wall patch can be sewn directly to viable margins of myocardium; however, with a recent acute infarct, pledgetted sutures should be placed 1 to 3 cm beyond the margins of necrotic myocardium in viable tissue for reinforcement.

Risk Factors Affecting Surgical Outcome

Among the many factors that affect outcome after CABG are the patient's state of health and the potential for complete revascularization. A CABG procedure in which revascularization is incomplete because of either severe distal coronary artery disease or inadequate conduits for bypass grafting is associated with a higher operative mortality rate and uncertain long-term outcome. Likewise, patients with concurrent medical problems, such as cerebrovascular, pulmonary, or renal insufficiency, are much more likely to sustain additional complications during coronary bypass surgery and carry a higher operative risk.

The primary factor that affects outcome after bypass surgery is the preoperative status of left ventricular function. As noted previously, it may be difficult to distinguish reversible left ventricular dysfunction from that which is irreversible. Operative risk is increased also when the patient requires any additional operative intervention, such as valve procedures. Furthermore, when left ventricular dysfunction is not improved by bypass grafting or when mitral valve replacement or ventricular plication are required because of complications of previous infarction, long-term outlook is noticeably worsened.

Elderly patients undergoing CABG have higher rates of morbidity and mortality. In one large study from the late 1970s, operative mortality in patients 70 years or older was nearly 8% compared with an overall estimated mortality rate in younger patients of about 3%. Recent studies emphasize the finding that much of the higher mortality rate among the elderly is due not to cardiac failure but to complications such as stroke, respiratory failure, renal failure, or sepsis. Nevertheless, there is a significant benefit in the late survival rate for patients older than 70 years who undergo successful bypass surgery.[8] Although age is an incremental risk factor for early death after coronary bypass surgery, advanced age should not be considered a contraindication to surgery.

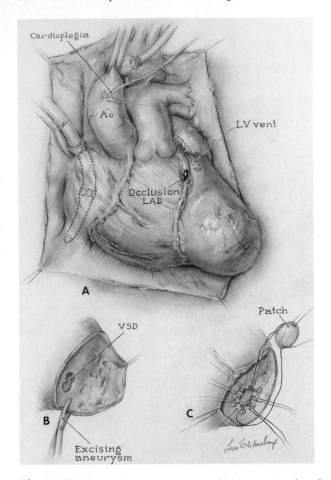

Fig. 16-6 Left ventricular aneurysm repair. Aneurysm arises from infarction of myocardium in territory of occluded coronary artery, here, the LAD *(A)*. Aneurysm is excised *(B)*, and any postinfarct ventricular septal defect *(VSD)* is repaired with prosthetic patch *(C and D)*. Teflon strips are used to buttress mural repair *(E and F)*.

The influence of the patient's gender on surgical outcome is less clear, despite several early reports suggesting a higher operative risk for women. This higher risk appears to be attributable to a greater prevalence of commonly accepted surgical risk factors, such as advanced age and severity of the anginal syndrome, in

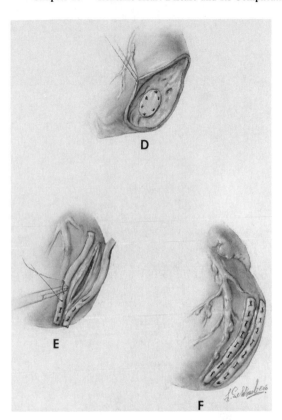

Fig. 16-6 cont'd.

women compared with men. It appears that long-term survival rates are similar for both groups despite a slightly lower vein graft patency rate and greater recurrence of angina in women.[3]

Other factors that are associated with an increase in the operative risk but that are not contraindications for bypass surgery include renal insufficiency, diabetes mellitus, peripheral vascular disease, cerebral vascular disease, respiratory insufficiency, and obesity. Most of these conditions are also associated with premature or accelerated atherosclerosis and a high incidence of generalized cardiovascular disease caused by hypertension, hyperlipidemia, and abnormal carbohydrate metabolism. Patients with end-stage renal disease have an increased operative morbidity rate, often due to bleeding and infection, and an increased mortality rate of at least 3% or 4%. Successful CABG, however, has been shown to improve the 5-year survival rate compared with other patients with end-stage renal disease. Furthermore, those patients with a functioning kidney transplant graft do better, in general, than patients requiring long-term hemodialysis.

Diabetic patients may have a similar operative mortality rate to nondiabetic patients, but infection risk is higher and long-term survival is poorer, with an estimated excess mortality rate of at least 1% per year when compared with nondiabetic patients. The severity of the diabetes at the time of operation is also a determinant of long-term survival.

Reoperative CABG has become increasingly more frequent during the past several years and now accounts for more than 5% of all CABG procedures carried out in the United States. Past series reporting the results of reoperations for coronary artery disease cited higher operative mortality rates compared with those associated with primary bypass procedures. Long-term survival rate, however, was similar in those patients in whom adequate revascularization at reoperation was achieved.

Short-term and long-term results

Controlled clinial trials have convincingly shown that surgical revascularization provides significant relief of anginal symptoms. Most series show initial elimination of angina in about 90% of patients, with about 70% of patients remaining symptom-free for 1 to 3 years. In a combined series from several coronary bypass studies, 77% of the patients were free of an ischemic event (defined as recurrence of angina, myocardial infarction, or sudden death) 5 years after surgery. By 10 years postoperatively only 50% of coronary bypass patients were free of ischemic events and only 15% of patients remained free of an ischemic event 15 years postoperatively.

Postoperative cardiac function

Several studies provide evidence that CABG enhances ventricular function both in the immediate postoperative period and late after surgery. The rate of ventricular diastolic relaxation, an energy-requiring process that is impaired by myocardial ischemia and that is a preload-independent measure of function, has been shown to improve significantly in the immediate and the early postoperative period. Despite some persistent controversy about long-term functional effects, especially of systolic function, in several controlled clinical trials, functional improvement has been documented both at rest and with exercise 8 months postoperatively. Moreover, a recent study demonstrated improvement in left ventricular ejection fraction attributable to improved contractility in myocardial regions in which ischemia had been demonstrable during exercise before surgery.

Graft patency

Clinical improvement after coronary bypass surgery, including the evaluation of angina, stabilization of ventricular function, and, most important, enhanced survival depend on short-term and long-term graft patency. In one study 82% of patients with at least one graft patent 12 months postoperatively were alive 12 years after surgery compared with only 42% of patients who had no patent grafts at 12 months. Early vein graft occlusion is likely due to poor blood flow, poor coronary arterial runoff, graft injury during preparation, or faulty surgical or anastomotic technique.

The occlusion rate for saphenous vein grafts is 5% to 20% during the first postoperative year and 2% to 4% annually for the next 4 years, for an approximate occlusion rate of 22% to 30% at 5 years. The rate then doubles to 5% per year, so that after 10 years 50% of vein grafts are occluded as a result of vein graft atherosclerosis.

IMA graft patency rates are 95% at 1 year, 94% at 8 years, and 85% at 10 years. This improved IMA graft patency has been reported for both pedicle and free IMA grafts. This excellent late IMA graft patency rate clearly correlates with increased patient survival, reduced recurrence of symptoms, and fewer reoperations.

Survival

The operative mortality rate is approximately 1% to 3% in elective cases. This increases to more than 5% for patients with poor preoperative left ventricular function, probably the most important determinant of operative risk.

About 90% of primary post-CABG patients survive for 5 years, 80% survive 10 years, and about 58% survive 15 years. Use of the IMA graft improves the rate of long-term survival to 89% at 10 years.

Reoperation

Approximately one fifth of patients undergoing CABG require reoperation after 10 years. Such cases generally make up 5% to 10% of the surgical case load, and this will probably increase. Patients undergoing reoperation have at least double the operative risk of primary elective CABG patients, because average age is higher and atherosclerotic disease is more advanced. Long-term results are also not as good, because revascularization is often not as complete and symptom relief is of shorter duration. Estimates for the rate of reintervention in all patients after primary CABG are 3% at 5 years, 10% at 10 years, and 39% at 15 years.

Emergency surgery

Emergency surgery clearly increases operative morbidity and mortality rates; however, because of factors of patient selection, timing of operation, and definition of emergent surgery, variation in estimates of risk is wide. A review of emergency CABG for PTCA failure reveals an operative mortality rate range of 0% to 11% with recent studies having more consistency with rates of 2.5% to 4%. Patients with acute papillary muscle rupture and mitral insufficiency have an operative mortality rate ranging from 15% to 60%. When this is analyzed further, however, it is apparent that younger, lower-risk candidates with moderate left ventricular dysfunction and coronary artery disease have a 90% 30-day postoperative survival rate and an 80% 5-year survival rate, whereas an older high-risk group with poor ventricular function and and severe coronary artery disease has a 30-day survival rate of only 55% and a 5-year survival rate of 27%.

Increased operative risk is often outweighed by a poorer prognosis for nonsurgical treatment. Acute ventricular septal defect has an operative survival rate of approximately 45% to 65%, yet the 2-year postoperative survival rate of 84% is far better than the 85% mortality rate at 2 months seen in nonsurgical patients. Long-term survival in these patients is enhanced with concomitant CABG.

Finally, emergency procedures in patients with cardiogenic shock carry an operative mortality rate of more than 50% and is estimated to increase risk by five times that of patients without cardiogenic shock. Some investigators advocate an aggressive surgical approach with either emergent operation, mechanical circulatory support with intraaortic balloon pump or ventricular assist device, or transplantation.

Left ventricular aneurysm

Operative mortality rate for resection or plication of a left ventricular aneurysm has a wide range of 2% to 20%, with approximately 60% of the mortality resulting from cardiac causes. The highest mortality rate is seen in patients with ventricular arrhythmias, congestive heart failure, renal failure, and cardiogenic shock; left ventricular function is the best predictor of survival. The patients who survive do relatively well, with an 85% to 93% 5-year survival rate. Patients with preoperative congestive heart failure have a significant improvement in function postoperatively; however, functional improvement in patients without congestive heart failure is controversial. Patients who have CABG together with left ventricular aneurysmectomy have a better survival rate than patients who have aneurysmectomy alone, although patients who also have a ventricular septal defect and require repair have a higher operative mortality rate.

Patients who undergo left ventricular aneurysm repair have a 76% to 79% 5-year and a 67% 10-year survival rate, compared with a 70% to 75% 3-year and a 90% 5-year mortality rate in patients with aneurysms that are not surgically corrected. Recurrence of left ventricular aneurysms is rare; instead, prognosis is determined by residual left ventricular function and severity of coronary artery disease.

REFERENCES

1. Braunwald E, Rutherford JD: Reversible ischemic left ventricular dysfunction: evidence for the "hibernating myocardium," *J Am Coll Cardiol* 8:1467, 1986.
2. Daugherty A, Schonfeld G: Roles of lipoproteins in the initiation and development of atherosclerosis, *Pharmacol Ther* 31:237, 1985.
3. Gardner TJ et al: Coronary artery bypass grafting in women: a ten year perspective, *Ann Surg* 201:780, 1985.
4. Gersh BJ, Califf RM, Loop FD et al: Coronary bypass surgery in chronic stable angina, *Circulation* 79(suppl I):46, 1989.
5. Gruppo Italiano per lo Studio della Streptochi-nasi nell'Infarto miocardico (GISSI): Long-term effects of intravenous thrombolysis in acute myocardial infarction: final report of the GISSI study, *Lancet* 2:871, 1987.

6. Heitmiller R, Jacobs ML, Daggett WM: Surgical management of postinfarction ventricular septal rupture, *Ann Thorac Surg* 41:683, 1986.
7. Hoffman JIE: Transmural myocardial perfusion, *Prog Cardiovasc Dis* 29:429, 1987.
8. Horneffer PJ et al: The effects of age on outcome after coronary bypass surgery, *Circulation* (suppl V):6, 1987.
9. Hultgren H, ed: Veterans Administration cooperative study of medical versus surgical treatment for stable angina: progress report, *Prog Cardiovasc Dis* 23:213, 1985.
10. Iskandrian AS, Hakki A: Thallium-201 myocardial scintigraphy, *Am Heart J* 109:113, 1985.
11. Killip T: Cardiogenic shock complicating myocardial infarction, *J Am Coll Cardiol* 14:47, 1989.
12. King SB III, Talley JD: Coronary arteriography and percutaneous transluminal coronary angioplasty: changing patterns of use and results, *Circulation* 79(suppl I):19, 1989.
13. Lazort L et al: Use of the multiple uptake gated acquisition for the preoperative assessment of cardiac risk. *Surg Gynecol Obstet* 167:234, 1988.
14. Patel B et al: Postischemic myocardial "stunning": a clinically relevant phenomenon, *Ann Intern Med* 108:626, 1988.
15. Rahimtoola SH: The hibernating myocardium, *Am Heart J* 117:211, 1989.
16. Varnauskas E: European Coronary Surgery Study Group: twelve year follow-up of survival in the randomized European Coronary Surgery Study, *N Engl J Med* 319:332, 1988.

17

Valve Replacement and Repair

Timothy S. Hall *and Bruce* A. *Reitz*

The original successful procedures to treat mitral stenosis were performed from 1925 to 1948. Commissurotomy and valvotomy were types of reparative procedures that were performed as closed heart operations because safe cardiopulmonary bypass did not exist at that time.[3,52,103] When cardiopulmonary bypass became available in the mid 1950s, more complex valve repair procedures became feasible. In 1960, a mechanical valve of the ball-in-cage design (Starr-Edwards) came into clinical use as a valve substitute.[50] The techniques for valve repair, which were not standardized or easily reproducible, then fell into disfavor. Subsequent developments included valves of animal or human tissue and other designs for prosthetic valves, with continually improving results.[23]

However, significant problems still exist. Anticoagulation remains a lifelong requirement for mechanical valves, and valve degeneration leading to failure is still the major problem for tissue valves. The challenges presented by these limitations, together with safer cardiopulmonary bypass and myocardial preservation, have contributed to a renewed interest in valve repair. This chapter discusses valvular diseases in adults, the indications for surgery, operative techniques, and specifics of postoperative care.

General Considerations

Surgery for valvular replacement is considered palliative. The hemodynamics of patients with symptoms are usually significantly improved after valve surgery, but patients are in turn subjected to the hazards of anticoagulation or gradual failure of a tissue valve, which may require reoperation. Because of these risks, intervention is usually delayed until patients have functionally significant heart failure (New York Heart Association [NYHA] III or IV) or a life-threatening complication such as embolization. With more sophisticated testing and safer surgical techniques, the indications for valvular surgery are changing, with an emphasis toward earlier surgery in certain subgroups and the aim of preserving ventricular function or preventing pulmonary disease.

Signs and Symptoms of Valve Disease

Patients with valvular lesions report tiredness, poor exercise capabilities, and difficulty lying flat, and many have chest pain or dizziness. The signs of heart failure may be present and include the following:

- Neck vein distention
- Pulmonary rales
- Peripheral coldness
- Hepatic congestion
- Peripheral edema
- Ascites and muscle wasting

Examination of the heart reveals pathologic changes. A systolic murmur usually accompanies aortic stenosis or mitral insufficiency. A diastolic murmur is present with aortic regurgitation and mitral stenosis. Mitral stenosis is often accompanied with an opening snap. Patients often have a gallop.[53]

Atrial and ventricular enlargement can usually be seen on the chest x-ray film. The electrocardiogram often shows ventricular hypertrophy and new onset of atrial fibrillation is not uncommon. Both cardiac catheterization and echocardiography may be used to estimate valve areas, gradients, and regurgitant flows.

Etiology

The major causes of valve degeneration include:

- Rheumatic heart disease
- Myxomatous degeneration
- Endocarditis

- Calcification
- Chordal rupture

These processes may result in stenosis, regurgitation, or a gradient. Other indications for valve surgery include endocarditis with either ongoing sepsis, conduction disturbance, or embolization. Coronary artery disease with unstable angina, arrhythmias, or myocardial infarction may be associated with papillary muscle dysfunction and may require valve replacement in combination with coronary artery bypass grafting for maximum benefit.

Choice of Prosthesis

The choice of the particular valve prosthesis is individualized to each patient. Young patients (<40 years old) and patients with chronic renal failure have an accelerated degeneration of tissue valves with early calcification of the leaflets. A mechanical valve is more appropriate for these patients. Exceptions include patients with severe coagulopathies and women expecting to become pregnant. Several mechanical valves have demonstrated a low rate of thromboembolic events and a low transvalvular gradient with exercise, which are compatible with an active lifestyle[10] (Table 17-1). Patients more than 70 years of age and those who cannot

Table 17-1   Valve Designs and Characteristics

Valve name	Type	Year
Starr-Edwards 1000, 6000	Caged ball	1960
Smeloff-Sutter	Caged ball	1964
Magovern-Conrad	Caged ball	1962
Hufnagel-Conrad	Caged disk	1965
Kay-Shiley	Caged disk	1966
Cooley-Cutter	Caged disk	1971
Gott-Daggett	Hinged leaflet	1964
Bjork-Shiley	Tilting disk	1969
Medtronic-Hall	Tilting disk	1977
Lillehei-Kaster	Tilting disk	1969
Kalke-Lillehei	Bileaflet	1968
St. Jude	Bileaflet	1977
Carpentier-Edwards	Tissue porcine	1976
Carpentier-Edwards	Bovine pericardium	1980
Hancock-Tissue	Porcine	1977

(history of major bleeding) or will not (unrealiable) take antico-agulants are candidates for a tissue valve. In addition to porcine xenografts, other tissue valves that are available include allografts (human donor valves) or autografts (the patient's own transplanted pulmonary valve). The problems with allografts include limitations of supply and a longer aortic cross-clamp time because of a more technically demanding operation. The benefit of allografts are thought to include greater durability than xenografts and significantly lower incidence of recurrent endocarditis when used for infected valves.[4] Pulmonary valve autografts may provide good long-term results, but the experience is limited and the operative procedure is significantly prolonged when compared with conventional valve replacement.[16]

Aortic Valve

Natural History and Indications

In a review of seven studies Ross and Braunwald[95] documented a rapid deterioration after the onset of symptoms in patients with aortic stenosis. Patients with syncope and angina with accompanying aortic stenosis have an average life expectancy of 3 years. Patients with the accompanying symptoms of congestive heart failure have an average survival time of 1.5 to 2 years (Fig. 17-1). Ten-year mortality rates ranged from 65% to 90% in patients with symptomatic aortic stenosis.[46,88] Wood[110] demonstrated a 7-year mortality rate of 30%. Seventy percent of these patients had angina, 33% syncope, and 45% heart failure.

The timing of therapy for aortic regurgitation is a more controversial problem because of the indolent nature of ventricular deterioration. Patients without symptoms have an 80% chance of remaining symptom free for 5 years.[9] However, the deterioration of left ventricular function continues and when symptoms arise, the patient's condition often deteriorates rapidly.[100] Rappaport[88] found a 75% 5-year survival rate with symptomatic aortic regurgitation (Fig. 17-2). Bland and Wheeler[6] demonstrated a 62% survival rate at 10 years. Indications for surgery on the aortic valve encompass the following:[49]

- Peak systolic gradient 50 mm Hg or greater
- Valve area 0.5 cm^2 or less
- Ventricular enlargement (systolic transverse axis dimension ≥5.5 cm or cardiothoracic ratio ≥0.55)

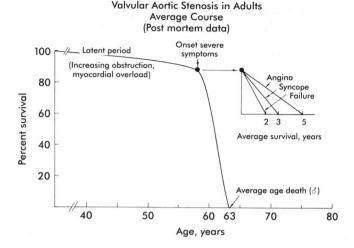

Fig. 17-1 Clinical course of patients with aortic stenosis as expressed in percent surviving in years. (From Ross J, Braunwald E: *Circulation* 37[5]:61, 1968.)

- Acute severe aortic regurgitation (endocarditis)
- Valvular disruption (aortic dissection)

Several studies demonstrated the importance of valve replacement before ventricular decompensation. Fioretti and colleagues[45] recorded better survival if surgery was performed before left ventricular dilation (end-systolic dimension >5.5 cm). Bonow and coworkers[8] showed an increased operative mortality rate if the period of preoperative left ventricular dysfunction is prolonged (>18 months). Several studies have shown a significant decrease in survival if the preoperative ejection fraction was depressed (>50%) or if end-systolic or diastolic volume was increased (55 mm and 90 mm, respectively).[9,53] Boucher and coworkers[11] have shown in patients undergoing valve replacement for aortic or mitral insufficiency that 67% with an ejection fraction greater than 60% have a normal ejection fraction early postoperatively as compared with 27% with a preoperative ejection fraction from 50% to 60%. Almost no patients with a preoperative ejection fraction less than 50% have a normal ejection fraction in the early postoperative period.

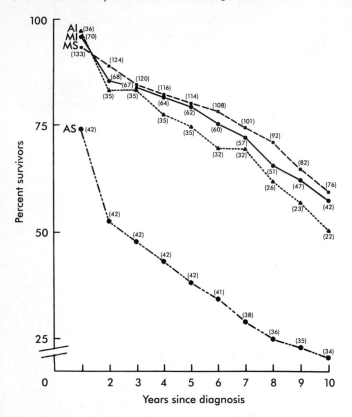

Fig. 17-2 Clinical course of patients with medically treated valvular disease as expressed in percent survival in years. *AI*, Aortic insufficiency; *AS*, aortic stenosis; *MI*, mitral insufficiency; *MS*, mitral stenosis. (From Rappaport E: *Am J Cardiol* 35:221, 1975.)

Therapeutic Options

Therapeutic options include percutaneous valvuloplasty, operative valvuloplasty or limited debridement, valve replacement (AVR), and extraanatomic conduit.

For patients with aortic stenosis percutaneous valvuloplasty is a rare therapeutic option. The associated mortality rate (2% to 7.5%) and high restenosis rate (50% to 75% at 6 months)[76,77] have led most clinicians to recommend this procedure only for truly nonsurgical patients.[76,86] Operative valvuloplasty represents a small percentage of patients (5%) in Western countries. Attempts at decalcifying valves, commissurotomy, and reconstruction of the aortic annulus may be useful in some patients but these limited procedures have not been proven to be comparable to valve replacement.[27,101] Preliminary studies of ultrasonic valvular decalcification have demonstrated poor results, with development of late regurgitation.[27]

Aortic Valve Replacement

The techniques involved in the operative procedure are demonstrated in Fig. 17-3.

Small aortic root

When a small aortic root is encountered, three easy alternatives include the following: (1) placing sutures from the ventricular side to the aortic side and seating the prosthesis on the top of the aortic annulus, which often gains one additional valve size; (2) placing

Text continued on p. 374

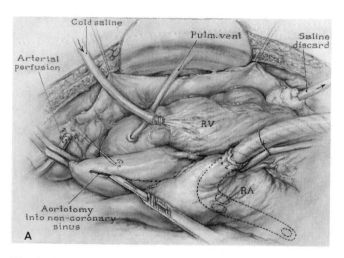

Fig. 17-3 A, Setup for aortic valve replacement. Cardiopulmonary bypass instituted with aortic cannula in ascending aorta and single two-stage right atrial cannula. Vent cannula is in main pulmonary artery. After one dose (500 ml) of crystalloid cardioplegia solution, hypothermia is maintained with topical iced saline solution. Initial aortotomy is demonstrated.

Continued.

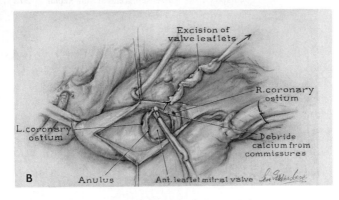

Excision of valve leaflets

R. coronary ostium

L. coronary ostium

Debride calcium from commissures

Anulus

Ant. leaflet mitral valve

B

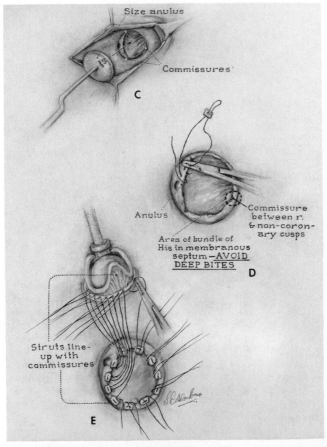

Size anulus

Commissures

C

Anulus

Commissure between r. & non-coronary cusps

Area of bundle of His in membranous septum—AVOID DEEP BITES

D

Struts line-up with commissures

E

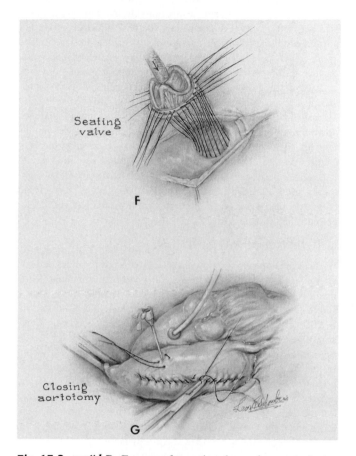

Seating
valve

F

Closing
aortotomy

G

Fig. 17-3, *cont'd* **B,** Exposure for aortic valve replacement. Aortotomy is extended down to noncoronary cusp. Calcification in aortic
annulus is debrided with fine-tip rongeurs. **C,** With annulus debrided,
orifice is measured with valve sizer. **D,** Horizontal everting pledgeted
mattress sutures are placed into the annulus. **E,** Sutures are then placed
in the valve sewing ring. **F,** Care is taken to seat the valve without
twisting any sutures, after which the sutures are tied. **G,** Aortotomy
is then closed with running 4-0 suture in two layers. Deairing needle
is used to evacuate intracardiac air.

the prosthesis in a tilted position with care taken to avoid the coronary ostia; and (3) using a small prosthesis, depending on the size and activity level of the patient. If these alternatives are not adequate, an opening in the annulus can be used to enlarge it. The opening can be placed in the noncoronary cusp and the initial aortic incision carried into the roof of the left atrium and onto the anterior mitral leaflet.[70] An alternative procedure is aortoventriculoplasty,[67] which involves an incision into the right coronary cusp to the left of the right coronary orifice. This incision extends down through the right ventricle, where it meets the aortic annulus into the right ventricular outflow tract. Both root-enlarging procedures require closure of both the annulus and adjoining cavity with either pericardium or a synthetic patch. Another less commonly used alternative that has been advocated by Brown and colleagues is the use of a valved conduit from the left ventricular apex to the thoracic aorta.[15]

Early postoperative care

The care of patients following AVR is the same for other patients after open heart surgery with several additional concerns. Postoperative hypertension should be avoided because of the aortic suture line. Keeping the systolic pressure less than 120 mm Hg or 20% less than the preoperative level is usually adequate. Early complications specific to aortic valve surgery involve the development of heart block, which is usually transient and easily controlled with temporary percutaneous pacing wires. Control of postoperative arrhythmias is also important. Ventricular hypertrophy creates the propensity for subendocardial ischemia and sustained ventricular ectopy. Ventricular arrhythmias are treated with lidocaine and with careful control of serum potassium and magnesium levels. Emboli can occur after valve replacement, and most surgeons employ anticoagulation even when tissue valves are used, because of the new sutures and exposed polyester on the prosthesis. Warfarin, 2 to 5 mg, is started on the first postoperative day and advanced to achieve a prothrombin time (PT) of 1.5 to 1.8 times control values. Without anticoagulation even the newer low-profile valves such as the St. Jude valve are associated with a high incidence of thromboemboli (10%) and a high rate of valve thrombosis (11%). If only antiplatelet agents are used, the risk of embolization is 4% yearly in comparison with 2% with warfarin anticoagulation.[30] With tissue valves anticoagulation is discontinued after 6 to 8 weeks.

Ventricular failure may be a particular problem postoperatively for patients with a low initial ejection fraction (<40%). Patients with severe aortic regurgitation may have adequate ejection fractions preoperatively and still have gradual ventricular failure. Afterload reduction, inotropic support, and intraaortic balloon assistance may be necessary while the ventricle adapts in the early postoperative period or recovers from the operative ischemic injury. During convalescence, aggressive diuresis is usually necessary to aid in pulmonary recovery, eliminate excess fluid administered during the operation, and treat symptomatic congestive heart failure symptoms. Continuous hemofiltration may be used to assist fluid mobilization in patients with renal compromise.

Late postoperative care and results

Late complications after valve surgery are related to the valve placed. Tissue valves start to show degeneration in most series at 7 years with a 50% deterioration rate at 13 years.[69] Recent studies have shown this is slightly lower in patients more than 70 years of age.[24] If a mechanical valve is used, lifelong warfarin therapy is necessary. The rate of significant bleeding complications (PT 1.5 to 2.0 times control values) are in the range of two to 12 per 100 patient years. The best level of anticoagulation is still controversial. As has been recently noted, it may be possible to improve the risk/benefit ratio of warfarin therapy in certain mechanical valves by lowering the PT time to ratios in the range of 1.5.[98]

Thromboembolism can occur in tissue valves or in mechanical valves despite anticoagulation. Except for the Bjork-Shiley valve, valve thrombosis is rare (1%). Embolic events, primarily cerebral, vary in occurrence according to the valve and its location, but range from two to 10 per 100 patient years. This rate is increased in elderly patients and in those with atrial fibrillation.[98]

The incidence of paravalvular leak ranges up to 17%.[75] It is important because it may represent the first sign of endocarditis and can contribute to hemolysis. The incidence of early endocarditis is approximately 1% in most series. The incidence of late endocarditis is 0.5 per 100 patient years. Rossiter and coworkers[96] showed that the rate of infection was slightly lower with tissue valves in the aortic position when compared with mechanical valves (2.2% vs 2.7%). Their study also demonstrated that a greater percentage of tissue valves with prosthetic endocarditis could be sterilized with medical therapy alone as compared with mechanical valves (68% vs 53%) with improved survival.

Overall, the 10-year survival rate after aortic valve replacement ranges from 65% to 80% and most patients are NYHA class I or II.[29,56,67] The incidence of freedom from valve-related problems is 50% at 5 years. The annual mortality rate ranges from 2% to 5%; 20% to 30% of which are valve related. Late deaths are predominantly cardiac related but not valve related: sudden death, myocardial infarction, and congestive heart failure.[67] Risk factors for poor outcome include increased age, depressed left ventricular function, and coronary artery disease.[29] Patients with acute aortic regurgitation represent a group at particularly high risk. The mortality associated with acute regurgitation with aortic dissection is 30%.[32] With endocarditis operation for congestive heart failure caused by acute aortic regurgitation is associated with a 7% to 50% mortality rate.[59]

Mitral Valve Therapy

Natural History

Because of the success of mitral valve repair as a procedure, the therapeutic options for a diseased mitral valve are more varied than for the aortic valve. Repair has yielded good long-term results with low operative mortality and morbidity rates. Long-term anticoagulation is not required (unless atrial fibrillation is present).

Mitral stenosis is a slow, progressive disease; when symptoms develop, patients have a 62% to 80% chance of surviving 5 years without surgery.[79,88] Embolization occurs in 20% of patients with mitral stenosis. The 5-year survival after the onset of symptoms in patients with mitral regurgitation is 80%[88] (Fig. 17-2) and is less with the combined lesions of insufficiency and stenosis (67%). When symptoms have progressed to moderate or severe, the 5-year survival rate drops to 55%.[51] Phillips and coworkers[84] have shown that increased age (>60 years) and an ejection fraction less than 40% correlated with a decreased survival rate 3 to 5 years after mitral valve replacement. Additionally, most patients recovered well but with a slight decrease in ejection fraction. Kennedy and coworkers[58] demonstrated that patients with mitral stenosis with or without some insufficiency have maintained preoperative ejection fractions with decreased ventricular volumes when evaluated 1 year postoperatively. Patients with primary insufficiency are more likely to have a drop in ejection fraction, suggesting less recovery of ventricular function. Schuler and coworkers[99] found that patients undergoing mitral valve replacement for mitral insufficiency have a fall in ejection fraction if they had a low normal or depressed ejection fraction ($<60\%$) preoperatively. This study indicated that preoperative increased end-diastolic or end-systolic dimensions (8.0 cm and 5.7 cm, respectively) suggested poor recovery.

Indications for surgery on the mitral valve include the following:

- Valve area less than 1.0 cm^2
- Valve gradient of at least 10 mm Hg
- Ventricular dilation (diastolic transverse axis dimension at least 6 cm)
- Acute insufficiency with a myocardial infarction not responsive to medical therapy

Other relative indications include the new onset of supraventricular arrhythmias. Additionally, a mild to moderately symptomatic patient with a stenotic valve, without calcification or insufficiency, may benefit from early open commissurotomy. A similar argument can be made for patients with mild symptoms and severe mitral regurgitation, if echocardiography suggests a reparable valve. A contraindication for valve surgery may include an ejection fraction of less than 20%.

Therapeutic Options

Therapeutic options for mitral valve procedures include percutaneous transseptal valvuloplasty, open or closed commissurotomy, valvular repair, and valvular replacement.

Percutaneous mitral valvuloplasty has been reported to be more successful than aortic valvuloplasty. Complications such as stroke (3% to 4%), acute insufficiency (30% to 40% mild, 2% severe), atrial septal defect, and cardiac tamponade (0.5%) have been reported.[86] The effectiveness of the procedure depends on proper patient selection.[76] With pliable noncalcific valves there is a 5% to 7% rate of recurrence at 18 months. In patients with thicker leaflets and calcific annuli, the symptomatic recurrence rate is 30% to 40%.[86] Open commissurotomy has shown a long-term success rate that is excellent for up to 5 years (90%) with a low operative mortality rate (1% to 2%).[54] Farhat and coworkers, in a study comparing open and closed commissurotomy, demonstrated a slightly better postoperative cardiac index and increase in valve

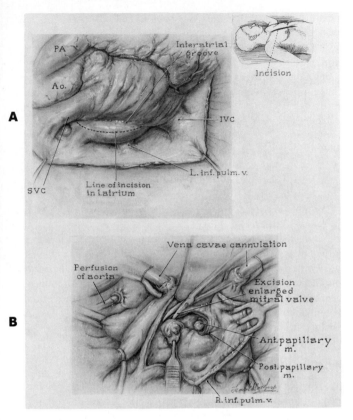

Fig. 17-4 A, Incision for left atriotomy starting at right superior pulmonary vein. **B,** On cardiopulmonary bypass with ascending aortic and bicaval connections, mitral valve is excised through left atriotomy.
Continued.

area[44] with open techniques. An additional advantage of the open procedure is the ability to remove left atrial clot. Valve repair and replacement are indicated for some anatomically deformed valves.

Mitral Valve Replacement

The technique of mitral valve replacement is illustrated in Fig. 17-4.

Several clinical[34,73] and experimental[104] reports emphasized the

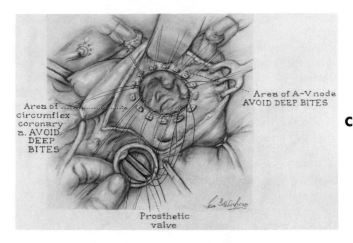

C

Fig. 17-4, *cont'd* C, Mitral valve placement with pledgeted everting horizontal mattress sutures. Placement of sutures should be avoided in *highlighted areas.*

importance of leaving the chorda tendineae intact when the mitral valve is replaced. To spare the cords but remove leaflet tissue that might obstruct the aortic outflow tract, a triangular incision can be used in the anterior leaflet. After reduction the leaflet remnants are plicated into the valve sutures, which pass through the annulus. This results in better preservation of ventricular function immediately after replacement and may help to prevent acute ventricular rupture.[73]

Early postoperative care

Important problems in postoperative management after mitral valve replacement are ventricular failure, pulmonary hypertension, and ventricular arrhythmias.

A dilated ventricle after valve replacement for mitral regurgitation may fail because of a marked increase in afterload caused by the loss of a low-pressure vent (unloading into a large left atrium). The dilation of the heart increases wall tension and increases energy and oxygen requirements and may result in ventricular failure and low cardiac output. Inotropic support and afterload reduction are very helpful. Patients with pure mitral insufficiency may require extended ventricular support. Intraaortic balloon counterpulsation or mechanical assistance may be required.

Pulmonary hypertension causing right ventricular failure can occur. Pulmonary vasodilators such as nitroglycerin, amrinone, or isoproterenol may be necessary. In cases where the pulmonary hypertension is not responsive to these medications, a pulmonary arterial infusion of prostaglandin E_1 with a concomitant infusion of norepinephrine into the left atrium for maintaining systemic pressure has been reported to be helpful.[31]

Patients with mitral regurgitation may have ventricular ectopy and may be prone to sudden ventricular fibrillation early after the operation. Careful attention to potassium and magnesium levels, an adequate arterial oxygen content, and adequate coronary artery perfusion pressure are helpful. Some surgeons advocate prophylactic lidocaine infusions in the first 24 hours after replacement or repair for insufficiency.

Ventricular rupture and tamponade have been reported as uncommon causes of low cardiac output during the immediate recovery from mitral surgery. The decreased cardiac index is accompanied by hemorrhage and death unless an immediate operative repair can be accomplished.[73]

Late postoperative care and results

The long-term complications of mitral valve replacement are similar to aortic replacement, although the patient survival rate is lower in most studies. The 5-year survival rate ranges from 45% to 85% with a decrease to 43% to 64% at 10 years.[12,64,65,83] Late mortality is predominantly from valve-related thromboembolism and non-valve-related cardiac problems such as ventricular failure, myocardial infarction, and sudden death. Improvement in cardiac output is more predictable after aortic valve replacement for insufficiency than for mitral valve replacement for insufficiency.[58,99]

Mitral Valve Repair

Evaluation

Mitral repair represents an alternative to valve replacement. Its proposed application in patients earlier in the disease process reflects its safety and effectiveness, as well as the absence of valve prosthesis—related morbidity. The renewed interest in valve repair techniques is also related to the new techniques used for evaluation of the repair, primarily intraoperative transesophageal echocardi-

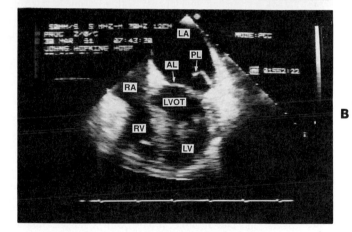

Fig. 17-5 A, TEE demonstrating left atrium *(LA)*, anterior leaflet mitral valve *(AL)*, posterior leaflet mitral valve *(PL)*, left ventricle chamber *(LV)*, and aortic outflow tract *(AO)*. **B,** TEE of prolapsing mitral valve.

ography (TEE). In both preoperative planning and postoperative assessment TEE (Fig. 17-5) has demonstrated significant value.

Lessana[65] evaluated subgroups of patients for mechanisms of mitral regurgitation and results of mitral repair. Patients with restricted valve motion and fibrosis had a greater morbidity rate (6%

vs 2.5%) and a higher rate of reoperation (22% vs 17%) when compared with patients with more pliable valves and prolapse.[65]

Technique for leaflet repair

Valve repair requires careful assessment of the leaflets, annulus, chordae, and prior ventricular wall injury. The valve leaflets must be pliable and have enough redundancy to coapt for valve closure. Leaflets that are fibrotic with commissural fusion can be trimmed and the commissures split with a knife to allow better mobility and leaflet coaptation. Posterior leaflet prolapse caused by chorda elongation or rupture can be treated by a rectangular excision of the abnormal leaflet with primary repair (Fig. 17-6, *A*). Small leaflet perforations such as those from endocarditis can be repaired with a simple stitch or pericardial patch. Annular dilation is common with regurgitant lesions. With mitral insufficiency the repair almost always includes an annuloplasty with a prosthetic ring to create a more anatomic orifice and better leaflet overlap (Fig. 17-6, *B*).[19]

Annuloplasty

Annuloplasty may entail sutures placed laterally in the annulus to narrow the orifice (Kay or Reed)[90] or a suture placed circumferentially in the annulus and pulled tight to the desired size (Kurlansky-DeVega, Shore).[63,102] Rigid rings such as those introduced by Carpentier and coworkers[20] can also be used to decrease and remodel the orifice shape and size (Fig. 17-7). Because the mitral annulus expands and contracts 20% to 34% during the cardiac cycle, a flexible ring was hypothesized to be more physiologic.[81,107] In a randomized study of 25 patients David and colleagues[35] showed better maintenance of ventricular function as measured by stroke volume and end-diastolic volume with a flexible mitral annuloplasty ring.

Chorda reconstruction

Attempts at limited resection of the anterior leaflet have led to poor results.[18] As a result techniques to control anterior leaflet prolapse with the use of chorda reconstruction have been developed. These techniques, which have been developed by Carpentier,[18] involve chorda fixation to secondary chordae or transposition of chordae from the posterior leaflet (with subsequent repair) to the area of the anterior leaflet that has prolapsed. Polytetrafluoro-

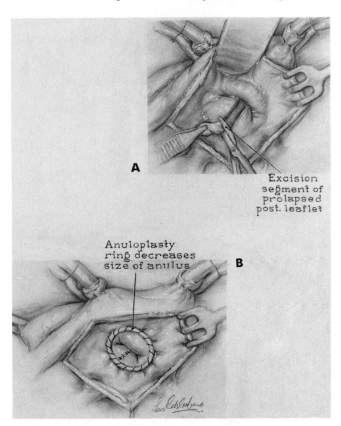

A

Excision
segment of
prolapsed
post. leaflet

Anuloplasty
ring decreases
size of anulus

B

Fig. 17-6 A, Excision segment of posterior mitral leaflet through left atriotomy. **B,** Flexible ring sewn into annulus with three running 3-0 sutures. Prior rectangular excision and repair of posterior leaflet are visualized.

ethylene suture or modified pericardium have also been used with success as chorda substitutes.[112] Chordae that are too long can be shortened by pulling the redundant chorda down and fixing it within the papillary muscle.[20] In cases where ventricular scar and aneurysms have developed around the posterior papillary muscle, a transventricular approach has been used with success for mitral repair and aneurysm resection.[87] In all patients excision of the left atrial appendage is recommended to help prevent embolization

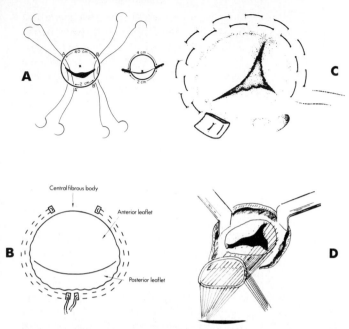

Fig. 17-7 A, Reed technique of annuloplasty with lateral plicating sutures measured from center of anterior leaflet. (**A** from Reed GE, Pooley RW, Moggio RA: *J Thorac Cardiovasc Surg* 79:321, 1980;) **B,** Shore technique with mitral valve plication with two semicircular pledgeted sutures. (**B** from Shore DF, Wong P, Paneth M: *J Thorac Cardiovasc Surg* 79:349, 1980;) **C,** Modification of DeVega tricuspid annuloplasty by Kurlansky to provide adjustment of orifice in beating heart. (**C** from Kurlansky P, Rose EA, Malm JR: *Ann Thorac Surg* 44:404, 1987;) **D,** Technique for placement of ring for tricuspid annuloplasty. (**D** from Carpentier A et al: *J Thorac Cardiovasc Surg* 67:53, 1974.)

should the patient revert to or remain in atrial fibrillation postoperatively.

Early postoperative care

The postoperative management of mitral repair is similar to mitral valve replacement with the proviso that these patients usually have a better maintained cardiac index with a lower left ventricular end-diastolic pressure[42] and fewer complications.[42,113] Some surgeons advocate anticoagulation because of the fresh suture line and the prosthetic ring used for annuloplasty. It is started on the second postoperative day and continued for 4 to 6 weeks if sinus rhythm is present. If atrial fibrillation is present, it is continued indefinitely. Rates for thromboembolic events and endocarditis range from 0% to 5% and 0% to 2%, respectively.[47] Comparative studies of repair versus replacement, although limited by the biases in patient selection, have shown better early results for valve repair with comparable long-term durability. In a review by Cosgrove and colleagues,[26] mortality with repair ranged from 0% to 5% as compared with 5% to 13% for mitral valve replacement.

Late postoperative care and results

Failure of valve repair occurs at a yearly rate similar to valve replacement (1% to 2%).[1,19,97,105] The rate of degeneration in studies from 9 to 14 years of follow-up ranged from 11% to 22% with some repairs intact at 14 years.[1,19,82,105] Besides improper initial repair, other causes for repair failure are annuloplasty ring dehiscence and overly aggressive annulus plication, leading to obstruction of the left ventricular outflow tract and systolic anterior leaflet motion of the mitral valve.[38] The 5-year survival rate after repair is uniformly better with mitral repair (76% to 96%) when compared with mitral replacement (45% to 85%).[19,26,80] Deloche and coworkers[38] reported a 15-year follow-up from the Carpentier group. Actuarial survival rate was 72% with 74% of patients in NYHA classes I and II. Seventy-six percent of patients surgically treated for rheumatic heart disease were free from reoperation after 15 years as compared with 93% of patients with degenerative valve disease.[38]

Ischemic Mitral Insufficiency

Patients with ischemic mitral insufficiency may have stable coronary artery disease with associated valve dysfunction or acute mitral regurgitation after infarction.

Indications

Patients with associated coronary artery disease (25% to 50%) should undergo coronary artery bypass concomitant with their valve procedures.[22,28] Short-term and long-term evaluation of mortality rates in most valve studies show nonvalve cardiac causes to be the major cause of long-term mortality.[19,24,56] Czer and colleagues[28] demonstrated that patients undergoing mitral valve replacement who do not undergo appropriate revascularization have a decreased long-term survival rate. Patients with acute mitral regurgitation after an infarction who undergo coronary bypass grafting should undergo mitral repair or replacement for the symptoms of moderate or severe mitral insufficiency. Mild mitral insufficiency, however, has not been shown to increase the operative mortality rate or to progress so as to require later valve surgery. Papillary dysfunction with associated wall dyskinesia has been associated with anterior leaflet arrest, which prevents normal coaptation and is often not amenable to repair.[66]

Postoperative Care

Ischemic mitral insufficiency represents a difficult problem. In a review of 19 studies mitral valve replacement caused by coronary artery disease was associated with an increased operative mortality rate of 21% (0% to 54%) as compared with 6% for patients undergoing mitral replacement or 12% for those undergoing mitral replacement with unrelated coronary artery bypass grafting.[92] The primary cause of death was ventricular failure. Emergent mitral replacement for ischemic disease was associated with a 38% operative mortality rate (0% to 54%) in six studies reviewed. In one study patients operated on earlier (1.7 days) demonstrated a better survival than patients who underwent operations later (9.3 days).[80]

Tricuspid Valve Procedures

Isolated tricuspid disease is a rare entity. Tricuspid stenosis occurs with rheumatic disease, usually with other associated valvular lesions. Tricuspid insufficiency can occur from organic causes such as endocarditis or from functional dilation caused by related mitral or aortic disease.

Indications

Indications for tricuspid repair include signs of right ventricular failure (hepatomegaly, ascites, peripheral edema), a dilated right ventricle on echocardiography with tricuspid regurgitation, and a transvalvular gradient greater than 4 mm Hg.

Some controversy remains regarding treatment of patients with the symptoms of right ventricular failure and an incompetent tricuspid valve related to mitral insufficiency. Studies have demonstrated that annular contraction (20% to 40%) before ventricular contraction is part of the mechanism of tricuspid competence implying the need for a small and functional annulus.[108] There is evidence that in patients with significant tricuspid insufficiency associated with other valvular disease the condition does not progress or may improve without adding the tricuspid repair to the other valve procedures.[13,85] However, other studies have shown a 40% to 53% incidence of symptomatic right ventricular failure if the tricuspid valve is not replaced or repaired.[14,60] King and coworkers[60] demonstrated a high operative mortality rate for later tricuspid replacement (25%), after mitral valve replacement, with only 50% of patients demonstrating significant improvement. Ubago and coworkers[109] estimated that functional regurgitation occurs when the annulus is dilated from 24 to 31 mm/m^2 body surface area and recommended annuloplasty with these dimensions. Carpentier and colleagues reported successful repair of the tricuspid valve together with mitral repair or replacement, with a 9.5% operative mortality rate and good postoperative tricuspid function in more than 90% of patients.[21] Tricuspid valve replacement (TVR) is usually indicated for stenosis related to rheumatic fever or on occasion for endocarditis (see next section).

Operative technique

A DeVega repair or Carpentier ring annuloplasty can be performed during rewarming after the end of ischemic arrest with no increase in cardiopulmonary bypass time (Fig. 17-7, *C* and *D*). Studies comparing the different TVR techniques have shown better results with a Carpentier ring annuloplasty than with the DeVega or Kay repairs[61,84] for functional insufficiency.

Postoperative care

Postoperative complications are few with TVR and are primarily related to ventricular failure, which is often associated with high pulmonary artery pressures or with progressive left ventricular failure. However, with tricuspid replacement, in addition to the increased mortality rate compared with repair, there is a 5% incidence of heart block.[74] A permanent epicardial pacemaker lead is usually placed after TVR because if heart block occurs postoperatively, the option to place a transvenous pacing wire is reduced because of the prosthetic valve in the tricuspid position.

Multiple Valve Procedures

Multiple valve procedures carry an increased risk because of the length and complexity of the operations and associated left ventricular injury caused by the extent of the valvular lesions. In a review of nine reports the mean operative mortality rate for combined aortic and mitral valve procedures was 14%.[39] Recent experience, including our own, suggests a lower operative mortality rate in the 5% to 10% range.[106] Patients with both aortic insufficiency and mitral insufficiency carry the worst prognosis; volume-overloaded, dilated hearts may not recover function. The primary postoperative risk is low cardiac output and pulmonary hypertension (present in 25% of patients). Other complications include ventricular arrhythmias, hemorrhage, and stroke. Patients with increased risk are those with long-standing symptoms, NYHA class IV (mortality rate as high as 50%), left atrial pressures greater than 30 mm Hg, and elevated end-diastolic pressures.[17,39,71,72]

Endocarditis

Endocarditis is defined as an infection involving tissues of a heart valve or an intracardiac structure. Patients with endocarditis may have fever (84% to 100% of patients), leukocytosis (40% to 60%), a new murmur (80% to 95%), and systemic emboli (10% to 20%).[17]

Patients at risk for endocarditis are those with a valvular lesion causing turbulence, such as those with rheumatic disease, mitral valve prolapse, congenital irregularity (such as a bicuspid aortic valve), or a prosthetic valve. Endocarditis can often be traced to an episode of bacteremia occasionally related to a dental procedure.

Physical evidence of endocarditis includes weight loss and lethargy; splenomegaly; and abscesses in the skin, brain (83%), lung, and liver. The mitral valve is involved in 86% of cases of native valve endocarditis in contrast to the right-sided lesions, which occur in less than 25% of cases and are often related to intravenous drug use. Native valve endocarditis is caused primarily by *Streptococcus, Staphylococcus aureus,* and gram-negative bacilli.[17]

Indications

Indications for urgent surgery include:
- Acute mitral or aortic regurgitation with heart failure or recurrent emboli (or high risk for further neurologic impairment)

- Intractable infection (fungi or resistant bacteria) despite administration of intravenous antibiotics
- Heart block or intracardiac fistula indicating continuing tissue destruction
- Early prosthetic valve endocarditis

Echocardiographic studies can provide serial measurements of valve regurgitation or ventricular function and the need for valve surgery. When vegetations are visualized on echocardiography, most patients eventually require surgery.[7,37] A vegetation alone, however, is not necessarily an indication for surgery. Embolization, *S. aureus* infection, and prosthetic valve endocarditis are associated with increased mortality rates.[17] Echocardiography (particularly TEE) is effective in detecting aortic root abscesses, which are present in 20% to 50% of patients with aortic valve endocarditis.[33,55,89]

Approximately 50% of patients do well with medical therapy. Progressive congestive heart failure from acute aortic or mitral insufficiency related to endocarditis carries a high mortality rate (45%) and is the most common indication for urgent surgery.[17,89] Operative mortality rates range from 7% to 40% with a 10% recurrence rate.[17]

Operative Technique

Surgical techniques include aggressive debridement of infected tissue, even if the valvular annulus is involved. Closure of ventricular defects may require a patch (synthetic or pericardial). Supraannular aortic valve translocation can also be used if the aortic annulus is believed to be irreparable.[91] Another preferred alternative is use of a valved conduit or an aortic homograft.[40,43] Aortic homografts have been reported to have a diminished reinfection rate.[78] Some reports indicate that a tissue valve is less likely to demonstrate annular abscesses. Recurrent infection in the tissue valve has been shown to be confined to leaflets.[25] Others have shown less infection with mechanical valves (5%) versus tissue valves (14%).[48]

For patients with tricuspid endocarditis simple valve excision has been recommended as initial treatment if pulmonary hypertension is not present. This allows for appropriate treatment of associated pulmonary septic emboli and is associated with a low mortality rate (96% survival rate at 10 years). Valve replacement may be needed in the future.[2]

Postoperative Care and Results

Postoperatively these patients are similar to other patients undergoing valve replacement, with the additional concerns of recurrent infection. Antibiotics should be continued for at least 4 weeks, and one report recommended treatment for at least 6 weeks, to limit further recurrent infections (6% vs 21%).[48]

David and coworkers[36] reported a 5-year actuarial survival rate of 79% with 96% of patients of NYHA classes I or II. Higher mortality rates were seen with prosthetic valve endocarditis, preoperative shock, and annular abscess.

Dreyfus and coworkers[41] reported results on valve repair for endocarditis that use Carpentier's techniques after excision of all infected valve tissue with pericardial replacement as necessary. Operative mortality rate was 2.5%. Reoperation was necessary in 2.5% of patients. However, no recurrences of endocarditis or further valve dysfunction was observed at 30 months.

Prosthetic Valve Endocarditis

Prosthetic valve endocarditis (PVE) represents a special entity. Early PVE is defined as infections less than 2 months after the operation, and late PVE as more than 2 months postoperatively. Early PVE is usually related to *Staphylococcus epidermidis, S. aureus,* fungi, or diphtheroids. Primary indications for surgery are ventricular failure, renal failure, embolization and sepsis.

Aggressive therapy is necessary in early PVE because of a high mortality rate (57% to 67%) primarily related to multisystem failure and sepsis.[5,68] Late PVE is similar to native valve endocarditis: it is caused by similar organisms (i.e., streptococci, *S. aureus,* gram-negative bacteria) and is associated with a lower mortality rate (active infection, 21%; healed, 8%) and lower recurrence rates.[5,68]

Medical therapy can be expected to cure 40% to 64% of patients with PVE. Patients with tissue valves and those with late endocarditis have a greater likelihood of responding to medical therapy. Conversely, patients with *S. epidermidis* infections, aortic root abscesses, fungal or pseudomonal infections, and early prosthetic valve infections are more likely to require surgical intervention.[5,57,68,93]

The 5-year survival rate is 54%, with successful rereplacement in patients with active PVE.[68] David and coworkers[36] reported a 12% operative mortality rate for this high-risk group of patients with a high complication rate. They reported a 5-year actuarial survival rate of 67%.

Summary

Current valve surgery has revisited old techniques of valve repair in response to the continuing shortcomings of valve replacement prostheses. Many mechanical valves last beyond 20 years but require constant anticoagulation and are associated with continued risks of thromboembolism and infection; the annual rate of morbidity from a prosthetic valve is approximately 1% to 3%. Tissue valves do not require long-term anticoagulation and are associated with less thromboembolism but begin degenerating after 7 years, with half requiring replacement by 13 years. Homografts are similar to tissue valves in their advantages, with perhaps a longer period before degeneration. The disadvantage of homografts is the limitation in supply. Valve repair represents a good alternative to valve replacement but unfortunately is not applicable to all patients. Long-term results of valve replacement show improved results primarily because of earlier operations performed before the onset of significant ventricular dysfunction. The perfect valve replacement prosthesis depends on future developments.

References

1. Angell W, Oury JH, Shah P: A comparison of replacement and reconstruction in patients with mitral regurgitation, *J Thorac Cardiovasc Surg* 93:665-675, 1987.
2. Arbulu A, Asfaw I: Tricuspid valvulectomy without prosthetic replacement: ten years of clinical experience, *J Thorac Cardiovasc Surg* 82:684-691, 1981.
3. Bailey CP: The surgical treatment of mitral stenosis, *Dis Chest* 15:377-397, 1949.
4. Barratt-Boyes BG: Long-term followup of patients receiving a free hand antibiotic sterilized homograft aortic valve. In Rabago G, Cooley DA, eds: *Heart valve replacement: current status and future trends,* Mt Kisco, NY, 1987, Futura.
5. Baumgartner WA et al: Surgical treatment of prosthetic valve endocarditis, *Ann Thorac Surg* 35:87-104, 1983.
6. Bland EF, Wheeler EO: Severe aortic regurgitation in young people: a long-term perspective with reference to prognosis and prosthesis, *N Engl J Med* 256:667-672, 1957.
7. Boda AJ, Zotz RJ, LeMire US, Bach DS: Prognostic significance of vegetations detected by two-dimensional echocardiography, *Am Heart J* 112:1291-1296, 1986.
8. Bonow RO et al: Reversal of left chronic aortic regurgitation: influence of duration of pre-operative left ventricular dysfunction, *Circulation* 70:570-579, 1984.

9. Bonow RO et al: The natural history of asymptomatic patients with aortic regurgitation and normal left ventricular function, *Circulation* 68:509-517, 1983.

10. Borkon AM, Reitz BA, Donahoo JS, Gardner TJ: St. Jude Medical valve replacement in infants and children. In Matloff JM, ed: *Cardiac valve replacement, current status,* Boston, 1985, Martinus Nijhoff.

11. Boucher CA et al: Early changes in left ventricular size and function after correction of left ventricular volume overload, *Am J Cardiol* 47:991-1004, 1981.

12. Bowen TE, Zajitchuk R, Brott WH, deCastro CM: Isolated mitral valve replacement with Kay-Shiley prosthesis, *J Thorac Cardiovasc Surg* 80:45-49, 1980.

13. Braunwald NS, Ross J Jr, Morrow AG: Conservative management of tricuspid regurgitation in patients undergoing mitral valve replacement, *Circulation* 35(suppl I):63, 1967.

14. Breyer RH et al: Tricuspid regurgitation: a comparison of non-operative management, tricuspid annuloplasty, and tricuspid valve replacement, *J Thorac Cardiovasc Surg* 72:867-870, 1976.

15. Brown JW et al: Apical-aortic on anastomosis: a method for relief of diffuse left ventricular outflow obstruction, *Surg Forum* 25:147, 1974.

16. Gula GA, Wain WH, Ross DN: Ten years' experience with pulmonary autograft replacements for aortic valve disease, *Ann Thorac Surg* 28:392-396, 1979.

17. Byrd RC, Cheitlin MD: Endocarditis. In Greenberg BH, Murphy E, eds: *Valvular heart disease,* Littleton, Mass, 1987, PSG Publishing.

18. Carpentier A: Cardiac valve surgery: the "French correction", *J Thorac Cardiovasc Surg* 86:323-387, 1983.

19. Carpentier A et al: Reconstructive surgery of mitral valve incompetence, *J Thorac Cardiovasc Surg* 79:338-348, 1980.

20. Carpentier A et al: Conservative management of the prolapsed mitral valve. *Ann Thorac Surg* 26:294-302, 1978.

21. Carpentier A et al: Surgical management of acquired tricuspid valve disease, *J Thorac Cardiovasc Surg* 67:53-65, 1974.

22. Cohn LH et al: Comparative morbidity of mitral valve repair versus replacement for mitral regurgitation with and without coronary artery disease, *Ann Thorac Surg* 45:284-290, 1988.

23. Cohn LH et al: Early and late risk of aortic valve replacement, *J Thorac Cardiovasc Surg* 88:695-705, 1984.

24. Cohn LH et al: Fifteen-year experience with 1678 Hancock porcine bioprosthetic heart valve replacements, *Ann Surg* 210(4):435-443, 1989.

25. Cooley DA: Surgical consideration in infective endocarditis, *Tex Heart Inst J* 16:263-269, 1989.

26. Cosgrove DM et al: Results of mitral valve reconstruction, *Circulation* 74(suppl I):82-87, 1986.

27. Craver JM: Aortic valve debridement by ultrasonic surgical aspirator: a word of caution, *Ann Thorac Surg* 49:746-753, 1990.

28. Czer LS et al: Mitral valve replacement: impact of coronary artery disease and determinants of prognosis after revascularization, *Circulation* 70(suppl I):198-207, 1984.

29. Czer LSC et al: Reduction in late death by concomitant revascularization with aortic valve replacement, *J Thorac Cardiovasc Surg* 95:390-401, 1988.

30. Czer LSC et al: The St. Jude valve: analysis of thromboembolism, warfarin-related hemorrhage, and survival, *Am Heart J* 114:389-397, 1987.

31. D'Ambra MN et al: Prostaglandin E_1 (PGE_1): a new therapy for refractory right heart failure and pulmonary hypertension after mitral valve replacement, *J Thorac Surg* 89:567-572, 1985.

32. Dalen JE et al: Dissection of the aorta: pathogenesis, diagnosis and treatment, *Prog Cardiovas Dis* 23:237-245, 1988.

33. Daniel WG et al: Improvement in the diagnosis of abscesses associated with endocarditis by transesophageal echocardiography, *N Engl J Med* 324:795-800, 1991.

34. David TE, Burns RJ, Bacchus CM, Druck MN: Mitral valve replacement for mitral regurgitation with and without preservation of chordae tendinea, *J Thorac Cardiovasc Surg* 88:718-725, 1984.

35. David TE, Komeda M, Pollick C, Burns RJ: Mitral valve annuloplasty: the effect of the type on left ventricular function, *Ann Thorac Surg* 47:524-528, 1989.

36. David TE et al: Heart valve operations in patients with active infective endocarditis, *Ann Thorac Surg* 49:701-705, 1990.

37. Davis RS et al: The demonstration of vegetation by echocardiography in bacterial endocarditis: an indication for early surgical intervention, *Am J Med* 69:57-63, 1980.

38. Deloche A et al: Valve repair with Carpentier techniques, *J Thorac Cardiovasc Surg* 99:990-1002, 1990.

39. Demots H: Multivalvular heart disease. In Greenberg BH, Murphy E, eds: *Valvular heart disease*, Littleton, Mass, 1987, PSG Publishing.

40. Donaldson RM, Ross DM: Homograft aortic root replacement for complicated prosthetic valve endocarditis, *Circulation* 70(suppl I):178-181, 1984.

41. Dreyfus G et al: Valve repair in acute endocarditis, *Ann Thorac Surg* 49:706, 1990.

42. Duran CG et al: Conservative operation for mitral insufficiency: critical analysis supported by post-operative hemodynamic studies of 72 patients, *J Thorac Cardiovasc Surg* 79:326-337, 1980.

43. Ergin MA et al: Annular destruction in acute bacterial endocarditis, *J Thorac Cardiovasc Surg* 97:755-763, 1989.

44. Farhat MB et al: Closed versus open mitral commissurotomy in pure noncalcific mitral stenosis: hemodynamic studies before and after operation, *J Thorac Cardiovasc Surg* 99:639-644, 1990.

45. Fioretti P et al: Echocardiography in chronic aortic insufficiency: is valve replacement too late when left ventricular end-systolic dimension reaches 55 mm? *Circulation* 67:216-220, 1983.

46. Frank S, Johnson A, Ross J: Natural history of valvular aortic stenosis, *Br Heart J* 3335:41-46, 1973.

47. Galloway AC et al: Current concepts of mitral valve reconstruction for mitral insufficiency, *Circulation* 78:1087-1098, 1988.

48. Gentry LO, Khoshdel A: New approaches to diagnosis and treatment of infective endocarditis, *Tex Heart Inst J* 16:250-257, 1989.

49. Greenberg B: Acquired aortic valve disease. In Greenberg BH, Murphy E, eds: *Valve heart disease,* Littleton, Mass, 1987, PSC Publishing.

50. Grunkemeier GL, MacManus Q, Thomas DR, Starr A: Regression analysis of late survival following mitral valve replacement, *J Thorac Cardiovasc Surg* 75:131-147, 1978.

51. Hammermeister KE et al: Prediction of late survival in patients with mitral valve disease from clinical, hemodynamic and quantitative angiographic variables, *Circulation* 57:341-349, 1978.

52. Harken DE, Ellis LB, Ware PF, Norman LR: The surgical treatment of mitral stenosis, *N Engl J Med* 239:801-809, 1948.

53. Henry WL et al: Observations in the optimum time for operative intervention for aortic valve replacement in symptomatic patients, *Circulation* 61:471-483, 1980.

54. Houseman LB et al: Prognosis of .patients after open mitral commissurotomy, *J Thorac Cardiovasc Surg* 73:742-745, 1977.

55. Jaffe WM et al: Infective endocarditis, 1983-1988: echocardiographic findings and factors influencing morbidity and mortality, *J Am Coll Cardiol* 156:1227-1233, 1990.

56. Jamieson WRE et al: The Carpentier-Edwards standard porcine bioprosthesis, *J Thorac Cardiovasc Surg* 99:543-561, 1990.

57. Karchner AW: Prosthetic valve endocarditis: mechanical valves. In Magilligan DJ, Quinn EL, eds: *Endocarditis: medical and surgical management,* New York, 1986, Marcel Dekker.

58. Kennedy JW, Doces JH, Stewart DK: Left ventricular function before and following surgical treatment of mitral valve disease, *Am Heart J* 97:592-598, 1979.

59. Kerriaks DJ, Ports TA: Emergencies in valve heart disease. In Greenberg BH, Murphy E, eds: *Valvular heart disease,* Littleton, Mass, 1987, PSG Publishing.

60. King BM et al: Surgery for tricuspid regurgitation late after mitral valve replacement. *Circulation* 70(suppl I):193, 1984.

61. Konishi Y et al: Comparative study of Kay-Boyd's, DeVega's, and Carpentier's annuloplasty in the management of functional tricuspid regurgitation, *Jpn Circ J* 47:1167-1172, 1983.

62. Konno S et al: A new method for prosthetic valve replacement in congenital aortic stenosis associated with hypoplasia of the aortic valve ring, *J Thorac Cardiovasc Surg* 70:909-919, 1975.

63. Kurlansky P, Rose EA, Malm JR: Adjustable annuloplasty for tricuspid insufficiency, *Ann Thorac Surg* 44:404-406, 1987.

64. Lepley D, Flemma RJ, Mullen DC: The Bjork-Shiley tilting disc valve in the mitral position. In Ionescu MI, Cohn LH, eds: *Mitral valve disease diagnosis and treatment,* London, 1985, Butterworths.

65. Lessana A et al: Mitral valve repair: results and the decision-making process in reconstruction, *J Thorac Cardiovasc Surg* 99:622-630, 1990.

66. Loperfidof F et al: Pulsed Doppler echocardiographic analysis of mitral regurgitation after myocardial infarction, *Am J Cardiol* 58:692-697, 1986.

67. Lund OL et al: Long-term prosthesis-related and sudden cardiac-related complications after valve replacement of aortic stenosis, *Ann Thorac Surg* 50:396-406, 1990.

68. Magilligan DJ: Bioprosthetic valve endocarditis. In Magilligan DJ, Quinn EL, eds: *Endocarditis: medical and surgical management,* New York, 1986, Marcel Dekker.

69. Magilligan AJ, Lewis JW, Stein P, Alton M: The porcine bioprosthetic heart valve: experience at 15 years, *Ann Thorac Surg* 48:324-330, 1989.

70. Manouguian S, Seybold-Epting W: Patch enlargement of the aortic valve ring by extending the aortic incision into the anterior mitral leaflet: new operative technique, *J Thorac Cardiovasc Surg* 78:402-412, 1979.

71. Melvin DB et al: Computer-based analysis of pre-operative and post-operative prognostic factors in 100 patients with combined aortic and mitral valve replacement, *Circulation* 46(suppl III):56-62, 1973.

72. Midell AI, DeBoer A: Multiple valve replacement: an analysis of early and late results, *Arch Surg* 104:471-476, 1972.

73. Miller DW, Johnson DD, Ivey TD: Does preservation of the posterior chordae tendinea enhance survival during mitral valve replacement? *Ann Thorac Surg* 28:22-27, 1979.

74. Mullany CJ et al: Repair of tricuspid valve insufficiency in patients undergoing double (aortic and mitral) valve replacement: perioperative mortality and long-term (1 to 20 years) follow-up in 109 patients, *J Thorac Cardiovasc Surg* 94:740-748, 1987.

396   The Johns Hopkins Manual of Cardiac Surgical Care

75. Murphy E: Prosthetic cardiac valves. In *Valvular heart disease*, Littleton, Mass, 1987, PSG Publishers.
76. Nishimura RA, Holmes DR, Reeder GS: Percutaneous balloon valvuloplasty, *Mayo Clin Proc* 65:198-220, 1990.
77. Nishimura RA et al: Doppler evaluation of results of percutaneous aortic balloon valvuloplasty in calcific aortic stenosis, *Circulation* 78:791-799, 1988.
78. Okitz Y et al: Early and late results of aortic root replacement with antibiotic sterilized aortic homograft, *J Thorac Cardiovasc Surg* 95:696-704, 1988.
79. Olesen KH: The natural history of 271 patients with mitral stenosis under medical treatment, *Br Heart J* 24:349-357, 1962.
80. Oliveira DBG, Dawkins KD, Kay PH, Paneth M: Chordal rupture II: comparison between repair and replacement, *Br Heart J* 50:318-324, 1983.
81. Ormiston JA, Shah PM, Tei C, Wong M: Size and motion of the mitral valve annulus in man. I. A two-dimensional echocardiographic method and findings in normal subjects, *Circulation* 64:113-119, 1981.
82. Pakrashi BC et al: Clinical and hemodynamic results of mitral annuloplasty, *Br Heart J* 36:768-780, 1974.
83. Perier P et al: Comparative evaluation of mitral valve repair and replacement with Starr, Bjork, and porcine valve prosthesis, *Circulation* 70 (suppl I):187, 1984.
84. Phillips HR et al. Mitral valve replacement for isolated mitral regurgitation: analysis of clinical course and late post-operative left ventricular ejection fraction, *Am J Cardiol* 48:647-654, 1981.
85. Pluth Jr, Ellis FH: Tricuspid insufficiency in patients undergoing mitral valve replacement, *J Thorac Cardiovasc Surg* 58:484-489, 1969.
86. Rahimtoola SH: Catheter balloon valvuloplasty of aortic and mitral stenosis in adults: 1987, *Circulation* 75:895-901, 1987.
87. Rankin JS et al: A clinical comparison of mitral valve repair versus valve replacement in ischemic mitral regurgitation, *J Thorac Cardiovasc Surg* 95:165-177, 1988.
88. Rappaport E: Natural history of aortic and mitral valve disease, *Am J Cardiol* 35:221-229, 1975.
89. Raychaudhurg T, Faichney A, Cameron EWJ, Walbaum PR: Surgical management of native valve endocarditis, *Thorax* 38:168-174, 1983.
90. Reed GE, Pooley RW, Moggio RA: Durability of measured mitral annuloplasty: seventeen-year study, *J Thorac Cardiovasc Surg* 79:321-325, 1980.
91. Reitz BA et al: Translocation of the aortic valve for prosthetic valve endocarditis, *J Thorac Cardiovasc Surg* 81:212-218, 1981.

92. Replogle RL, Campbell CD: Surgery for mitral regurgitation associated with ischemic heart disease, *Circulation* 79(suppl I):122-125, 1989.

93. Richardson JV, Karp RB, Kirklin JW, Dismukes WE: Treatment of infective endocarditis: a ten year comparative analysis, *Circulation* 58:589-597, 1978.

94. Rivera R, Duran E, Ajuria M: Carpentier's flexible ring versus DeVega's annuloplasty, *J Thorac Cardiovasc Surg* 89:196-223, 1985.

95. Ross J, Braunwald E: Aortic stenosis, *Circulation* 37: (suppl 5):61-67, 1968.

96. Rossiter SJ et al: Prosthetic valve endocarditis: comparison of heterograft tissue valves and mechanical valves, *J Thorac Cardiovasc Surg* 76:795-803, 1978.

97. Sand ME et al: A comparison of repair and replacement for mitral valve incompetence, *J Thorac Cardiovasc Surg* 94:208-219, 1987.

98. Saour JN, Sieck JO, Mamo LAR, Gallus AS: Trial of different intensities of anticoagulation in patients with prosthetic heart valves, *N Engl J Med* 332:428-432, 1990.

99. Schuler G et al: Temporal response left ventricular performance to mitral valve surgery, *Circulation* 59:1218-1231, 1979.

100. Segal J, Harvey WP, Hufnagel C: A clinical study of one hundred cases of severe aortic insufficiency, *Am J Med* 2:200-210, 1956.

101. Shapira N et al: Aortic valve repair for aortic stenosis in adults, *Ann Thorac Surg* 50:110-120, 1990.

102. Shore DF, Wong P, Paneth M: Results of mitral valvuloplasty with a suture plication technique, *J Thorac Cardiovasc Surg* 79:349-357, 1980.

103. Souttar HS: Surgical treatment of mitral stenosis, *Br Med J* 2:603-606, 1925.

104. Spence PA et al: Toward a better understanding of the etiology of left ventricular dysfunction after mitral valve replacement: an experimental study with possible clinical implications, *Ann Thorac Surg* 41:363-371, 1986.

105. Spencer FC, Colvin SB, Culliford AT, Isom OW: Experiences with the Carpentier techniques of mitral valve reconstruction in 103 patients (1980-1985), *J Thorac Cardiovasc Surg* 90:341-350, 1985.

106. Stassano P et al: Double valve implantation: long-term evaluation of 8 different bioprostheses, *Tex Heart Inst J* 18:34-40, 1991.

107. Tsakiris AG, Sturm RE, Wood EH: Experimental studies on the mechanisms of closure of cardiac valves with use of roentgen videodensitometry, *Am J Cardiol* 32:136-143, 1973.

108. Tsakiris AG et al: Motion of the tricuspid valve annulus in anesthetized intact dogs, *Circ Res* 36:4348, 1975.

109. Ubago JL et al: Analysis of the amount of tricuspid valve annular dilatation required to produce functional tricuspid regurgitation, *Am J Cardiol* 52:155-158, 1983.

110. Wood P: Aortic stenosis, *Am J Cardiol* 1:553-71, 1983.

111. Yacoub M et al: Surgical treatment of mitral regurgitation caused by floppy valves: repair versus replacement, *Circulation* 64 (suppl II):210-215, 1981.

112. Zussa C et al: Artificial mitral valve chordae: experimental and clinical experience, *Ann Thorac Surg* 50:367, 1990.

Diseases of the Aorta

18

Michael A. Acker, Eloise J. Wagner, G. Melville Williams, and Vincent L. Gott

Although diseases of the thoracic aorta are among the most serious and challenging problems with which the cardiothoracic surgeon deals, remarkable progress has been made in the last few years so that the current overall surgical results are extremely gratifying.

There is now a general consensus among cardiovascular surgeons regarding the management of the various problems of the the thoracic aorta. Considerable disagreement, however, remains in the literature regarding the etiology and pathophysiology of the various disease entities of the aorta. For example, the term *cystic medionecrosis* as originally described by Erdheim[12] in 1930 is not completely accurate and yet it has been used to describe the pathologic process that occurs in most patients with aortic root aneurysm. More recently it has been determined that necrosis is almost never present in these aneurysmal segments, and although elastin fragmentation of fibers may be present in the media, cystic degeneration is fairly rare. Fortunately, with the recent development of sophisticated biochemical assays for aortic wall collagen and the use of scanning electron microscopy, the pathophysiology of aortic aneurysms and dissections is gradually being clarified.

Pathology

Arteriosclerotic aneurysm

Arteriosclerotic aneurysms present with almost equal frequency in the ascending and descending thoracic aorta. More rarely this type of aneurysm may involve the aortic arch and the complete extent of the thoracoabdominal aorta. These aneurysms ordinarily have a fusiform shape that at least in the ascending aorta distinguishes them from the pear-shaped aortic root aneurysms seen in patients with Marfan syndrome and nonspecific myxomatous degeneration.

Aneurysms Resulting from Marfan Syndrome and Nonspecific Myxomatous Degeneration

In the great majority of patients with Marfan syndrome a sizable aneurysm of the aortic root (annuloaortic ectasia) develops by 20 years of age. In fact, without surgical intervention approximately 90% of these patients die as a result of a cardiovascular mishap.

In patients with Marfan syndrome aneurysms and dissections can also develop in other areas of the aorta, but this is infrequent compared with the ascending aorta.

Histologic examination of the involved aortic wall in these Marfan patients demonstrates fractured elastin fibers in the media, resulting in marked reduction in the tensile strength of the wall.[30] Biochemical assays of the aortic wall in these same patients also demonstrate a quantitative reduction of elastin content.[30]

Patients who do not have Marfan syndrome may also have sizable aneurysms of the aortic root. These patients could be designated as having nonspecific annuloaortic ectasia resulting from myxomatous degeneration of the aortic media. The aneurysms in these patients are at the same risk of dissection and rupture as in the Marfan patient and they need to be dealt with in an equally aggressive manner.

Aortic Dissection

All the aneurysms that have been discussed can be the forerunner of a dissection process, although it is somewhat rare for this to occur in the arteriosclerotic aneurysm. On the other hand, it is possible on rare occasions to have a dissection that commences in the ascending aorta without an actual aneurysm or even mild dilation in this area.

The most common classifications used in discussing aortic dissection have been devised by DeBakey and colleagues[10] (Fig. 18-1) and the cardiovascular surgeons at Stanford University[24] (Fig. 18-2). In the older DeBakey classification the type I dissection involves the ascending aorta together with the transverse arch and possibly the distal aorta. If the dissection involves only the ascending aorta, it would be classified as a DeBakey type II dissection. Dissections that involve the aorta distal to the left subclavian

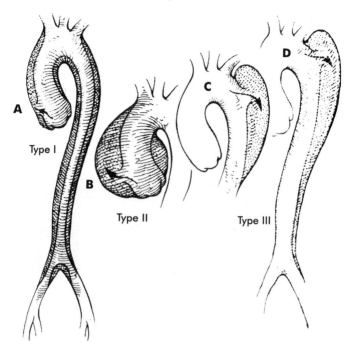

Fig. 18-1 DeBakey classification of thoracic aortic dissections. See text for details. (From DeBakey ME et al: Dissection and dissecting the aorta: *Surgery* 92:1118, 1982.)

artery are classified as DeBakey type III. More recently the first two DeBakey groups have been classified by Stanford cardiac surgeons as type A, and the type III aneurysm is classified as type B. Although both these classifications are excellent, the senior author of this chapter prefers the DeBakey classification because it more precisely delineates the extent of the dissection, and this in turn relates directly to the natural course and prognosis of the disease process.

One of the most outstanding recent discussions of aortic dissection has been presented by our senior cardiovascular pathologist, Dr. Grover Hutchins, and his associate Dr. Stephen Wilson.[39] In their report Hutchins and Wilson reviewed the histories of all patients who underwent postmortem examinations at The Johns

Type A   Type B

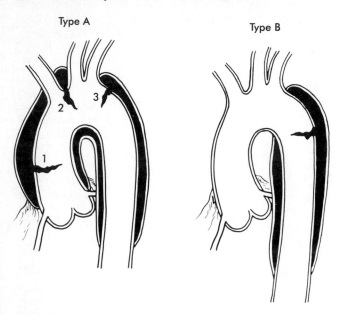

Fig. 18-2 Stanford classification of thoracic aortic dissections. See text for details. (From Miller DC et al: Operative treatment of aortic dissections, *J Thorac Cardiovasc Surg* 78:365, 1979.)

Hopkins Hospital (JHH) between 1889 and 1980 with a diagnosis of aortic dissection. Briefly, Hutchins and Wilson reviewed the autopsy records of the 204 patients with aortic dissection during that 91-year period and compared them with age-, race-, and sex-matched control subjects. Their results revealed that in the group with aortic dissection the mean age was 55 years, 65% were men, 53% were black, and, most important, 69% were hypertensive as compared with only 29% in the control group. The intimal tear was located in the ascending aorta in 50% of the patients, in the area of the ligamentum ductus in 34%, other sites in 7%, and unlocated in 13%. Arteriosclerosis was slightly more prevalent in the patients with dissection than in the matched control subjects. Also "cystic medial necrosis" was slightly more prevalent in the patients with dissection, but only 10% of the overall group of 204 patients with dissection had this pathologic entity. This excellent study of Hutchins and Wilson clearly demonstrated that aortic dissection occurs mainly in elderly hypertensive men. Most important, the data indicate that cystic medionecrosis is ordinarily not a pathogenic lesion in aortic dissection and confirms the earlier suggestion by Schlatmann and Becker,[33,34] and Hirst and Gore,[18] that the actual dissection process most frequently results from degeneration of elastic fibers of the media as a result of long-standing hypertensive injury.

Traumatic Aneurysm

Traumatic aneurysm of the thoracic aorta can result from either penetrating or blunt injury. A penetrating injury more often occurs in the ascending aorta than in the descending aorta, and a high percentage of these injured persons die within minutes after the trauma has occurred.

High-impact deceleration injuries can cause disruption of the ascending aorta; however, these persons seldom survive long enough to reach the operating room. In patients who do survive a disruption of the aorta from a deceleration injury the tear usually occurs at the level of the ligamentum arteriosum. This appears to be the usual site of disruption with deceleration injuries because the aorta distal to the ligamentum is tethered to the posterior portion of the chest wall by intercostal vessels, and proximal to this point the velocity of movement of the aortic arch can be high as a result of sudden deceleration of the heart and mediastinal structures.

Clinical Considerations and Diagnosis

Arteriosclerotic Aneurysm

Most arteriosclerotic aneurysms are found in patients more than 60 years of age. Typically, thoracic arteriosclerotic aneurysms are associated with aneurysms at other sites and general evidence of occlusive arteriosclerotic disease. Most thoracic arteriosclerotic aneurysms are asymptomatic and present as a mediastinal mass on routine chest x-ray films. When symptoms and signs are found, they are usually related to rapid growth, with pressure or obstruction of related structures. Pain is the most common symptom at presentation. Usually the pain is chronic and dull, and gradually becomes more unrelenting. This may be related to a gradual increase in aneurysmal size or pressure on the chest wall. Precordial pain radiating to the jaw or neck is associated with ascending aortic aneurysms whereas back pain is associated with descending thoracic aortic aneurysms. Occasionally, acute sharp pain signals sudden expansion or rupture.

The symptoms and signs of a thoracic arteriosclerotic aneurysm depend on its size and exact location. Large aneurysms can produce hoarseness by compression of the recurrent laryngeal nerve; wheezing, cough, hemoptysis, or pneumonitis by tracheal or bronchial compression, and dysphagia by esophageal compression. Aortic insufficiency is rarely caused by arteriosclerotic aneurysms of the ascending aorta, although this is commonly associated with aortic dissection.

History and physical examination are usually notable not for the aneurysm but rather for manifestations of arteriosclerotic disease, including signs of coronary artery disease, carotid and femoral bruits, aneurysms of the abdominal aorta, and femoral and popliteal arteries.

The chest x-ray film is the most useful initial screen for arteriosclerotic aneurysms of the thoracic aorta. Thoracic computed tomographic (CT) scan with contrast distinguishes the aneurysm from nonvascular mediastinal masses and determines its exact size. It is the best method for evaluating aortic wall intergrity and for observing the aneurysm for a period of time. If surgery is being contemplated, an aortogram is indicated to provide the details of vascular anatomy. Magnetic resonance imaging (MRI) has recently been found to be extremely useful in the preoperative evaluation of these patients. This type of scan can determine blood flow without contrast, provide better definition of vascular anatomy than the CT scan, and provide anatomic information on the heart. Akins and coworkers[1] found MRI evaluation definitive for descending thoracic aortic aneurysms, although the aortogram remains necessary for ascending and arch aneurysms. Further workup before surgery should include a complete cardiac evaluation, noninvasive carotid studies, and evaluation of lower extremity circulation.

Arteriosclerotic aneurysms of the descending thoracic aorta have a tendency to increase gradually in size and rupture. Pressler and McNamara[31] found a mean survival time of less than 3 years and a 44% rupture rate. Bickerstaff and coworkers[3] found the 5-year actuarial survival rate of 19% and a 51% rupture rate in patients followed up medically without surgery for descending thoracic aneurysms.

Treatment of these patients is based on the relative risk of surgery versus the risk of rupture. Frequent complications of operative repair include myocardial infarction, stroke, and pulmonary and renal failure. Absolute indications for surgical repair include all symptomatic aneurysms, rapid increase in size, and asymptomatic aneurysms greater that 10 cm in diameter.[26] If the aneurysm is small (i.e., >6 cm in diameter) or if the patient is at particularly high risk, observation with frequent CT or MRI follow-up to assess aneurysmal growth is justified. Some surgeons recommend elective surgery in all patients who have arteriosclerotic thoracic aneurysms and are at reasonable risk. Crawford and coworkers[6] reported a 58% 5-year actuarial survival rate in patients who had their aneurysms surgically treated versus a 19% survival rate with medical treatment. They recommend total replacement of all aortic disease, because any remaining aortic aneurysmal disease is primarily responsible for late death.

Aneurysms Resulting from Marfan Syndrome and Nonspecific Myxomatous Degeneration

The major cause of preoperative death in patients with Marfan syndrome is aortic disease resulting in either dissection on aneurysmal rupture.[32] In patients with a Marfan aneurysm (or any type of nonspecific annuloaortic ectasia) any symptoms that possibly could suggest acute dissection warrant an aggressive workup, including CT scan, MRI, or aortogram.

Although the entire aorta can potentially be involved, aortic root dilatation is the most common manifestation. The aortic root in all Marfan patients must be monitored closely from the time of diagnosis with serial echocardiograms to document progression of disease. Previous expectant nonoperative management of Marfan syndrome with ascending aortic aneurysm was associated with frequent dissection, rupture, and generally poor prognosis. Elective repair of ascending aortic aneurysms can be done relatively safely, and this has led to the recommendation that all aneurysms 6 cm or greater in size be prophylactically repaired.[13] A recent article from our cardiac group reported a 1% hospital mortality rate in 100 consecutive Marfan patients undergoing a composite graft of an ascending aortic aneurysm. The one death occurred in a patient who arrived in the operating room (OR) with a frank rupture and a myocardial infarction.[14]

Preoperative evaluation should include aortogram, and CT scan or MRI. The aortogram defines the extent of dissection, the severity of sinus Valsalva dilatation, the degree of cephalad displacement of the coronary ostia, the involvement of brachycephalic vessels with aneurysmal change or dissection, and the severity of aortic insufficiency. Because of potential involvement, the entire aorta must be studied. CT scan or MRI provides precise information on aneurysm size and is useful as a baseline for postoperative comparison. Presently we prefer preoperative MRI over CT scan because of its ability to provide coronal and sagittal sections of the entire aorta without the need for contrast.

Crawford's excellent results in the repair of all cardiovascular manifestations of the Marfan syndrome including arch, descending and thoracoabdominal aneurysms, and dissections suggest that a more aggressive approach to all aortic problems in Marfan patients, in addition to the ascending aortic aneurysm, may permit better long-term survival.[9,35]

Aortic Dissection

Acute thoracic aortic dissections are seen typically in persons either with a history of long-standing hypertension or with annuloaortic ectasia. Ascending aortic dissections occur at a somewhat younger age (55 years) than descending dissections (63 years).[3] Dissections in Marfan syndrome occur at a particularly young age, with the average age at death being 32 years in one series of untreated patients.[27]

Clinically the hallmark of acute aortic dissection is the sudden onset of pain. The pain is characteristically sharp and severe, and is initially located in the retrosternal or midscapular location. As the dissection progresses, the pain typically migrates down the back. The onset can be heralded by syncope, diaphoresis, and hypotension. Further manifestations depend on variations in the location, extent, and complications associated with the dissection. Aortic rupture leading to cardiac tamponade or exsanguination into the chest or abdomen is the most common cause of death. Branch vessel obstruction resulting from the dissection can lead to stroke; myocardial infarction; paraplegia; and intestinal, renal, and lower extremity ischemia. Neurologic defects, signs of an acute abdomen, or a pulse deficit may be noted. Signs of total aortic obstruction may also be noted if the false lumen protrudes to obstruct the true lumen. If the dissection detaches the aortic valvular apparatus, the patient will have a new diastolic murmur of aortic insufficiency and acute left-sided heart failure. The myriad of variations in the presentation and course of aortic dissection make the differential diagnosis extensive. It must be differentiated from an acute myocardial infarction, pulmonary embolus, stroke, acute abdomen, acute paralysis, or limb ischemia.

If acute aortic dissection is suspected clinically and by initial chest x-ray film, then urgent confirmation of the diagnosis is made by aortogram and/or chest CT scan or MRI. A normal electrocardiogram helps to rule out an acute myocardial infarction. A CT scan is useful as an initial study in an atypical presentation or to differentiate a dissection from a myocardial infarction. The double-channel aortic lumen with intimal flap and extralumenal hematoma, if present, is visualized on a CT scan. The diagnosis of an acute dissection can also be made by MRI, but in the acute setting this method remains cumbersome. If we strongly suspects a dissection, we still prefer the aortogram as our definitive test. It ordinarily defines the exact site of intimal tear and provides details of vascular anatomy. Additional information on extent of dissection, involvement of major visceral branches, and the presence of aortic insufficiency is also provided. In the stable older patient with a type A dissection it is also important to obtain coronary angiography.

In patients suspected of having acute aortic dissection, arterial and central venous catheters should be placed for continous pressure monitoring. In addition, urine output, level of consciousness, and peripheral circulation must be carefully monitored. During evaluation hypertension must be meticulously controlled with sodium nitroprusside. In addition, intravenous esmolol is used to reduce myocardial contractility (dP/dt).

Dissections involving the ascending aorta have been shown to carry an improved survival rate if immediately corrected surgically. The management of descending aortic dissections (i.e., type III or type B) remains controversial. Most centers, given the general unsatisfactory results of early surgical repair, recommend aggressive medical treatment with nitroprusside and β-blockers to stabilize these dissections. Indications for early repair include evidence of dissection extension, compromise of major vascular branches, impending rupture, or inability to control pain. This aggressive medical regimen halts the progression of the descending hematoma, and an 80% hospital survival rate can be expected. Patients with dissections that are stabilized medically can be operated on later, when tissues are less friable, with a lower operative mortality rate.[11,19] The Stanford group, however, continues to advocate early repair. They point to their present 13% operative mortality rate and to their belief that if the operation is postponed until complications occur, operative risk will increase.[25]

Traumatic Aneurysm

Penetrating injury to the thoracic aorta is relatively rare in comparison with blunt injury. Most persons who sustain such an injury die before reaching the hospital. Those who do arrive usually have severe hypotension resulting from ongoing hemorrhage. A few patients may arrive in the emergency room with apparent hemodynamic stability and evidence of a widening mediastinum or chest x-ray film. A pulse deficit may be present if an injury to a branch vessel has occurred. In the stable patient CT scan and/or aortogram may be of value. Most often, however, the diagnosis must rest only on a high suspicion based on the condition of the patient and the location of the wound.

Traumatic aortic disruption resulting from blunt trauma is usually a result of a deceleration injury and occurs most commonly in the area of the ligamentum arteriosum. In the vast majority of cases this injury is immediately fatal. In 10% to 15% of patients, however, the disruption is contained temporarily by the adventitial layer and mediastinal structures, allowing the patient to survive long enough to reach the hospital. Risk of rupture is greatest immediately after the injury. It is estimated that 40% rupture within 2 days. A high index of suspicion as to all patients with a history of severe deceleration injury or chest trauma is needed to make the correct diagnosis. Severe multisystem trauma is frequently associated with this injury. Symptoms and signs associated with traumatic aortic disruption include intrascapular back pain, retrosternal chest pain, unexplained hypotension, upper extremity hypertension, bilateral femoral pulse deficits, and initial chest tube output greater than 750 ml.

A few persons with blunt trauma injury of the thoracic aorta may arrive at the hospital in an asymptomatic condition. The chest x-ray film is the first diagnostic test. Mediastinal widening of greater than 8 cm is a sensitive but nonspecific sign of traumatic aortic disruption. Other findings on chest x-ray film correlating with traumatic aortic disruption include blurring of the aortic knob, deviation of the trachea, and left hemothorax. If an aortic injury is suspected, an immediate aortogram is indicated for definitive diagnosis and to delineate specific anatomy. Once the diagnosis is made, immediate operation is indicated in most patients.

Operative Management

Aneurysms and Dissections of the Ascending Aorta and Aortic Arch

Most disease processes of the ascending aorta and aortic arch can be categorized for the purpose of operative repair into one of three distinct pathologic processes. These include fusiform aneurysms (arteriosclerotic), type I or II (type A) dissection, and annuloaortic ectasia.

Fusiform aneurysm (arteriosclerotic)

As mentioned previously, fusiform aneurysms of the ascending aorta are normally the result of arteriosclerotic degeneration of the aortic wall; these are the most straightforward of the ascending aortic lesions with which the cardiothoracic surgeon has to deal.

Standard cardiopulmonary bypass as described in Chapter 4 is used. The operative approach from the standpoint of cannulation and venting is similar to that used for aortic valve replacement, but normally the fusiform aneurysm precludes use of the distal ascending aorta for arterial cannulation. In this situation the arterial cannula is placed in the common femoral artery.

The patient's temperature is normally lowered to a rectal temperature of 27° C. The distal portion of the ascending aorta is cross-clamped, and potassium cardioplegic arrest is achieved with 1000 ml of potassium chloride solution. Normally for a standard fusiform aneurysm the aorta is completely transected above and below the aneurysm and a simple sleeve graft (low-porosity Dacron) is placed with 3-0 Prolene sutures. The graft can be preclotted by coating it with 5% albumin and then baking in an autoclave for 5 minutes.

These patients with fusiform aneurysm of the ascending aorta may also have significant aortic valve disease necessitating valve replacement, or they may have coronary arteriosclerosis and may need to have an internal mammary artery or saphenous vein graft placed to one or more coronary vessels.

Aortic dissection (type A, or type I and II)

Ordinarily the dissections that commence in the ascending aorta present as an acute process and require urgent or emergency surgery. Unless there is a major contraindication to surgery, patients with an acute dissection of the ascending aorta should ordinarily be moved directly from the catheterization laboratory to the OR for their procedure. The majority of these patients with a dissection of the ascending aorta have concomitant aortic insufficiency requiring valve replacement. The majority also have annuloaortic ectasia, although dissections of the ascending aorta can occur without aortic root enlargement. The surgical management of ascending aortic dissection resulting from annuloaortic ectasia is addressed in the next section. If this latter pathologic process has not occurred, then the operative approach is somewhat similar to that described previously for fusiform aneurysm. The main difference, however, is that dissection of the ascending aorta ordinarily occurs within very friable tissue, and we believe that some type of Teflon felt reinforcement is normally required at each anastomotic suture line. The felt strips used for this type of reinforcement are approximately 1 cm wide and can be placed either in the medial dissection plane or external to the adventitial layer. Occasionally the aortic wall tissue is so friable that a double layer of felt strips are required, one within the lumen and one on the exterior of the aortic wall.

Frequently the aortic insufficiency that accompanies dissection of the ascending aorta can be dealt with by resuspension of the three commissures of the aortic valve. More often than not the dissection starts from a transverse tear in the intima in the lower portion of the ascending aorta. A strip of Teflon felt can be placed in the medial dissection plane, and with the inner and outer layer of the aorta oversewn to include this felt the normal architecture of the aortic valve is restored and thus becomes competent. If this cannot be achieved, then the valve must be replaced.

It is of course essential in the operative repair of a dissection of the ascending aorta to resect the aorta at the site of the intimal tear. By completely transecting the aorta just proximal to the innominate artery and obliterating the false lumen with a whipping 3-0 Prolene suture that incorporates a Teflon felt strip, the false channel is normally eliminated. If this is the case, then the ascending aorta is replaced with a sleeve graft of low-porosity polyester that has been coated with albumin and baked as described in the foregoing section on fusiform aneurysms.

One of the most challenging problems that the cardiothoracic surgeon faces is a type I (type A) dissection that commences in the ascending aorta and spirals into the arch and descending aorta with multiple fenestrations in the partitioning septum. If the surgeon is fortunate enough to have a patient with a chronic dissection of this type, circulatory arrest can be used (described in Annuloaortic Ectasia) and the septum, which may contain fenestrations, is simply resected as far as need be, at least to the proximal portion to the descending thoracic aorta. We have been gratified with the results in patients with chronic type I dissection in whom we have been able to resect this partitioning septum in the aortic arch with circulatory arrest.

For patients who have the serious problem of an acute type I dissection with a spiraling tear or fenestrations in the arch, ordinarily the ascending aorta and arch must be replaced.

Annuloaortic ectasia (with involvement of the ascending aorta or aortic arch)

Before the description by Bentall and DeBond[2] in 1968 of the composite graft repair of large aneurysms of the aortic root, the operative results for this problem were extremely poor. During the past 20 years with the use of composite graft repair of aneurysms of the aortic root, the hospital mortality rate has been normally reported at 5% or less. The results of this operation are so satisfactory that it is generally agreed that all patients with an aortic root aneurysm that is greater than 6 cm in diameter should have prophylactic composite graft repair even if they are completely asymptomatic.

The operative approach for these patients with aneurysms of the aortic root is similar to that described in the foregoing two sections on the fusiform aneurysms and aortic dissection (Fig. 18-3). The femoral artery is routinely cannulated for the patient with aortic root aneurysms, and the operative repair is normally carried out as depicted in Fig. 18-3. One thousand milliliters of potassium chloride cardioplegic solution is injected either into the aortic root if there is no insufficiency or directly into the coronary arteries if there is insufficiency. If the coronary ostia have migrated more than 15 mm from the annulus, annular 2-0 Tevdek sutures are

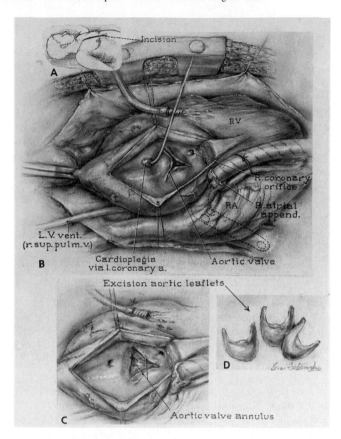

Fig. 18-3 Bentall's method of composite graft replacement of ascending aorta for patients with annuloaortic ectasia. See text for details. (From Gott VL et al: *Ann Thorac Surg* 52:38-45, 1991.)

placed as everting mattress sutures with the Teflon pledgets above the annulus. If the coronary ostia have not migrated sufficiently, the annular sutures are placed with the pledgets below the annulus so that there is no eversion of this structure and therefore no shortening of the distance between the annulus and the coronary ostia (Fig. 18-3, *E*). With this technique proposed by Helseth and colleagues[16] direct anastomosis can usually be carried out as in

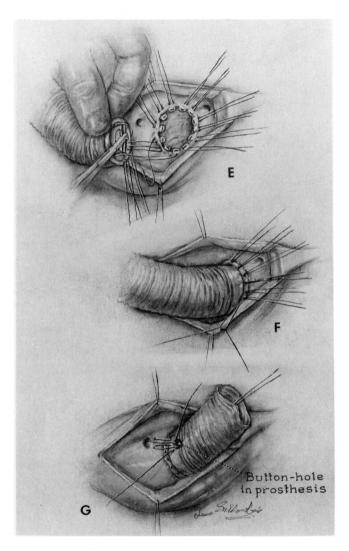

Fig. 18-3 *cont'd*. See legend on opposite page.

Continued.

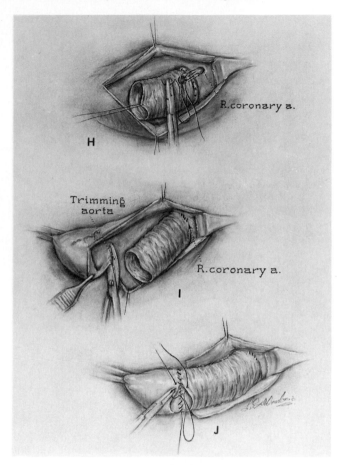

Fig. 18-3 cont'd. See legend on p. 412.

See legend on p. 412.

Fig. 18-3, *G* and *H*, even if the coronary ostia are fairly low. Cabrol and coworkers[4] and Crawford and coworkers[9] routinely use an interposed 10 mm graft between the coronary ostia and the composite graft as depicted in Fig. 18-4. We have used this technique frequently in the past but currently prefer not to use it routinely. In fact, if we are dealing with extremely low-lying coronary ostia, we normally excise the ostia with a button of aortic wall, and mobilize and then implant them in an appropriate place

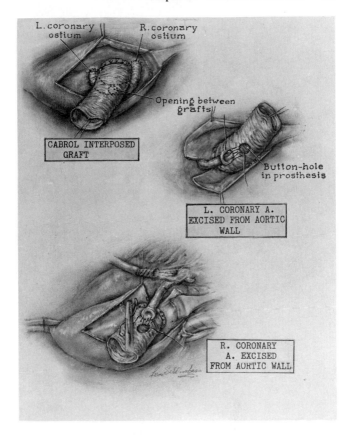

Fig. 18-4 Methods for dealing with low-lying coronary ostia during composite graft repair. See text for details. (From Gott VL et al: *Ann Thorac Surg* 52:38-45, 1991.)

on the composite graft (Fig. 18-4). The aorta is then transected distally as in Fig. 18-3, *I* and a running anastomosis is created with a 4-0 Prolene suture (Fig. 18-3, *J*). It has been our preference for many years to use the aneurysm wall as a wrap as described by Bentall and DeBono in their original article. Because of a potential problem of hypertensive hematoma between the composite graft and the aneurysm wrap, we have for the last 2 years followed the advice of Kouchoukos and colleagues[22] and have not

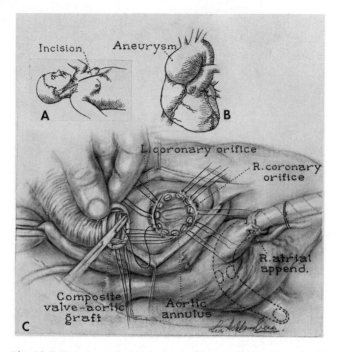

Fig. 18-5 Technique of replacing ascending aorta and aortic arch with deep hypothermia and total body circulatory arrest. See text for details.

used the inclusive wrap but simply tacked the redundant aneurysm wall over the graft so that it is not blood-tight.

Normally for most patients with annuloaortic ectasia the standard Bentall composite graft works well. Sometimes, however, the aneurysm extends into the proximal aortic arch or involves the entire aortic arch. In this situation we prefer the technique of circulatory arrest as first described by Griepp and coworkers[15] and popularized by Ott and coworkers.[29] This technique has greatly simplified the surgeon's approach to the aortic arch. Because no vascular clamps are needed, excellent exposure can be obtained of the complete aortic arch and the proximal portion of the descending thoracic aorta. If we anticipate that we will be resecting a portion of the aortic arch, we have our perfusionist cool the patient's body to a rectal temperature of 18° C. During this period

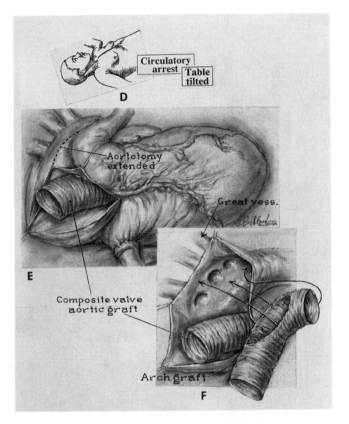

Fig. 18-5 cont'd. See legend on opposite page.   *Continued.*

of cooling we proceed with the composite graft replacement (Fig. 18-5, *C*) of the ascending aorta, and when the proper level of hypothermia has been achieved, we then place the patient in deep Trendelenburg position, drain off any excess blood to the heart-lung machine, turn off the pump, and proceed with resection of the diseased portion of the aortic arch and graft replacement of this segment (Fig. 18-5, *D* to *G*). This cooling technique appears to provide 45 minutes of safe circulatory arrest for an operative procedure on the aortic arch. When this aspect of the operation is completed, the pump is turned back on, the aortic arch graft is clamped proximally, reperfusion of the head vessels is achieved,

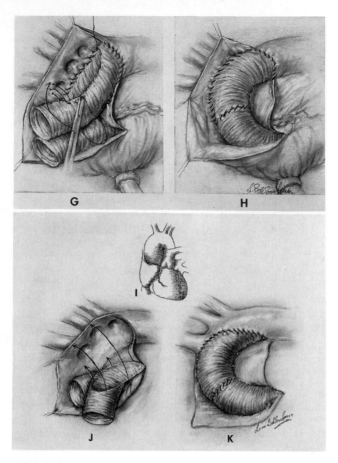

Fig. 18-5 cont'd. See legend on p. 416.

and we continue then with the composite graft repair and subsequently anastomose the two grafts together (Fig. 18-5, *H*). Patients with an aneurysm of the proximal arch do not require as extensive a resection of the aorta as depicted in Fig. 18-5, *I* to *K*.

Aneurysms and Dissections of the Descending Thoracic Aorta and Thoracoabdominal Aorta

All aneurysms and dissections of the descending thoracic aorta and the thoracoabdominal aorta require a left thoracotomy with single-lung anesthesia. For aneurysms involving the upper thoracic aorta the fourth inner space or bed of the fifth rib is the optimal site of entry. Aneurysms involving the lower thoracic aorta require a correspondingly lower thoracotomy. Extensive thoracoabdominal aneurysms normally require lengthening of the incision across the costal margin into a midline or a paramedial abdominal incision. Alternatively the long thoracoabdominal skin incision may be used and the chest and flank entered through two separate incisions. We have come to prefer this approach in elderly patients; we excise the fifth rib to gain proximal control and go through the ninth inner space to obtain exposure of the abdominal aorta. The diaphragm is incised peripherally and the kidney and abdominal contents retracted anteriorly. The upper intercostal incision is used to obtain aortic control and to perform the proximal anastomosis. The lower incision is used for intercostal artery attachment when necessary and for the attachment of renal and visceral vessels, concluding with aorta-to-aorta anastomosis inferiorly.

There has been considerable debate about the relative benefits of shunt or pump bypass versus a no-shunt technique, but studies such as those by Katz and coworkers[20] seem clearly to indicate that the is risk of paraplegia is time related when the descending thoracic aorta is cross-clamped for more than 30 minutes (Fig. 18-6). Most cardiothoracic surgeons do not operate on the descending thoracic aorta frequently enough to permit them to carry out a major aortic resection and graft replacement within 30 minutes. A shunt or pump bypass permits an unhurried proximal anastomosis in all cases and of course can be sustained throughout the operation in aneurysms limited to the upper two thirds of the descending thoracic aorta.

In our early experience with surgery of the descending thoracic aorta (1965 to 1975) the TDMAC-heparin shunt was favored for most of these cases[36] (Fig. 18-7). The vascular grafts available at that time were extremely porous, and the perioperative bleeding that accompanied full heparinization for left atrial–femoral bypass carried a very significant morbidity and mortality rate. Use of the heparin shunt eliminated the need for systemic heparinization and the need of a bypass pump. From 1975 to 1988 we favored femoral vein–femoral artery bypass with a pump-oxygenator. This technique permitted simple cannulation of the femoral artery and femoral vein and theoretically provided the best possible protection to the spinal cord and abdominal organs. Even with complete heparinization the problem of perioperative bleeding was greatly min-

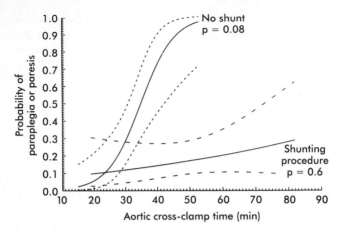

Fig. 18-6 Nomogram relating probability of spinal cord injury (paraplegia or paresis) to aortic cross-clamp time (minutes) for patients in whom no shunting procedure was used and for those in whom it was used. All patients were operated on at University of Alabama Medical Center and had acute traumatic aortic transection. *Dashed lines* are 70% confidence limits. (From Katz NM et al: *J Thorac Cardiovasc Surg* 81:669, 1981.)

imized with improved low-porosity grafts and improved suture material.

Commencing in 1988 our preferred technique has been left atrial–femoral artery bypass with the BioMedicus centrifugal pump[17,28] (Fig. 18-8). This technique of left atrial–femoral bypass has several advantages over femoral vein–femoral artery pump-oxygenator bypass. Most important, the heparin dose can be reduced by two thirds to 100 U/kg and the overall pump bypass circuit is much simpler in that the BioMedicus pump can be placed close to the operative field with short inflow and outflow lines. We place a 2-0 Tevdek purse-string suture in the waist of the left auricle and cannulate the left atrium with a 28F cannula. The lines and the pump are filled with blood, and this is returned to the patient through a cannula in the left common femoral artery. This simple type of left atrial–femoral artery pump bypass not only provides the best possible perfusion of the abdominal organs and lower spinal cord but also decompresses the left ventricle in a satisfactory manner. Direct aortic cannulation is carried out when

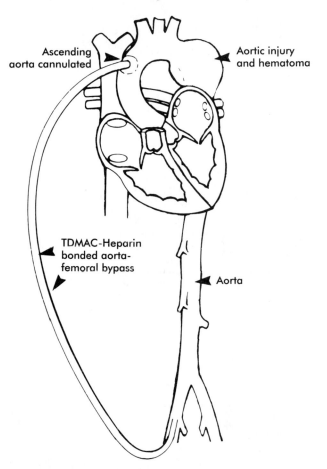

Fig. 18-7 Technique of aortic–femoral artery shunting with TDMAC-heparin–bonded shunt. (From Olivier HF Jr et al: *Ann Thorac Surg* 38:586, 1984.)

the aneurysm extends from the middle of the thoracic aorta or below to the abdomen, and the left atrium is not easily accessible.

Traumatic aneurysms

These aneurysms, whether acute or chronic, occur almost routinely at the level of ligamentum ductus and normally require a

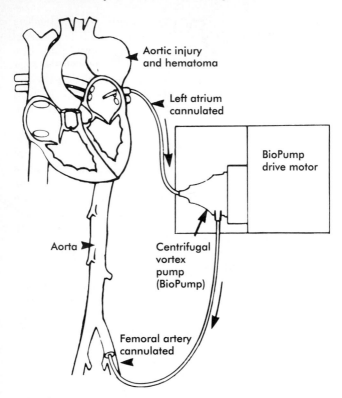

Fig. 18-8 Technique of left atrial–femoral artery bypass with interposed BioMedicus pump. (From Olivier HF Jr et al: *Ann Thorac Surg* 38:586, 1984.)

sleeve graft replacement with a low-porosity Dacron polyester graft. As with graft replacement of the ascending aorta, we preclot the graft with 5% albumin and then bake it in the steam autoclave for 5 minutes. The rare traumatic aneurysm or aortic transection can be directly reanastomosed without a graft when a short segment is involved. Although we prefer to use left atrial–femoral pump bypass for these traumatic aneurysms, if massive bleeding is present when the chest is opened, we simply clamp the aorta above and below the site of the aortic tear and proceed with a graft replacement of this segment of the aorta. Unfortunately, this particular problem of acute traumatic transection of the descending thoracic aorta has been one of the most active areas in cardiothoracic surgery for generating litigation. We feel, however, that there are occasions in the presence of massive bleeding when it is imperative that the surgeon proceed with a clamp-and-sew technique, which, as noted earlier in the study by Katz and coworkers,[20] carries an increased risk of paraplegia with more prolonged cross-clamp times.

Although some surgeons still preferentially use the TDMAC-heparin shunt for all descending thoracic aortic resections,[37] we believe that it probably should be reserved for a situation when a head injury or a serious soft tissue injury is present, where systemic heparinization would be detrimental to the patient. Temporary aortic bypass with a pump appears to offer greater control and flexibility in managing perfusion in the upper and lower regions of the body.

Type III (type B) dissection

The critical feature of operative repair of either acute or chronic dissection of the descending thoracic aorta involves the elimination of the site of entry, which most frequently occurs within 2 inches of the ligamentum ductus. As indicated in this chapter under Pathology, these dissections can be a result of elastin fragmentation as part of Marfan syndrome or from a nonspecific myxomatous degeneration. More rarely dissections of the descending thoracic aorta or abdominal aorta can result from arteriosclerosis.

Again, as with the traumatic aneurysms of the descending thoracic aorta, a sleeve graft replacement of the site of entry of the acute dissection is essential. Ordinarily, we would use left atrial–femoral artery pump bypass for this type of surgery. However, with antihypertensive medical management fewer acute type B dissections require repair. When the type B dissections expand chronically, they usually have multiple entry points and extensive repair of the thoracoabdominal aorta is necessary.

Fusiform and saccular aneurysms

These aneurysms of the descending thoracic aorta and thoracoabdominal aorta are most often of arteriosclerotic origin. Saccular aneurysms limited to the thoracic aorta are repaired simply by achieving proximal and distal control and by placing a sleeve graft within the aneurysm sac with the inclusion technique. More extensive fusiform aneurysms of the thoracoabdominal aorta demand techniques permitting rapid attachment of the critical arteries to the graft, and ischemia. When the fusiform aneurysm involves the complete thoracoabdominal aorta, extensive graft replacement according to the techniques developed primarily by Crawford and coworkers[5,8] must be used (Fig. 18-9). As noted in the illustration

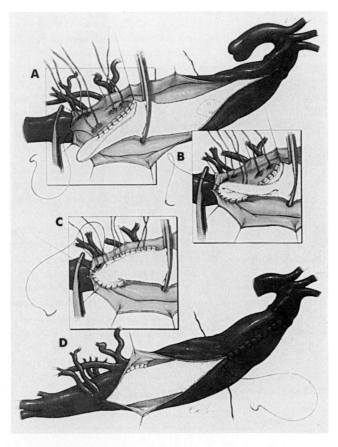

Fig. 18-9 Method of polyester graft replacement of extensive thoracoabdominal aneurysm. See text for details. (From Crawford ES, Crawford JL: *Diseases of the aorta*, Baltimore, 1984, Williams & Wilkins.)

the use of the balloon catheters within the major abdominal branches limits blood loss and is very helpful. All these cases also require the use of the cell saver and the rapid infuser.

The most significant complication attending repairs of thoracoabdominal aneurysms is paraplegia. Although our understanding of the mechanisms leading to paraplegia remains incomplete, ultimately it is caused by perturbations in spinal cord blood supply.

Normally the spinal cord receives its blood supply from four sources of varying importance:

- Neck: Branches of the vertebral, thyrocervical, and costocervical arteries
- Upper thoracic aorta: The thoracic radicular branch of an intercostal artery
- Lower thoracic and upper abdominal aorta: A lumbar or intercostal artery having as a branch the artery of Adamkiewicz or greater radicular artery (GRA); considered by most experts to be the artery critical to spinal cord viability
- Internal iliac artery: Small branches assumed to supply the end of the spinal cord and cauda equina

Because the spinal cord blood supply is segmental, the greater the extent of aorta replaced, the greater the chance of spinal cord ischemia. In the large experience of Crawford and colleagues, the replacement of the entire abdominal aorta or of small sections of the thoracic aorta results in an incidence of neurologic disturbance of only 3%.[7] However, when most of the descending thoracic and most of the abdominal aorta requires repair, the incidence of these neurologic problems increases to 28%. Although many of these patients had only partial paralysis (paraparesis), rendering the operation worthwhile as a life-saving procedure, the mechanisms responsible for paralysis, particularly that which occurs hours or days after surgery, remain unknown and apparently uninfluenced by intraoperative aortic bypass and/or spinal fluid drainage.

Intuitively, knowledge of spinal cord blood supply in each patient at high risk might direct surgical therapy more accurately and rapidly, and might provide a prognosis for the patient. However, most surgeons are fearful of spinal angiographic studies because paraplegia has been reported after aortography itself. However, the use of less toxic contrast media and digital subtraction techniques encourage us[38] and Kieffer and colleagues[21] to employ selective catheterization of intercostal and lumbar vessels to define which lower intercostal and upper lumbar arteries were present and whether any of these contributed importantly to the GRA. Angiographic complications in both studies were related to atheroembolization and occurred in two of 50 patients of Kieffer and coworkers and in one of our 47 patients.

In our experience the incidence of paraplegia and paresis after surgery was the greatest in patients having a patent GRA arising from an intercostal artery situated in the center of the aneurysm. Conversely, when the critical intercostal artery supplying blood to the spinal cord could be retained as part of the beveled posterior aortic wall, neurologic outcome was significantly better.

Laschinger and coworkers[23] demonstrated that spinal cord function could be monitored intraoperatively by somatosensory evoked potentials (SEPs). This technique and its modifications have been challenged for their particular value by the surgeon who is operating just as rapidly as possible in all these procedures. However, we believe that the use of SEPs is highly important because their absence signifies at what stage of the operation or during recovery damage occurs to the spinal cord. For example, we have lost SEPs within 15 minutes of thoracic cross-clamping in two patients, and the SEPs never returned. Both these patients had large GRAs originating directly from a large intercostal artery in the center of the aneurysm. This means that some patients are so dependent on the GRA that no technique currently available can avoid spinal cord ischemia. More correlations must be established between anatomy, procedure, and the time of injury if we are to improve results in this group of patients.

The complex and poorly understood mechanisms responsible for paraplegia should not obscure established facts. First, repairs of aneurysms limited to the upper thoracic aorta usually have a successful outcome irrespective of whether partial bypass is used. We prefer partial bypass with a BioMedicus pump because it provides more control for the surgeon, particularly under circumstances where aortic tissue does not hold stitches readily. Second, the repair of aneurysms involving the entire abdominal aorta and a portion of the thoracic aorta have results that are equally good. In these cases bypass is useful only during the performance of the proximal anastomosis. Even so, it eliminates at least 10 to 15 minutes of ischemia to the liver, kidneys, and intestines. Only the more extensive aneurysms require individual management. To treat this group more appropriately we need more information, and we will continue to use all currently advocated adjuncts to develop clinical-pathologic correlations that will help future patients.

Special Postoperative Measures

The postoperative care after aortic surgery is not dissimilar to that given after all major cardiovascular operations. Cardiac output is maximized by maintaining optimal filling pressures, preferably with colloidal solutions or red blood cells, and afterload reduction by sodium nitroprusside or nitroglycerin. Inotropic agents are used if needed. A special effort is made to avoid postoperative hypertension with afterload reduction and β-blockers if needed. Hypertension postoperatively can lead not only to bleeding from fragile aortic suture lines but also predisposes in patients operated on for dissection the development of redissection or rupture of the retained false channel. In all aortic dissections and for Marfan syndrome oral β-blockers are begun on the second postoperative day. Broad-spectrum antibiotics are continued for 48 hours. Careful monitoring of neurologic functioning is an important part of the postoperative course. Evaluation and identification of any paresthesia or change in the patients' level of consciouness are important during the recovery process.

Patients who have had their descending thoracic aorta clamped during surgery are at special risk for acute tubular necrosis (ATN). A high urine output is optimal in these patients and is achieved by maintaining an adequate preload and by using renal doses of dopamine if needed. In addition to avoiding ATN, the maintenance of an optimal cardiac output with an adequate preload may help to avoid postoperative paraplegia.

Patients sustaining traumatic aortic disruptions commonly have associated multisystem trauma. Postoperative care of major central nervous system injuries, pulmonary failure, renal failure, major orthopedic injuries, and infection often are of primary importance after repair of the initial aortic injury.

Careful long-term follow-up of all patients with aortic dissections and Marfan patients is essential. Control of hypertension decreases late aneurysm formation in remaining false channels and the ever-present risk of new dissection. Patients are followed up with serial CT scans or MRI examinations. Enlarging false channel aneurysms are resected before they become too large. Marfan patients are especially prone to the development of aneurysms and dissections in the residual aorta, which then requires further surgical correction. We recommend for all Marfan patients long-term β-blockers for maintenance, to decrease the progression of aortic disease.

Patients with resection of arteriosclerotic aneurysms are at special risk for postoperative myocardial infarction and rupture of distant aortic aneurysms. Careful management of hemodynamics, electrolytes, and gas exchange can decrease the immediate risk from heart disease. Crawford and colleagues[9] have shown that an aggressive surgical approach to the second aneurysm both in diagnosis and in subsequent prophylactic resection has decreased both early and late postoperative mortality rates. The second aneurysm is usually resected at a 6-week interval when cardiac, pulmonary, and renal function have been optimized.

Results

Ascending Aorta and Aortic Arch Aneurysms and Dissections

In the period between January 1983 and December 1990, 229 patients underwent surgical repair of their ascending aorta and aortic arch at JHH. A breakdown of the different disease processes is presented in Fig. 18-10. Approximately half the patients undergoing operative repair in this group came to surgery with a Marfan aneurysm of the ascending aorta and in some cases the aortic arch. Twenty-five percent of the overall group of 229 patients required surgery for a non-Marfan dissection, with the majority of these patients having an acute process. Fifty-four of the patients were operated on for an arteriosclerotic aneurysm or an aneurysm

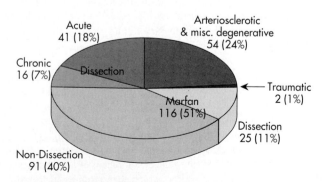

Fig. 18-10 Distribution of disease processes for 229 patients undergoing surgery of ascending aorta and aortic arch.

resulting from a miscellaneous degenerative process. Only two patients in the group had a traumatic aneurysm of the ascending aorta.

In Table 18-1 two hospital deaths are noted among the 116 patients undergoing composite graft repair of a Marfan aneurysm of the ascending aorta, or an overall mortality rate within the hospital of 1.7%. Both these patients arrived in the OR with an acute dissection and rupture of the ascending aorta. Both died in the OR.

Table 18-2 presents a breakdown of the 25 patients with Marfan syndrome who came to surgery with a dissection. Twelve of the patients had an acute dissection with the two operative deaths mentioned in the last paragraph, and 13 of the patients had a chronic dissection with no mortality within the hospital.

The late mortality rate in this group of 116 Marfan patients has been low, with only five late deaths (late mortality rate 4.3%).

The operative results in 54 patients undergoing repair of aneurysms of arteriosclerotic or miscellaneous degenerative origin of the ascending aorta and arch are presented in Table 18-3. Overall the hospital mortality rate was 8.1% among the 54 patients in this group.

Eighty-two patients have been operated on at JHH in 1983 and 1990 for a type A dissection (Fig. 18-11). Fifty-seven of these patients had a non-Marfan dissection, and 25 had a dissection resulting from Marfan syndrome. The hospital's overall mortality

Table 18-1   Composite Graft Repair of Marfan Aneurysm of Ascending Aorta (JHH, 1983-1990)

Patients (no.)	Deaths (no.)	Mortality rate (%)
116	2	1.7

Table 18-2   Incidence of Aortic Dissection Among 116 Marfan Patients Receiving Composite Grafts

Dissection	Patients (no.)	Deaths (no.)	Mortality rate (%)
Acute	12	2	16.6
Chronic	13	0	0
TOTAL	25	2	8.0

Table 18-3 Aneurysms Resulting from Arteriosclerotic and Miscellaneous Degenerative Disease (Ascending Aorta and Aortic Arch; JHH, 1983-1990)

Operation	Patients (no.)	Deaths (no.)	Mortality rate (%)
Urgent	7	1	14.3
Elective	47	3	6.4
TOTAL	54	4	8.1

rate was 18% for the 82 patients, and most of these deaths occurred in patients with acute dissections. Eight of the 10 hospital deaths in the non-Marfan acute dissection category had frank rupture, and both the Marfan patients who died came to the OR with a ruptured aorta. Therefore the hospital's mortality rate was 23% among the 53 patients who came to the OR with acute dissection and only 10% among the 29 patients with a chronic dissection.

Forty-six patients having operative repair of the ascending aorta also had a resection of a portion or all their aortic arch. The classification of disease processes for these 46 patients is presented in Fig. 18-12. Twenty of the 46 patients underwent replacement of the proximal aortic arch, and the remaining 26 patients had most or all the aortic arch replaced (Table 18-4). Total body circulatory arrest with systemic hypothermia was used for all these patients. Four hospital deaths occurred among the 20 patients undergoing proximal arch replacement. Three of these patients came to the OR with an acute dissection and rupture of the ascending aorta. Surprisingly, no hospital deaths occurred among the 26 patients undergoing major arch replacement.

Descending Thoracic Aortic Aneurysm and Dissections (Excluding Thoracoabdominal Operative Procedures)

Fig. 18-13 presents the overall breakdown on the disease processes seen among 43 patients undergoing surgery of the descending thoracic aorta at JHH between 1983 and 1990.

The operative results among 19 patients undergoing surgery of the descending thoracic aorta for an arteriosclerotic or miscellaneous degenerative process are presented in Table 18-5. Table 18-6 presents the results among 22 patients undergoing an operative procedure for a dissection of the descending thoracic aorta.

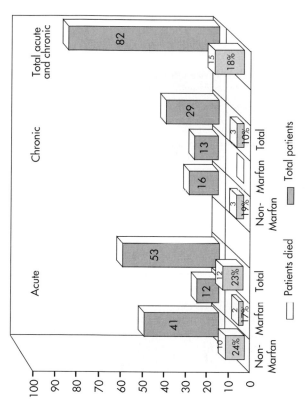

Fig. 18-11 Operative results for 82 patients undergoing surgery for type A dissection of thoracic aorta. Fifty-three patients underwent surgery for acute dissection and 29 patients for chronic dissection. Hospital mortality rate for each group of patients is presented.

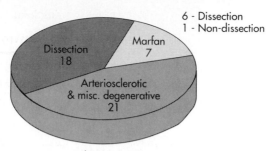

6 - Dissection
1 - Non-dissection

Total Patients = 46

Fig. 18-12 Distribution of disease processes among 46 patients having resection of portion or entire aortic arch with deep hypothermia in combination with total body circulatory arrest.

Table 18-4   Aortic Arch Repair with Total Body
Circulatory Arrest

Arch replacement	Patients (no.)	Arrest time (min)		No. (%) of hospital deaths
		Mean	Range	
Proximal	20	30	18-44	4 (20)
Major	26	32	19-57	0 (0)
TOTAL	46			4 (8.7)

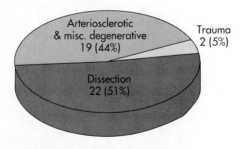

Total Patients = 43

Fig. 18-13 Distribution of disease processes for 43 patients undergoing surgery on descending thoracic aorta.

Table 18-5   Aneurysms Resulting From Arteriosclerotic and
Miscellaneous Degenerative Disease
(Descending Thoracic Aorta, JHH, 1983-1990)

Operative status	Patients (no.)	No. of deaths (%)	Spinal cord injury	
			Paresis	Paralysis
Urgent	13	4 (30.8)	3	0
Elective	6	1 (16.7)	1	0
TOTAL	19	5 (26.3)	4	0

Table 18-6   Dissection of the Descending Thoracic Aorta:
Operative Results (JHH, 1983-1990)

Dissection	Patients (no.)	No. of deaths (%)	Spinal cord injury	
			Paresis	Paralysis
Acute	10	2 (20)	1	3
Chronic	12	0 (0)	0	2
TOTAL	22	2 (9.1)	1	5

All but two of the 43 patients operated on for aneurysms and
dissections of the descending thoracic aorta had some type of spinal
cord protection during the operation. The data related to mortality
and spinal cord injury are presented in Table 18-7. Only two of
the patients had aortic clamping, with one sustaining paresis. In
the remaining 41 patients some type of spinal cord protection was
employed. It is apparent that even with attempts at protecting the
spinal cord blood supply with a variety of bypass techniques,
ischemic injury may still occur. In most instances this results from
permanent interruption of a critical spinal cord nutrient artery arising from the resected segment of the aorta.

Only two patients were operated on at our hospital between
1983 and 1990 for a traumatic aneurysm of the descending thoracic
aorta; both these patients survived.

Thoracoabdominal Aortic Aneurysms

Before the institution of all of the monitoring and therapeutic
measures discussed in this chapter under Operative Management,
our patients with extensive thoracoabdominal aneurysms did not

Table 18-7   Type of Aortic Bypass for Lesions of the Descending Thoracic Aorta: Hospital Mortality Rate and Spinal Cord Injury

	Clamp only	Heparin shunt	CPB-CA	Femoral-femoral bypass	LA-femoral bypass	Total
Arteriosclerosis						
Urgent						
Patients (No.)	2			9	2	13
Mortality (%)				4		4
Paresis (No.)	1			2		3
Paralysis (No.)				—		—
Elective						
Patients (No.)				4	2	6
Mortality (%)				1		1
Paresis (No.)				1		1
Paralysis (No.)				—		—
Dissection						
Acute						
Patients (No.)		1		6	3	10

Mortality (%)			—	2	2
Paresis (No.)	1		—		1
Paralysis (No.)			2	1	3
Chronic					
Patients (No.)		1	9	2	12
Mortality (%)			—		
Paresis (No.)			—		
Paralysis (No.)			2		2
Trauma (acute)					
Patients (No.)	1		1		2
Mortality (%)					
Paresis (No.)					
Paralysis (No.)					
Total					
Patients (No.)	2	1	29	9	43
Mortality (%)	1		5	2	7
Paresis (No.)			3		5
Paralysis (No.)			4	1	5

CPB-CA, Cardiopulmonary bypass–circulatory arrest; LA, left atrial.

fare well; only 9 of 22 survived neurologically intact. After the application of these adjunctive measures in 1988, 14 of 18 patients undergoing repair of equally extensive thoracoabdominal aneurysms survived neurologically intact. (This is a significant difference [$p < 0.05$].)

Because patients with these extensive aneurysms are uncommon, the inescapable conclusion must be that such patients should be referred to a center with acknowledged investigational concerns to achieve better results through understanding of the mechanisms leading to these devastating neurologic complications.

Concluding Thoughts on the Results of Surgery for Thoracic and Thoracoabdominal Aneurysms

If one looks at the foregoing results of surgery for thoracic and thoracoabdominal aneurysms, they seem to be representative of results obtained in other major cardiovascular centers. The proportion of patients with a Marfan aneurysm is slightly greater because of the very active Marfan clinic in our hospital. On the other hand, we had a disproportionately small number of patients with traumatic aneurysm of the aorta, principally because the major adult trauma center in our city is located in another hospital.

Overall, the results of surgery for aneurysms and dissections of the ascending aorta and arch have been good. However, the mortality rate is still fairly high among patients coming to the OR with an acute dissection of the ascending aorta, particularly when there is a frank rupture.

The low incidence of morbidity and mortality has been gratifying in the patients undergoing replacement of a portion or all the aortic arch with the technique of total body circulatory arrest with systemic hypothermia. This particular technique has greatly simplified surgery of the aortic arch and is the principal reason for the improved survival rate seen in these patients in the last 7 years.

The hospital mortality rate for patients undergoing surgery of the descending thoracic aorta is still significant, particularly for those patients requiring an urgent operative procedure for an aneurysm of arteriosclerotic or miscellaneous degenerative origin. Despite our attempt to use some means of spinal cord protection for these patients, a moderate incidence of spinal cord injury still exists. We do believe that left atrial–femoral bypass or femoral-femoral bypass is indicated whenever possible for these patients. Occasionally though, the technique of clamp-and-sew has to be used, particularly for massive bleeding that can accompany an acutely rupturing aneurysm.

Finally, the operative results obtained in patients with thoracoabdominal aneurysms have been gratifying during the last several years. Clearly there seems to be significant advantage in using left atrial–femoral bypass in this group of challenging patients.

References

1. Akins EW et al: Preoperative evaluation of the thoracic aorta using MRI and angiography; *Ann Thorac Surg* 44:449-507, 1987.

2. Bentall H, DeBono A: A technique for complete replacement of the ascending aorta; *Thorax* 23:338-339, 1968.

3. Bickerstaff LK et al: Thoracic aortic aneurysms: a population-based study; *Surgery* 92:1103-1108, 1982.

4. Cabrol C et al: Complete replacement of the ascending aorta with reimplantation of the coronary arteries; *J Thorac Cardiovasc Surg* 81:309-315, 1981.

5. Crawford ES et al: Progress in treatment of thoracoabdominal and abdominal aortic aneurysms involving celiac, superior mesenteric, and renal arteries; *Ann Surg* 188:404-422, 1978.

6. Crawford ES et al: Aortic arch aneurysm; *Ann Surg* 199:742-752, 1984.

7. Crawford ES et al: Thoracoabdominal aortic aneurysms: preoperative and intraoperative factors determining immediate and long-term results of operations in 605 patients; *J Vasc Surg* 3:389-404, 1986.

8. Crawford ES et al: The impact of distal aortic perfusion and somatosensory evoked potential monitoring on prevention of paraplegia after aortic aneurysm operation; *J Thorac Cardiovasc Surg* 95:357-367, 1988.

9. Crawford ES et al: Diffuse aneurysmal disease (chronic aortic dissection, Marfan, and mega-aorta syndromes) and multiple aneurysms: treatment by subtotal and total aortic replacement emphasizing the elephant trunk operation; *Ann Surg* 211:521-537, 1990.

10. DeBakey ME et al: Dissection and dissecting aneurysm of the aorta: twenty-year follow-up of five hundred twenty-seven patients treated surgically; *Surgery* 92:1118-1134, 1982.

11. Doroghazi RM et al: Longterm survival of patients with treated aortic dissections; *J Am Coll Cardiol* 3:1026-1034, 1984.

12. Erdheim J: Medionecrosis aortae idiopathica aptica: *Arch Pathol Anat* 276:187-229, 1930.

13. Gott VL et al: Surgical treatment of aneurysm of the ascending aorta in the Marfan syndrome: results of composite-graft repair in 50 patients; *N Engl J Med* 314:1070-1074, 1986.

14. Gott VL et al: Composite graft repair of Marfan aneurysm of the

ascending aorta: results in 100 patients; *Ann Thorac Surg* 52:38-45, 1991.

15. Griepp RB et al: Prosthetic replacement of the aortic arch; *J Thorac Cardiovasc Surg* 70:1051-1063, 1975.

16. Helseth HK et al: Results of composite graft replacement for aortic root aneurysms; *J Thorac Cardiovasc Surg* 80:754-759, 1980.

17. Hess RJ et al: Traumatic tears of the thoracic aorta: improved results using the Bio-Medicus pump; *Ann Thorac Surg* 48:6-9, 1989.

18 Hirst AE, Gore I: Is cystic medionecrosis the cause of dissecting aortic aneurysm? *Circulation* 53:915-916, 1976.

19. Jex RK et al: Early and late results following repair of dissections of the descending thoracic aorta; *Vasc Surg* 3:226-237, 1986.

20. Katz NM et al: Incremental risk factors for spinal cord injury following operation for acute traumatic aortic transection; *J Thorac Cardiovasc Surg* 81:669-674, 1981.

21. Kieffer E et al: Preoperative spinal cord arteriography in aneurysmal disease of the descending thoracic and thoracoabdominal aorta: preliminary results in 45 patients; *Ann Vasc Surg* 3:34-46, 1987.

22. Kouchoukos NT, Marshall WG Jr, Wedige-Stecher TA: *J Thorac Cardiovasc Surg* 92:691-705, 1986.

23. Laschinger JC et al: Experimental and clinical assessment of the adequacy of partial bypass in maintenance of spinal cord blood flow during operations on the thoracic aorta; *Ann Thorac Surg* 36:417-426, 1983.

24. Miller DC et al: Operative treatment of aortic dissections; *J Thorac Cardiovasc Surg* 78:365-382, 1979.

25. Miller DC et al: Independent determinants of operative mortality for patients with aortic dissections; *Circulation* 70(suppl I):153-164, 1984.

26. Moreno-Cabral CE et al: Degenerative and atherosclerotic aneurysms of the thoracic aorta; *J Thorac Cardiovasc Surg* 88:1020-1032, 1984.

27. Murdock JL et al: Life expectancy and causes of death in the Marfan syndrome; *N Engl J Med* 286:804-808, 1972.

28. Olivier HF Jr et al: Use of the BioMedicus centrifugal pump in traumatic tears of the thoracic aorta; *Ann Thorac Surg* 38(6):586-591, 1984.

29. Ott DA, Frazier UH, Cooley DA: Resection of the aortic arch using deep hypothermia and temporary circulatory arrest; *Circulation* 58(suppl I):227-231, 1978.

30. Perejda AJ et al: Marfan's syndrome: structural, biochemical, and mechanical studies of the aortic media; *J Lab Clin Med* 106:376-383, 1985.

31. Pressler V, McNamara JJ: Thoracic aortic aneurysm; *J Thorac Cardiovasc Surg* 79:489-498, 1980.

32. Pyeritz RE, McKusick VA: The Marfan syndrome; *N Engl J Med* 300:772-779, 1979.

33. Schlatmann TJ, Becker AE: Histologic changes in the normal aging aorta: implications for dissecting aortic aneurysm; *Am J Cardiol* 39:13-20, 1977.

34. Schlatmann TJ, Becker AE: Pathogenesis of dissecting aneurysm of aorta; *Am J Cardiol* 39:21-26, 1977.

35. Svensson LG et al: Impact of cardiovascular operation on survival in the Marfan patient; *Circulation* 80(suppl I): 233-242, 1989.

36. Valiathan MS et al: Resection of aneurysms of the descending thoracic aorta using a GBH-coated shunt bypass; *J Surg Res* 81:197-205, 1968.

37. Verdant A et al: Surgery of the descending thoracic aorta: spinal cord protection with the Gott shunt; *Ann Thorac Surg* 46:147-154, 1988.

38. Williams GM et al: Angiographic localization of spinal cord blood supply and its relationship to postoperative paraplegia; *J Vasc Surg* 13:23-35, 1991.

39. Wilson SK, Hutchins GM: Aortic dissecting aneurysm; *Arch Pathol Lab Med* 106:175-180, 1982.

Surgery for the Cardiac Arrhythmias

19

Levi Watkins, Jr., and Eric Taylor

The development of electrophysiologic evaluation in the workup of patients with cardiac arrhythmias has advanced the understanding of the mechanisms underlying these arrhythmias and has facilitated identification of populations at high risk of sudden death. The surgical assault on medically refractory life-threatening arrhythmias has progressed considerably in the last decade. This chapter reviews the current surgical management of the major cardiac arrhythmias.

Supraventricular Arrhythmias

For many years medical management has been the mainstay of treatment for supraventricular tachyarrhythmias (SVTs). Pharmacologic therapy, however, is not always successful and may be associated with deleterious side effects. Newly developed surgical techniques have provided not only ways of enhancing control of these arrhythmias but also methods for ablating them. Recent years have seen the introduction of percutaneous radiofrequency ablation catheters for treatment of various SVTs. These techniques are safe and effective and hence have emerged as the procedure of choice for certain supraventricular arrhythmias. Surgery is indicated in lethal arrhythmias refractory to non-operative therapy. This section reviews the surgical management of three types of SVTs: Wolff-Parkinson-White syndrome, automatic atrial tachycardia, and atrioventricular (AV) nodal tachycardia.

Wolff-Parkinson-White Syndrome

The underlying disease of accessory pathway arrhythmias is ventricular preexcitation resulting from the presence of accessory AV connections.[1] Although the precise incidence is unknown, approximately 0.1 to 3 of 1000 electrocardiograms (ECGs) demonstrate some form of preexcitation.[2,3] The goal of surgical therapy is interruption of these abnormal pathways while normal physiologic conduction is maintained.

Preoperative assessment

Surface ECGs may be normal or may demonstrate the tachycardia. Frequently evidence of preexcitation with delta waves may be present.

Routine cardiac catheterization is usually not necessary but is performed when other cardiac disease requires definition (e.g., coronary heart disease).

Electrophysiologic testing is essential in defining the anatomic location of the accessory tract and in determining the presence of multiple pathways.

Indications for surgery

Patients refractory to medical therapy, particularly those with 1:1 conduction and rapid ventricular response, are candidates for surgery.

Operative procedure

Direct surgical interruption

Direct surgical interruption through an endocardial approach is used for division of accessory pathways.[4,6] After standard sternotomy, epicardial mapping is performed. If preexcitation is present and stable, the mapping can be done in sinus rhythm. If not, atrial pacing is used to stimulate tachycardia. Usually, intraoperative mapping correlates well with the preoperative data. Occasionally pacing and attempts to induce tachycardia result in hypotension; in such cases mapping is completed after initiation of cardiopulmonary bypass.

Left free-wall pathways are approached through the left atrium. An incision is made just above the annulus posterior to the mural leaflet of the mitral valve (Fig. 19-1). Care is taken to avoid the circumflex marginal artery and the coronary sinus. The incision is carried through the atrial wall down to the epicardial reflection. Superficial myocardial fibers attached to the annulus are also divided. The annular incision and the atriotomy are closed in a continuous fashion (Fig. 19-2). The heart is rewarmed, and the patient is weaned from cardiopulmonary bypass. Electrophysio-

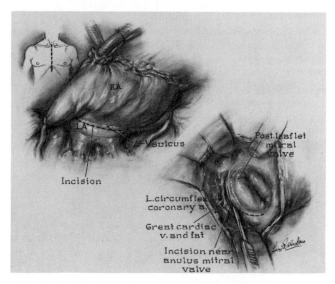

Fig. 19-1 Supraannular incision posterior to mural leaflet of mitral valve for interruption of left free-wall pathway.

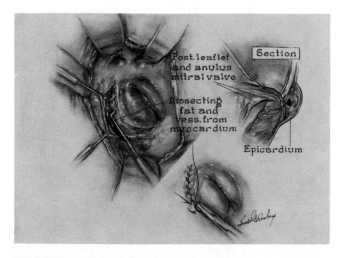

Fig. 19-2 Dissection of epicardial fat and superficial myocardial fibers attached to annulus.

logic assessment is then performed. The ECG is examined for evidence of preexcitation. Antegrade and retrograde pacing should no longer induce tachycardia. The Wenckebach phenomenon occurs with pacing.

Alternately the pathway may be divided from the epicardial approach without the use of cardiopulmonary bypass.[5,7,8]

Cryoablation

Successful cryoablation of accessory pathways has been achieved.[10] In this procedure the pathway is cooled to $-60°$ C for 120 seconds with a cryoprobe. The advantages of the procedure are that surgical dissection is minimized and cardiopulmonary bypass is often not required.

Results

Successful division of accessory tracts occurs in 95% to 98% of patients with free-wall pathways and in 80% with septal pathways.[4,6] The overall operative mortality rate is approximately 1%. Postoperatively, heart block occurs in less than 1% of patients, depending on the location of the AV connection.

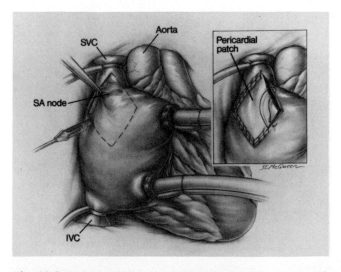

Fig. 19-3 Excision of sinoatrial node and surrounding tissue with pericardial repair. (Courtesy of Dr. Lowe, Duke University, Durham, N.C.)

Automatic Atrial Tachycardia

This arrhythmia accounts for 2% to 3% of SVTs in adults and 10% in children.[9,11] The underlying mechanism is either a single extranodal automatic focus or heightened automaticity of the sinoatrial node. Historically this arrhythmia has been less amenable to surgery. However, the recent development of innovative electrophysiologically guided surgical procedures have made it possible to treat medically refractory automatic atrial tachycardia.

Preoperative assessment

Surface ECG may show incessant, narrow complex SVT. In patients with increased automaticity of the sinus node the ECG may demonstrate homogenous P waves, whereas in that arising from a single extranodal focus, the ECG tends to show a morphologically different P wave from that seen during sinus rhythm.

Cardiac catheterization is usually not necessary unless other disease is suspected.

Electrophysiologic mapping is done to identify the site of ectopic activity and also to exclude AV node reentrant tachycardia or concealed extranodal bypass tracts.

Indications for surgery

Candidates for surgery are usually symptomatic with syncope, palpitations, and/or congestive heart failure.

Operative procedure

After standard sternotomy with individual cannulation of the superior vena cava and the inferior vena cava, cardiopulmonary bypass is begun. Epicardial mapping is performed to identify the site of ectopic activity. If the underlying case is increased automaticity of the sinus node, then treatment consists of excision of the node and placement of a pericardial patch (Fig. 19-3). When the underlying problem is chronic ectopic atrial tachycardia, treatment depends on the location of the ectopic site. Essentially the surgical procedure consists of excision of the area surrounding the ectopic focus. Defects are then repaired either by oversewing or by use of a rotational flap (Fig. 19-4).

Results

The surgical treatment of automatic atrial tachycardia has an overall success rate of 87%.[14] Postoperative complications include heart block with requirement for AV pacing.[14]

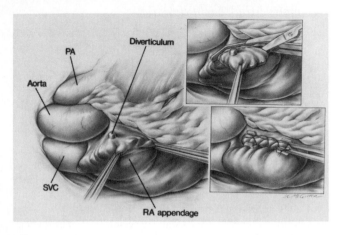

Fig. 19-4 Atrial diverticulum representing ectopic focus, which is excised and oversewn. (Courtesy of Dr. Lowe, Duke University, Durham, N.C.)

AV Nodal Tachycardia

AV nodal tachycardia is the most common type of supraventricular arrhythmia, constituting 63% to 87% of SVTs.[13,15] AV nodal reentrant tachycardia is characterized by tachycardia with a QRS complex of supraventricular origin and regular rhythm. Until recently the only effective treatment for refractory AV nodal tachycardia was surgical ablation of the His bundle.[12] This method, although successful, results in another problem: heart block. Consequently, other methods were sought to interrupt the reentry circuit responsible for the tachycardia without blocking normal AV conduction.

Preoperative evaluation

AV nodal tachycardia is recognized electrocardiographically by a regular ventricular rhythm and a normal QRS complex. Typically the P waves are buried in the QRS complex and the heart rate is usually between 150 to 250 beats/min.

Preoperative electrophysiologic testing is necessary to characterize the tachycardia and to determine the presence of extranodal accessory pathways.

Indications for surgery

Surgical candidates usually have syncope, light-headedness, or dizziness and are refractory to medical therapy.

Operative procedures

Reentrant circuits may be interrupted with cryosurgical interruption or with surgical skeletonization of the AV node.

Cryosurgical interruption

The principal objective of the procedure is to ablate as much of the perinodal tissue as possible without causing permanent AV conduction block. The operative approach is by median sternotomy. Under normothermic cardiopulmonary bypass and during atrial pacing with constant monitoring of AV nodal conduction, nine separate cryolesions ($-60°$ C for 2 minutes) are placed at selected sites around the triangle of Koch in the lower right atrial septum (Fig. 19-5). This effectively ablates most of the perinodal tissue without causing permanent injury to the AV node.[16]

Skeletonization of the AV node

The principal objective of skeletonization of the AV node is to dissect the node from most of the atrial inputs with the intent of altering perinodal substrate and averting reentry. The surgical approach is median sternotomy. After right atriotomy the exposed AV node is dissected free from surrounding tissue (Fig. 19-6). On completion of AV node skeletonization the superficial and posterior atrial inputs to the node are separated. The deep atrial inputs are left intact.[17]

Results

To date, cryosurgical interruption has been 100% successful in 76 cases and no operative deaths have been reported.[16] Skeletonization of the node has been successful in 90% to 94% of cases and no operative deaths have been reported. The incidence of heart block is 3% to 6% of cases.[17]

Right Ventricular Arrhythmias

The underlying disease of right ventricular arrhythmias consist of right ventricular dysplasia, cardiomyopathy, or both. Islands of diseased tissue surrounded by viable myocardium provide a sub-

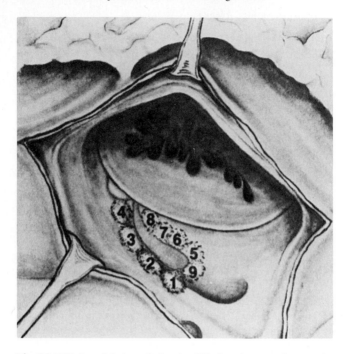

Fig. 19-5 Right atrial view of triangle of Koch and surrounding cryolesions.

strate for reentrant tachycardia. The substrate may involve the entire right ventricle. The goal of surgery is to isolate these areas from the remainder of the heart.[18]

Preoperative Assessment

Unless tachycardia is present, the ECG in fact may be normal. Echocardiography typically demonstrates a dilated, hypocontractile right ventricle. The left ventricle is usually normal.

Catheterization is done to assess potential coronary disease and usually confirms the echocardiography.

Electrophysiologic testing typically demonstrates polymorphic ventricular tachycardia originating in the right ventricle, often near the outflow tract.

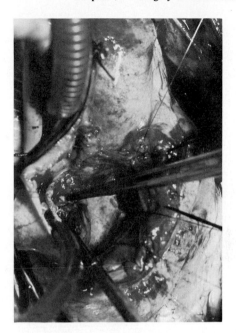

***Fig.* 19-6** Right atrial septal wall has been mobilized and AV node skeletonized (pointed out by forceps). (Courtesy of Dr. Guiradon, London, Ontario, Canada.)

Operative Procedure

Right ventricular disconnection is used to isolate the arrhythmogenic foci from the left ventricle. After standard sternotomy with individual cannulation of the superior and inferior venae cavae, cardiopulmonary bypass is initiated. Normothermia is maintained to facilitate epicardial mapping. The procedure is performed on the beating, nonworking heart. A longitudinal ventriculotomy in the right ventricle is made parallel to the interventricular septum; it is extended superiorly to the pulmonary valve annulus, then inferiorly to the tricuspid valve annulus (Fig. 19-7). The posterior wall of the right ventricle is incised from the endocardial surface. Cryolesions are placed at the pulmonary valve and tricuspid valve annuli, completing the isolation. The ventricle is then repaired in a single-layered fashion (Fig. 19-8).

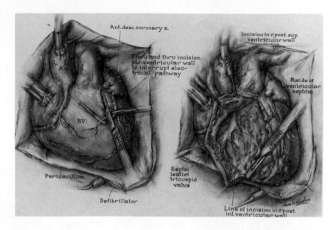

Fig. 19-7 Right ventricular disconnection: Longitudinal ventriculotomy extending from pulmonary annulus to tricuspid annulus.

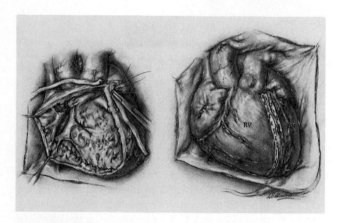

Fig. 19-8 Repair of right ventriculotomy.

Results

Although right ventricular disconnection is limited in use, arrhythmia control has now been reported without fail in more than 15 patients without operative mortality. Postoperative complications include long-term right-sided heart failure and the need for AV pacing.[18]

Left Ventricular Arrhythmias

The most common cause of ventricular tachycardia and fibrillation is coronary heart disease and its complications (i.e., left ventricular aneurysm formation and myocardial fibrosis). The underlying pathologic mechanism in these arrhythmias is interventricular reentrant circuits that usually include endocardial scar. Myocardial ischemia may also play a role, the extent of which is not clear. Current operative procedures are designed to interrupt or ablate reentrant circuits, thereby obliterating associated arrhythmias.

Preoperative Assessment

Cardiac catheterization is done to determine the extent of coronary disease. Ventriculography permits assessments of regional wall motion, which is important in determining operative risk. Candidates with active remaining wall segments have relatively low risks independent of aneurysmal size. Those with hypokinetic function of the remaining walls have substantially higher risk.

Programmed electrical stimulation determines the presence or absence of sustained ventricular tachycardia. In addition, catheter endocardial mapping localizes the anatomic site of origin of the arrhythmia.

Indications for Surgery

Surgical candidates are refractory to medical therapy and usually have clearly defined and mapped ventricular tachycardia.

Operative Procedures

Electrically guided endocardial resection is the procedure of choice for these arrhythmias.[19] After sternotomy and standard cardiac cannulation, cardiopulmonary bypass is instituted. Normothermia is maintained to facilitate intraoperative mapping. After ventriculotomy sustained ventricular tachycardia is induced with programmed electrical stimulation. A hand-held probe is used for endocardial mapping (Fig. 19-9). In the event ventricular tachycardia cannot be induced or if rapid deterioration to ventricular defibrillation occurs, blind resection of the entire endocardial scar is performed, taking into account the preoperative map. After determining the site of earliest ventricular activation, the heart is cooled to 25° C and arrested with potassium cardioplegia solution. The endocardium is widely resected at this site (Fig. 19-10). Any additional scar is also resected. For inferior aneurysms, in addition

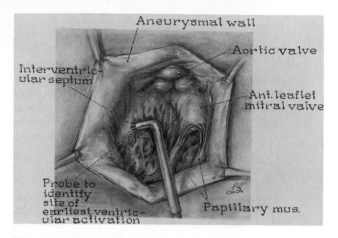

Fig. 19-9 Left ventriculotomy and hand-held probe used for endocardial mapping.

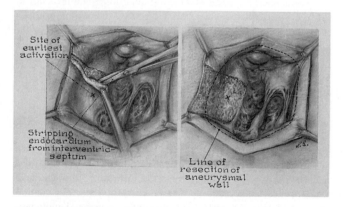

Fig. 19-10 Septal focus of earliest ventricular activation and surrounding endocardial resection.

to surgical resection, cryoablation is also used. When indicated, aneurysmectomy and coronary artery bypass grafting are performed. Implantation of the automatic defibrillator is indicated in some patients.[20,21]

An alternative procedure is encircling endocardial ventriculotomy.[22,25] After initiation of cardiopulmonary bypass, the left ventricle is opened through the aneurysm and a standard aneurys-mectomy is performed. The border between endocardial fibrosis at the base of the aneurysm and normal myocardium is identified. A circumferential incision is made just outside the endocardial fibrosis. This incision is perpendicular to the endocardial wall and carried down to the epicardial surface, leaving the epicardium intact. If a posterior location or papillary muscle site of origin is identified, the procedure can be limited to encircling the posterior papillary muscle and posterior wall of the left ventricle.

Results

With endocardial resection arrhythmia control is achieved in approximately 90% of patients and the operative mortality rate is 5% to 10%.[19]

Automatic Implantable Cardioverter Defibrillator

Despite advances in antiarrhythmic pharmacologic agents and in directed surgical therapy, a sizable population of patients remains who are best treated with the automatic implantable cardioverter defibrillator (AICD). Patients with end-stage cardiomyopathy of various causes are prime examples of such a population. The AICD is a totally implantable device that provides continuous monitoring of cardiac rhythm and defibrillation capability for persons remaining at high risk for malignant arrhythmias.[23,24,26,29]

The Device

The device (Fig. 19-11) consists of an intrathoracic lead system connected to a generator implanted in an abdominal pocket. The lead system is composed of a bipolar rate-sensing electrode and a set of defibrillating electrodes. The cathode is located at the left ventricular apex in the form of a rectangular patch. The anode is either a second patch positioned over the right atrium or a spring electrode positioned in the superior vena cava. The generator is encased in titanium and hermetically sealed. It is powered by lithium batteries, which last approximately 24 months. The AICD is capable of delivering approximately 50 discharges. The system detects malignant tachyarrhythmias by two mechanisms: (1) the probability density function and (2) rate detection capability. The probability density function describes the time that the differentiated transcardiac electrogram remains at the isoelectric line. Es-

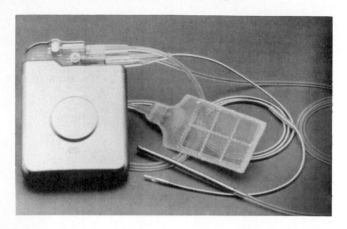

Fig. 19-11 AICD, pulse generator, and attached lead system.

sentially, on occurrence of a malignant arrhythmia the AICD senses it within 5 to 10 seconds, charges a capacitor in another few seconds, and delivers a shock of approximately 30 J. The energy may vary somewhat depending on which unit is employed.

Indications

Current candidates are all refractory to antiarrhythmic medications; they have usually survived a single cardiac arrest and most often have inducible ventricular tachycardia.

Preoperative Assessment

Conventional cardiac catheterization is performed to establish the presence and extent of cardiac disease. Electrophysiologic testing is done to evaluate inducibility and to determine response to specific antiarrhythmic drug therapy.

Operative Procedures

Placement of the Endotak lead system utilizes a nonthoracotomy technique that requires little surgery. It consists of an intravascular electrode with two coils and a sensing lead and a large subcutaneous patch.

The *subxiphoid approach* is used in patients without previous cardiothoracic surgery. Although the entire system can be implanted epicardially with this approach, we position the right ven-

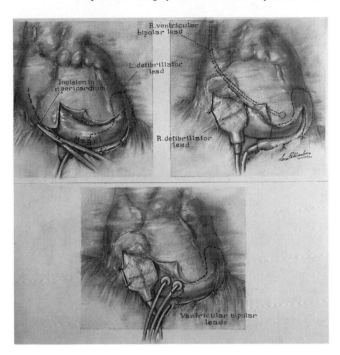

Fig. 19-12 Subxiphoid AICD implant with epicardial patches.

tricular electrode percutaneously in the apex of the right ventricle and then implant a dual-patch defibrillating lead system at surgery (Fig. 19-12). These patches are most often placed intrapericardially, but recently we have placed them *extrapericardially* in persons who may require open heart surgery in the future.[28]

Anterolateral thoracotomy[27] is used in patients with previous cardiac surgery to avoid scar tissue associated with sternotomy and previous surgery. Before surgery the superior vena caval electrode is positioned under fluoroscopy, and at surgery the heart is approached through a small anterolateral thoracotomy. The left apex is dissected extrapericardially (Fig. 19-13). The apical electrode is sutured to the apex, a pocket is developed, and the device is tested after appropriate thresholds have been determined.[27,30]

Median sternotomy[27] is used when AICD implantation is used together with corrective open heart procedures. An all-epicardial system is implanted after the primary procedure is completed (Fig.

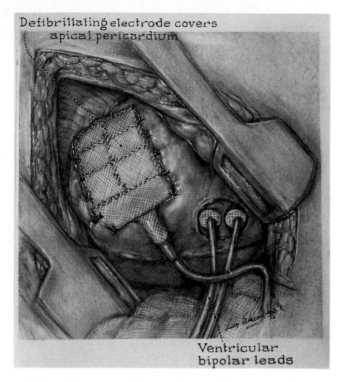

Fig. 19-13 Anterolateral thoracotomy for AICD implantation.

19-14). Ventricular bipolar leads are screw-on electrodes placed in the right ventricular myocardium. Two-patch electrodes are then sutured to the heart. A pocket is developed as previously described. Defibrillatory thresholds and testing of the device are performed *postoperatively* in the catheterization laboratory under more physiologic conditions.[27,30]

With the *subcostal technique,* after a subcostal incision (Fig. 19-15) the costal attachments of the diaphragm are taken down, exposing the pericardium. The pericardium is then opened. A dual-patch electrode is positioned over the left ventricle together with a bipolar lead. The system is then tested as described previously.

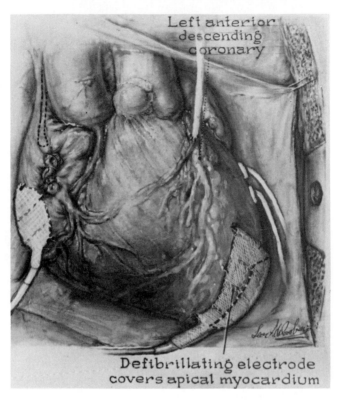

Fig. 19-14 Median sternotomy for AICD implantation.

Results

For AICD implantation the overall operative mortality rate is 2.7%. The most serious postoperative complication is infection.[31,36] This has occurred in 4.7% of our patients. In half these patients the infection was limited to the pocket. In the remaining half the infection involved the entire system. When the infection is confined to the pocket it can be handled by excision of only the generator. When it involves both the leads and the pocket, the entire system must be explanted.

Control of arrhythmias is fairly successful, with the sudden

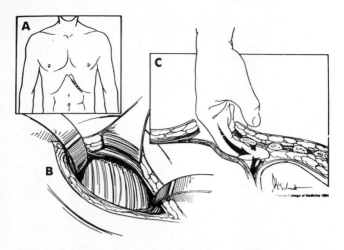

Fig. 19-15 Subcostal technique for AICD implantation. (Courtesy of Dr. Lawrie, Baylor University, Waco, Tex.)

death rate approximating 2% annually in patients with the implanted device.

References

1. Bellet S: *Clinical disorders of the heart beat,* ed 3, Philadelphia, 1971, Lea & Febiger.
2. Borbola J et al: The automatic implantable cardioverter defibrillator: clinical experience, complications and follow-up in 25 patients, *Arch Intern Med* 142:70, 1988.
3. Chung KY, Walsh TJ, Massie E: Wolff-Parkinson-White syndrome, *Am Heart J* 69:1, 1965.
4. Cox JL, Gallagher JJ, Underleider RM: Encircling endocardial ventriculotomy for refractory ischemic ventricular tachycardia. IV. Clinical indications, surgical technique, mechanism of action and results, *J Cardiovasc Surg* 83:865, 1982.
5. Cox JL, Holman WL, Cain ME: Cryosurgical treatment of atrioventricular node reentrant tachycardia, *Circulation* 76:1329, 1987.
6. Cox JL et al: Right ventricular isolation procedures for nonischemic ventricular tachycardia, *J Thorac Cardiovasc Surg* 90:212, 1985.
7. Echt DS et al: Clinical experience, complications, and survival in 70 patients with the automatic implantable cardioverter-defibrillator, *Circulation* 71:289, 1985.

8. Farshidi A et al: Electrophysiologic characteristics of concealed bypass tracts: clinical and electrical correlates, *Am J Cardiol* 41:1052, 1978.

9. Gallagher JJ et al: Cryosurgical ablation of accessory atrioventricular connections: a method for correction of the pre-excitation syndrome, *Circulation* 55:471, 1977.

10. Gallagher JJ et al: Epicardial mapping in the Wolff-Parkinson-White syndrome, *Circulation* 57:854, 1978.

11. Goodman LR et al: Complications of automatic implantable cardio-verter-defibrillator: radiographic, CT, and echocardiographic evaluation, *Radiology* 170(2):447, 1989.

12. Guiraudon GM et al: Surgical repair of Wolff-Parkinson-White syndrome: a new closed-heart technique, *Ann Thorac Surg* 37:67, 1984.

13. Guiraudon GM et al: Closed-heart technique for Wolff-Parkinson-White syndrome: further experience and potential limitations, *Ann Thorac Surg* 42:651, 1986.

14. Guiraudon G et al: Encircling endocardial ventriculotomy: a new surgical treatment of life-threatening ventricular tachycardias resistant to medical treatment following myocardial infarction, *Ann Thorac Surg* 26:438, 1978.

15. Guiraudon GM et al: Surgical treatment of supraventricular tachycardia: a five year experience, *PACE* 9:1376, 1986.

16. Guiraudon GM et al: Skeletonization of the atrioventricular node for AV node reentrant tachycardia: experience with 32 patients, *Ann Thorac Surg* 49:565, 1990.

17. Hendry PJ et al: Surgical treatment for automatic atrial tachycardias, *Ann Thorac Surg* 49:253, 1990.

18. Josephson ME, Harken AII, Horowitz LN: Endocardial excision: a new surgical technique for the treatment of recurrent ventricular tachycardia, *Circulation* 60:1430, 1979.

19. Kelly PA et al: The automatic implantable cardioverter-defibrillator: efficacy, complications and survival in patients with malignant ventricular arrhythmias, *J Am Coll Cardiol* 11(6):1278, 1988.

20. Kelly PA et al: Postoperative infection with the automatic implantable cardioverter-defibrillator: clinical presentation and the use of the gallium scan in diagnosis, *PACE* 11(8):1220, 1988.

21. Klein GJ et al: Surgical correction of the Wolff-Parkinson-White syndrome in the closed heart using cryosurgery: a simplified approach, *J Am Coll Cardiol* 3:405, 1984.

22. Marchlinski FE et al: The automatic implantable cardioverter-defibrillator: efficacy, complications, and device failures, *Ann Intern Med* 104:481, 1986.

23. Mirowski M et al: Termination of malignant ventricular arrhythmias with an implanted automatic defibrillator in human beings, *N Engl J Med* 303:322, 1980.

24. Mirowski M et al: The automatic defibrillator: new modality for treat-

ment of life threatening ventricular arrhythmias, *PACE* 5:384, 1982.

25. Mirowski M et al: The automatic implantable cardioverter-defibrillator: an overview, *J Am Coll Cardiol* 6:461, 1985.

26. Platia EV et al: Treatment of malignant ventricular arrhythmias with endocardial resection and implantation of the automatic implantable cardioverter-defibrillator, *N Engl J Med* 314:213, 1986.

27. Sealy WC: The evolution of the surgical methods for interruption of right free wall Kent bundles, *Ann Thorac Surg* 36:29, 1983.

28. Sealy WC, Gallagher JJ: The surgical approach to the septal area of the heart based on experiences with 45 patients with Kent bundles, *J Thorac Cardiovasc Surg* 79:542, 1978.

29. Sealy WC, Gallagher JJ, Kasell J: His bundle interruption for control of inappropriate ventricular responses to atrial arrhythmias, *Ann Thorac Surg* 32:429, 1981.

30. Veltri EP et al: Clinical efficacy of the automatic implantable cardioverter-defibrillator: six-year cumulative experience, *Circulation* 74(suppl):109, 1986.

31. Watkins L Jr et al: Implantation of the automatic defibrillator: the subxiphoid approach, *Ann Thorac Surg* 34:515, 1982.

32. Watkins L Jr et al: Automatic defibrillation in man: the initial experience, *J Thorac Cardiovasc Surg* 82:492, 1981.

33. Watkins L Jr et al: Surgical techniques for implanting the automatic implantable defibrillator, *PACE* 7:1357, 1984.

34. Watkins L Jr et al: The treatment of malignant ventricular arrhythmias with combined endocardial resection and the implantation of the automatic defibrillator: a preliminary report, *Ann Thorac Surg* 37:60, 1984.

35. Wellens HJJ, Durrer D: The role of an accessory atrioventricular pathway in reciprocal tachycardia: observations in patients with and without the Wolff-Parkinson-White syndrome, *Circulation* 52:58, 1975.

36. Wu D et al: Clinical, electrocardiographic and electrophysiologic observations in patients with paroxysmal supraventricular tachycardia, *Am J Cardiol* 41:1045, 1978.

Heart and Lung Transplantation and Cardiomyoplasty for End-Stage Cardiopulmonary Disease

20

Sharon M. Augustine, William A. Baumgartner, R. Scott Stuart, and Michael A. Acker

Transplantation of the heart has evolved from an experimental procedure done by a limited number of persons to a recognized therapeutic modality performed in more than 150 hospitals in the United States. This explosion in heart transplantation is illustrated in the most recent report from the Registry for the International Society of Heart Transplantation.[11] The initial postoperative care of the recipient after heart or lung transplantation is generally similar to those patients undergoing major open heart or thoracotomy procedures, provided organ function is good in the initial postoperative period. This chapter summarizes the preoperative characteristics of these patients and the particular preoperative signs or symptoms that might lead to difficulties in the postoperative period, briefly describes the operation, and emphasizes the areas of postoperative care that are unique to a patient undergoing transplantation.

Preoperative Evaluation

Patients are referred for transplant evaluation for a variety of reasons. Table 20-1 lists the most common diagnoses for which pa-

Table 20-1   Common Diagnoses Requiring Transplantation

Heart	Heart-Lung
Idiopathic dilated cardiomyopathy*	Primary pulmonary hypertension*
Ischemic heart disease*	Eisenmenger's syndrome*
Congenital heart disease	Cystic fibrosis
Valvular heart disease	Emphysema
Retransplantation	Pulmonary fibrosis
Double-Lung	Single-Lung
Emphysema*	Pulmonary fibrosis*
Cystic fibrosis*	Emphysema*
Pulmonary fibrosis	Primary pulmonary hypertension
Primary pulmonary hypertension	Eisenmenger's syndrome
Eisenmenger's syndrome	

*Primary diagnostic indication.

tients undergo heart and lung transplantation procedures. Although these represent the majority of diagnoses, several other patients have undergone transplant operations for less common diagnoses such as amyloidosis.[9] As can be seen in the table, there is considerable overlap of diagnoses with regard to type of operation, which is indicative of the rapidly evolving field of lung transplantation.

The criteria for acceptance of a heart recipient and a lung recipient in the majority of programs are summarized in Tables 20-2 and 20-3, respectively. Several programs have abandoned a strict age limit for patients but rather use a "physiologic" age for evaluation.

Absolute contraindications to thoracic organ transplantation are systemic infection, fixed pulmonary vascular resistance greater than 6 Wood units (isolated heart only), and irreversible kidney or liver disease. Several other conditions can be difficult to gauge with regard to reversibility after operation. The following conditions can represent potential management problems in the postoperative period:

• Cachexia
• Muscular atrophy
• Elevated pulmonary vascular resistance (isolated heart only)
• Pulmonary emboli, or infarction

***Table* 20-2**   Recipient Acceptance Criteria for Heart
Transplantation

End-stage heart disease not amenable to medical or other surgical therapy
N.Y. Heart Association class III-IV symptoms during optimal medical therapy
Prognosis for 1 yr survival <75%
Age generally <60 yr
Healthy other than heart disease
Emotionally stable, well motivated to resume active lifestyle
History of compliance with medical advice
Supportive family and friends willing and able to make similar long-term commitments

From Achuff SC: Clinical evaluation of potential heart transplant recipients. In Baumgartner WA, Reitz BA, Achuff SC, eds: *Heart and heart-lung transplantation,* Philadelphia, 1990, WB Saunders.

***Table* 20-3**   Recipient Acceptance Criteria for Lung
Transplantation

Life expectancy ≤12-18 mo
No other major systemic disease
Steroids (prednisone ≤10 mg/day)
No chronic or recurrent infection in retained lungs for single-lung transplants
No pleurodesis or major thoracic surgery involving transplant field
History of compliance with medical regimens
Emotionally stable, well motivated to resume active lifestyle
Supportive family and friends willing and able to make similar long-term commitments
Age generally ≤50 yr for heart-lung; ≤55 yr for double-lung; ≤60 yr single-lung

- Hepatomegaly
- Renal dysfunction
- Gastrointestinal disease
- Infection
- Pulmonary problems stemming from amiodarone administration

Cachexia

Various degrees of cachexia can decrease the patient's response to infection and limit the degree of rehabilitation in the early post-operative period. Patients who are nutritionally depleted have more difficulty overcoming postoperative complications.

Muscular Atrophy

Muscular atrophy coexists with cachexia and also limits the patient's ability to be physically rehabilitated. The administration of prednisone potentiates the problem of muscle weakness, compounding the ability of the patient to participate fully in the rehabilitation program.

Elevated Pulmonary Vascular Resistance

Severe pulmonary hypertension is one of the few absolute contraindications to heart transplantation. A normal donor heart is incapable of maintaining adequate right ventricular stroke work against a fixed and elevated pulmonary vascular resistance. Preoperatively this is measured in various ways, but the traditional value of more than 6 Wood units without response to vasodilators is the limit beyond which orthotopic heart transplantation is indicated. A potential alternative is placement of the heart in a heterotopic position. This effectively allows the right ventricle of the recipient to provide the forward output to the lungs and the donor heart's left ventricle to provide systemic output.

Pulmonary Emboli and Infarction

Patients with cardiomyopathy with dilation are often prone to forming intracardiac thrombi caused by low cardiac output and obligatory periods of bed rest. For this reason many of these patients receive chronic warfarin (Coumadin) anticoagulation at the time of transplantation. Sometimes difficult to diagnose, a pulmonary abnormality other than vascular congestion seen on the chest x-ray film should prompt further investigation. The presence of a pulmonary infarct can often lead to the development of a pulmonary infection in the area of the infarction after transplantation.

Hepatomegaly

Severe liver dysfunction is sometimes difficult to characterize objectively. Those patients with marked elevations of serum bilirubin and enzyme levels should be closely examined. On the other hand, mild elevations of enzymes and serum bilirubin are often seen in preoperative patients as a result of congestive hepatomegaly caused by heart failure. The combination of hepatomegaly and preoperative warfarin contribute to bleeding disorders immediately after the operation. After successful transplantation hepatomegaly usually resolves quickly.

Renal Dysfunction

Irreversible changes in the renal parenchyma are also often difficult to evaluate preoperatively. Patients with congestive heart failure undergo severe diuresis in the months preceding transplantation. This is often manifested in elevated serum levels of urea nitrogen and creatinine. Because renal function is further depressed with cardiopulmonary bypass and the concomitant administration of cyclosporine, patients with elevated levels of blood urea nitrogen and creatinine should be carefully examined because renal failure requiring dialysis after cardiopulmonary bypass is associated with a high mortality rate.

Gastrointestinal Disease

Many transplant programs perform routine upper gastrointestinal series, barium enema, and abdominal ultrasound on all potential transplant candidates more than 50 years of age, to assess organ disease. These problems can usually be identified in the postoperative period by maintaining a high index of suspicion.[1]

Infection

The presence of systemic infection represents another absolute contraindication to heart transplantation. Infiltrates on chest x-ray film, however, can be obscured by the alveolar pattern observed with congestive heart failure.

Amiodarone

Patients receiving amiodarone are subject to pulmonary problems after routine open heart surgery. In addition, heart transplant recipients taking amiodarone preoperatively often require prolonged ventricular pacing while awaiting an adequate sinus rate to resume.

Operation

Potential operative problems can influence the initial postoperative care. In a recent report from the Registry of the International Society of Heart Transplantation,[6] cardiac failure represented a

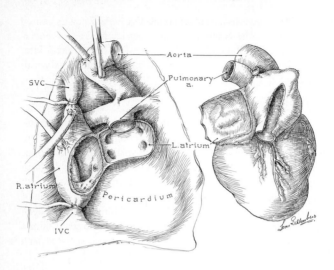

Fig. 20-1 Operative technique of orthotopic heart transplantation. Anastomoses include left atrium, right atrium, pulmonary artery, and aorta.

significant cause of early perioperative mortality. The immediate failure of the donor heart can be due to inadequate preservation, elevated pulmonary vascular resistance of the recipient, or injury of the donor heart incurred during the brain death process.

A particular operative problem unique to this procedure is kinking of the pulmonary artery.[2] This is due to redundant pulmonary artery tissue and results in exaggerated right-sided pressures and a fall in cardiac output despite good left ventricular function. This is usually recognized in the operating room and repaired at that time.

Sinus node dysfunction is a frequent problem in the early postoperative period. This is usually not due to direct sinus node injury from surgical trauma but rather related to ischemia and the preservation process.

The operative technique itself has been modified only minimally from its original description in 1960.[12] Fig. 20-1 depicts the current technique. Four anastomoses are required, starting with the left atrium and followed by the right atrium, pulmonary artery, and aorta. Table 20-4 lists several operative problems associated with heart transplantation.

***Table* 20-4**   Operative Problems Associated with Heart Transplantation

---

Right ventricular failure
  Pulmonary hypertension
  Poor preservation
Left ventricular failure
  Poor preservation
  Donor-related variables
    High inotropic support
    Hypertension
    Hypotension
    Hormonal alterations
Bradyarrhythmias
  Ischemic injury
  Amiodarone administration
Technical aspects
  Hemostasis
  Pulmonary artery kinking
  Deairing of the heart

Hemostasis is of paramount importance in heart and lung transplantation. In patients with a history of cardiac surgery who receive warfarin therapy, early administration of 4 to 6 U of fresh-frozen plasma (after protamine administration) results in satisfactory and expeditious control of bleeding.

As with heart transplantation, the lung or lungs can be injured while in the donor or as a result of the preservation process and subsequent reperfusion. The majority of preservation techniques for lung transplantation that are used result clinically in adequate preservation for 4 to 5 hours after the operation. Inadequate preservation is usually manifested by hypoxia and roentgenographic findings of increased interstitial markings. In addition to respiratory insufficiency caused by inadequate preservation, the heart-lung, double-lung, and single-lung transplant patient can be subject to the following intraoperative nerve injuries:

- Vagus nerve injury, resulting in gastric retention
- Recurrent laryngeal nerve injury, resulting in hoarseness
- Phrenic nerve injury, resulting in paralyzed diaphragm

With recent advances in surgical technique these injuries are relatively uncommon today.[15] Fig. 20-2 depicts the operative technique for heart-lung transplantation. It consists of three anasto-

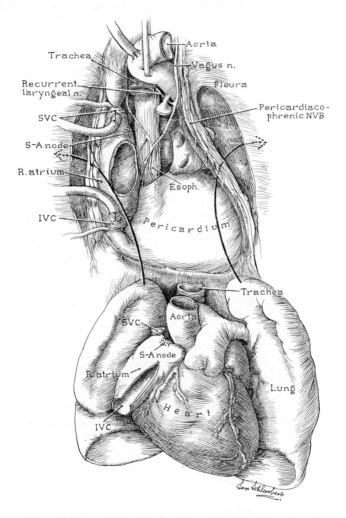

Fig. 20-2 Operative technique of heart-lung transplantation. Anastomoses consist of trachea, right atrium, and aorta.

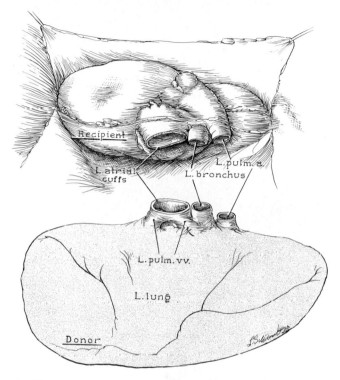

Fig. 20-3 Operative technique of single lung transplantation. Anastomoses include bronchus, pulmonary artery, and left atrium.

moses beginning with the trachea and followed by the right atrium and aorta. Fig. 20-3 and 20-4 depict the operative techniques for single-lung and double-lung transplantation.

Postoperative Recovery

Isolation

Most transplant centers have liberalized the criteria for isolation of transplant patients. Although a few centers still maintain complete reverse isolation, most centers employ handwashing, a mask, and a private room. Some centers, however, have no special precautions and report comparable morbidity and mortality.[4,7]

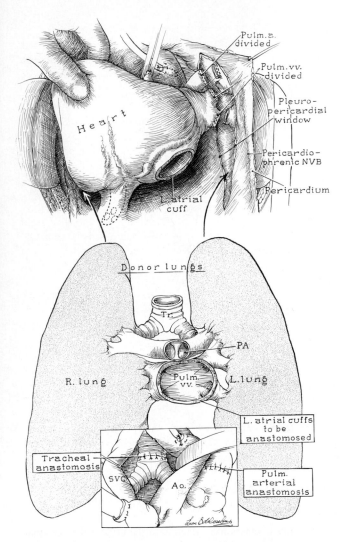

Fig. 20-4 Operative technique of double lung transplantation. Anastomoses consist of trachea, left atrium, and pulmonary artery.

Initial Patient Resuscitation

Transfer of the patient from the operating suite to the intensive care unit occurs in an orderly manner as outlined in Chapter 5. The patient's mediastinal and pleural tubes, intravenous lines, and pacing wires are sorted and appropriately managed. Central venous lines, used for monitoring and the administration of drugs, are seldom needed for more than 3 or 4 days. The radial artery monitoring line is usually removed on the second postoperative day after extubation unless needed for frequent arterial blood gas sampling or blood pressure management.

Mediastinal and pleural tubes are removed after 24 hours when drainage is reduced to less than 25 ml/hr. It is often efficacious to delay tube removal until drainage substantially subsides because of the development of pleural and pericardial effusions in the early postoperative period. Preoperative fluid overload or renal dysfunction after the operation may contribute to formation of pericardial and pleural effusions. Pericardial effusions have been observed more frequently in cyclosporine-treated patients.

Laboratory Tests / Chest X-ray Films

Routine laboratory tests similar to those outlined in Chapter 5 are ordered after heart and lung transplantation. Chest x-ray films may be obtained more frequently in patients undergoing lung transplantation. In addition to the routine tests, specific transplant-related laboratory tests need to be considered. These include cyclosporine blood levels, serologic tests, cultures, and assays for OKT3 and rabbit antithymocyte globulin (RATG)/rabbit antithymocyte serum (RATS).

Cyclosporine Levels

A variety of methods for measuring cyclosporine concentration are now available. We recently switched to a monoclonal antibody radioimmunoassay that is specific for the parent compound (Cyclo-Trac SP ^{125}I RIA Kit, INCSTAR, Stillwater, Minn.). With this technique therapeutic trough levels in the immediate postoperative period are 200 to 400 ng/ml. If cyclosporine is being administered intravenously, a steady-state level of 250 to 300 ng/ml is regarded as therapeutic immunosuppression. The dose of cyclosporine should be modulated on the basis of its corresponding level and the patient's serum creatinine level, to reduce nephrotoxicity.

Serologic Tests

Cytomegalovirus, toxoplasmosis, herpes simplex virus, and Epstein-Barr virus titers are drawn once during the hospital course before discharge. The results of these titers are compared with the patient's preoperative levels and are also used as a baseline for future analysis.

Cultures

Multiple routine cultures were obtained in the initial experience with heart transplantation, but recent evidence suggests that cultures should be obtained only if prompted by fever or by a particular symptom or sign.

Assays for OKT3 and RATG/RATS

OKT3 is used in our transplant program to treat resistent rejection. Daily blood is sent for the assessment of T3 cells, which should be suppressed to essentially zero within 24 hours of initiation of treatment. After the initiation of OKT3 a blood sample is drawn, ideally at day 21, for the assessment of monoclonal antibodies. The antibody analysis is presently being performed by Orthopharmaceuticals (Raritan, N.J.). When antithymocyte serum products are used, total circulating T cells are measured. The therapeutic threshold is a reduction of T cells to less than 25 cells/mm^3.

Immunosuppression

Numerous protocols are in existence for maintenance immunosuppression. The majority of programs use a variation of a triple-drug immunosuppressive protocol. Our protocol is listed in Table 20-5. Patients are given cyclosporine, 6 to 10 mg per kilogram of body weight preoperatively, on the basis of the preoperative serum creatinine level. Steroid administration is initiated in the operating room, with 500 mg of methylprednisolone given after the administration of protamine. Postoperatively patients receive cyclosporine at approximately 10 mg/kg/day (divided into two equal doses by mouth or through an oral gastric tube). If a rising creatinine level develops, we favor switching cyclosporine to the intravenous route. The dosage required for adequate levels is generally in the range of 1 to 2 mg/kg/day given as a constant intravenous infusion. Methylprednisolone (125 mg intravenously) is adminis-

Table 20-5 Immunosuppressive Protocol

	Methylprednisolone	Prednisone	Azathioprine	Cyclosporine	RATS
Preoperatively				10 mg/kg	
Intraoperatively	500 mg				
Immediately post-operatively	125 mg every 8 hr for 3 doses	1 mg/kg tapered to 2 mg/kg to 0.4 mg/kg*		10 mg/kg	1 vial for 3 days†
Long-term		0.2 mg/kg	1-3 mg/kg	5 mg/kg	

*Administration delayed 2 weeks after transplant for heart-lung recipients.
†Added for lung transplant patients.

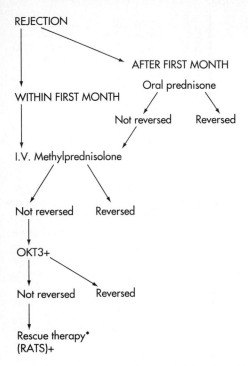

REJECTION

AFTER FIRST MONTH

Oral prednisone

WITHIN FIRST MONTH

Not reversed   Reversed

I.V. Methylprednisolone

Not reversed   Reversed

OKT3+

Not reversed   Reversed

Rescue therapy*
(RATS)+

*For severe rejection, concomitant administration of Methylprednisolone
+ Rabbit antithymocyte serum

Fig. 20-5 Treatment of rejection. *, For severe rejection, concomitant
administration of methylprednisolone. †, RATS, rabbit antithymocyte
serum.

tered every 8 hours for three doses in the immediate postoperative
period. After the third dose of methylprednisolone, prednisone is
given orally starting at 1 mg/kg/day and tapered to 0.4 mg/kg/
day by 2 weeks. Azathioprine (Imuran) is given at approximately
2 mg/kg/day and adjusted to maintain the white blood cell count
in the range of 4000 to 5000/mm^3.

Patients undergoing lung transplantation receive one vial of
RATS intravenously for 3 postoperative days. Steroids are also
withheld for 1 to 2 weeks.

Table 20-6   Administration of Drugs Used for Rejection

Prednisone	100 mg/day for 3 days followed by 5 mg/day taper until baseline is reached
Methylprednisolone	1 g/day for 3 days
OKT3	5 mg/day to eliminate T3 marker cells for 10-14 days
RATS	1 vial/day to reduce T cell count to ≤ 25 mm³ for 10-14 days

Fig. 20-5 demonstrates the algorithm we use for treatment of rejection. The highest incidence of rejection has been found to occur within the first 3 months after transplantation. In our experience 84% of patients have at least one episode of rejection during this period. However, the majority of episodes (80%) have been reversed by treatment with a short course of oral or intravenous corticosteroids. When corticosteroids are unsuccessful, the monoclonal antibody OKT3 or antithymocyte serum are used. The doses and administration of these drugs to treat rejection are listed in Table 20-6.

Special Postoperative Concerns

The following require special attention in the postoperative period:
- Autonomic nervous system (denervation)
- Hemodynamics
- Respiratory system
- Renal system
- Infection
- Psychosocial aspects
- Nutrition
- Physical therapy

Effects of Denervation

Adrenergic mechanisms (chronotropic and inotropic) through sympathetic release of norepinephrine increase heart rate and contractility. Parasympathetic fibers, through branches of the vagus nerve, inhibit both the impulses originating in the sinoatrial (SA) node and conduction through the atrioventricular (AV) node. This parasympathetic inhibitory effect is usually dominant; however, the absence of parasympathetic stimulation caused by denervation results in a somewhat faster resting heart rate in the transplanted heart. Pope and coworkers[14] and Stinson and coworkers[19] reported the average resting heart rate in the denervated heart to be in the range of 90 to 100 beats/min.

Response to exercise is also affected by the transplanted heart's denervation. Because the direct stimulation through sympathetic fiber release of norepinephrine to the SA node and heart muscle cannot occur, the denervated heart is dependent on other mechanisms. Initially, cardiac output increases because of muscular activity that increases venous return. Later in exercise, heart rate and cardiac output increase in response to inotropic and chronotropic effects of circulating catecholamines released from noncardiac sites.[3,5,13,14,16,19]

Orthostatic hypotension may occur because of the lack of compensatory tachycardia when venous pooling decreases preload. This is an important concept when the patient is assisted out of bed or when vasodilatation occurs for any reason. The lack of heart rate response also may be misleading in initial assessment of cardiovascular stress states such as hypoxia, hemorrhage, or hypovolemia. An elevated remnant SA node rate can be suggestive of problems unobservable by monitoring the donor heart rate.[3,5,13,16,17]

Hemodynamics

Global myocardial depression of a variable extent may occur as a result of the following:
- The period of ischemia or inadequate preservation before implantation is protracted
- Prolonged administration of high levels of vasopressors, including dopamine, before cardiectomy may result in myocardial catecholamine depletion, further impairing ventricular performance
- A variety of poorly understood homeostatic alterations may occur in the donor that contribute to myocardial depression
- Right ventricular dysfunction after reimplantation may occur as a result of elevated pulmonary vascular resistance in the recipient

Sinus node dysfunction may result from ischemia, atrial stretch, or direct intraoperative trauma. In the absence of sinus node function a slow junctional rhythm usually occurs, which can be over-ridden with bipolar atrial pacing or accelerated by the administration of chronotropic drugs such as isoproterenol or dobutamine. The heart rate is maintained in the range of 90 to 110 beats/min to maximize cardiac output during the first several days after the operation. Often patients who have been receiving amiodarone preoperatively have a delay in restoration of an adequate rate. This delay may last for up to 4 weeks but in our experience has not resulted in the need for a permanent pacemaker implantation. Patients with sustained bradycardia should be given a trial of theophylline ethylenediamide (aminophylline). The administration of this drug has often resulted in the prolonged acceleration of the heart rate.

Systolic blood pressure is generally maintained in the range 90 to 110 mm Hg by means of afterload reduction with nitroprusside or nitroglycerin, thereby further maximizing cardiac function. Nitroglycerin may provide a greater reduction of pulmonary vascular resistance than nitroprusside and may have less tendency to inhibit the pulmonary hypoxic vasoconstrictor reflex.

In the majority of patients, cardiac function after transplantation is good. Patients are generally receiving isoproterenol, dopamine, and nitroglycerin for maintenance of heart rate, urine output, and cardiac output, respectively. Cardiac function generally returns to normal within 3 to 4 days, during which time the patient can be weaned from these supplemental medications. Supplemental oral antihypertensive agents, particularly calcium channel blockers (nifedipine) allow reduction in dose of intravenous vasodilators.

Respiratory

After heart transplantation, ventilation and weaning protocols are similar to those for other patients undergoing open heart surgery. However, several preexisting problems may interfere with respiratory management and should be recognized. Hepatomegaly may retard metabolism of anesthetic agents and muscle relaxants, thereby prolonging the need for mechanical ventilation. Right-sided heart dysfunction may be a reflection of elevated pulmonary vascular resistance, which might inhibit ventilatory weaning. As mentioned, pulmonary effusions are also commonly observed after transplantation.

Patients undergoing lung transplantation are treated similarly to those patients undergoing isolated heart transplantation. They are allowed to wake up from anesthesia and are weaned from the ventilator on the basis of established protocols (see Chapter 8). Close attention is given to fluid balance to avoid overhydration and to encourage diuresis because of the routine fluid accumulation after cardiopulmonary bypass. Bronchoscopy is occasionally necessary if severe atelectasis is present. When bronchoscopy or suctioning is performed, extreme care should be taken to avoid excessive trauma to the tracheal or bronchial suture line. Because dissection of both phrenic nerves occurs with the heart-lung and bilateral lung operations, inability to wean the patient should prompt evaluation of diaphragmatic movement by fluoroscopy.

Renal Function

Some degree of renal dysfunction is usually seen in the postoperative heart or lung transplant patient. This is a result of preoperative factors related to congestive heart failure and inadequate kidney perfusion and compounded by cardiopulmonary bypass and the administration of cyclosporine. Cyclosporine is generally administered in an oral form unless evidence of increasing renal dysfunction is present. Intravenous cyclosporine may ameliorate renal failure to some extent by avoiding the peaks seen with oral administration. Dopamine is often used (2 to 3 µg/kg/min) to improve renal blood flow.

Because many of these patients have been receiving high doses of diuretics preoperatively, they may not respond to routine doses generally administered after conventional open heart surgery. Increased doses of furosemide or additional agents may be necessary to promote vigorous diuresis. The use of bumetanide (Bumex) and ethacrynic acid (Edecrin) has often been successful when standard diuretics are inadequate. The excessive use of loop diuretics should be avoided because of otic nerve toxicity. Renal dysfunction resulting from cyclosporine reverses as the dose is reduced. Occasionally dialysis may be necessary because of poor renal function observed preoperatively.

Infections

Assessing for signs and symptoms of infection is often clouded by immunosuppression. The antiinflammatory effects of steroids often restrict the ability of patients to produce pyrogens. Normal body temperature tends to be lower, and therefore very small increases in temperature should be noted. Aggressive fever work-ups should be performed for any temperature greater than 38° C.

A variety of bacterial infections can occur in the transplant patient. Table 20-7 illustrates the site and cause of infections in transplant patients.[8] The overall incidence of infections is 0.06 episodes per patient-month. Common organisms are *Streptococcus, Staphylococcus,* and gram-negative bacteria.

The most frequent infections after transplantation are those associated with viral illnesses. Patients are at an increased risk of herpes simplex as well as cytomegalovirus (CMV) infection. The latter infection can occur as a result of transmission from the donor heart or through blood transfusions in the recipient who is sero-negative before transplantation, or reactivation of a latent virus can occur in a patient with a preoperative positive titer. Because of the limited ischemic time for donor hearts, time does not always permit appropriate CMV matching. All seronegative transplant recipients therefore receive seronegative blood. CMV infections are usually subclinical, manifested by a drop in white blood cell count, slight elevation of liver function parameters, or a syndrome of leukopenia, fever, and malaise. However, it can contribute directly to mortality and significant morbidity as manifested by retinitis and pneumonia, especially in lung transplant patients. It also predisposes the patient to superinfection with bacteria or fungi and has been linked to the postoperative development of coronary artery disease. For only CMV mismatch, ganciclovir 9(1,3-dihydroxy-2-propoxymethyl)-guanine (ganciclovir) is administered postoperatively as prophylaxis for 2 to 4 weeks. Prophylaxis is continued on an outpatient basis with acyclovir.

The majority of early infections are related to bacterial and viral pathogens. Opportunistic pathogens such as *Toxoplasma, Pneumocystis carinii,* and fungi generally do not occur during the early postoperative period but become prevalent 1 to 6 months after transplantation. For CMV-seronegative recipients who receive CMV-positive organs, ganciclovir is administered postoperatively as prophylaxis for 2 to 4 weeks. Prophylaxis is continued on an outpatient basis with acyclovir.

The diagnosis and treatment of suspected infections should be carried out aggressively and expeditiously. Workup of a lung infiltrate involves sputum culture, needle aspirate of the infiltrate, or bronchoscopic examination with culture. Bacterial infections

Table 20-7 Infections in Cardiac Transplant Recipients

Early Posttransplant Infections (First Month)	Late Posttransplant Infections (after First Month) and Duration of Immunosuppression
Pneumonia: GNB	
Mediastinitis	
Staphylococcus epidermidis	Viral
Staphylococcus aureus	CMV
GNB	Herpes simplex
IV lines	Varicella-zoster
S. epidermidis	Non-A, non-B hepatitis
S. aureus	Bacteria
GNB	*Listeria*
Candida albicans	*Nocardia*
Urinary tract infections	*Legionella*
GNB	*Mycobacterium*
Enterococcus	Fungi
C. albicans	*Aspergillus*
Skin	*Cryptococcus*
Herpes simplex virus	*Candida*
	Mucor (Phycomycetes)
	Protozoa
	Pneumocystis carinii
	Toxoplasma gondii

From Horn JE: Infectious complication following heart transplantation. In Baumgartner WA, Reitz BA, Achuff SC, eds: *Heart and heart-lung transplantation*, Philadelphia, 1990, WB Saunders.
GNB, Gram-negative bacilli.

are treated with the appropriate antibiotics. Serious CMV infections can be treated with 9(1,3-dihydroxy-2-proproxymethyl)-guanine (ganciclovir).[10-18,20] The cutaneous or pharyngeal lesions of herpes simplex can be treated with acyclovir, 200 mg four or five times daily. The prevalence of specific organisms is influenced by idiosyncratic nosocomial infection patterns of individual institutions and by antibiotic usage practices.

Psychosocial Support

The emotional and psychosocial support provided to transplant recipients begins in the evaluation process. Patients and their families are seen by a dedicated social worker, and this care is continued through the hospital course and during long-term follow-up. Patients and families are prepared for discharge from the hospital through continued education by the transplant coordinator and nursing staff on issues of medications, side effects, activity levels, and other health concerns. Interaction with the coordinator, staff, and social worker provides patients with the reassurance that they are equipped with adequate knowledge of the medical regimen to leave the transplant center environment. Emotional lability is often seen in patients because of the stress of the operation and the administration of steroids.

Nutrition

An oral diet can usually be started on the second postoperative day and advanced as tolerated. In general, an increase in appetite develops as a result of steroid administration. Emphasis is placed on dietary instructions to reduce the serum cholesterol level in hopes of diminishing development of late graft arteriosclerosis. Occasionally recipients are cachectic as a result of their long-standing heart or heart-lung disease. These patients often require diet supplementation, especially if their caloric intake is limited in the early postoperative period.

For patients undergoing isolated heart transplantation, diet can often be supplemented with total parental nutrition during the early postoperative period. Patients undergoing lung transplantation are susceptible to fluid overload. Enteral feeding with a small nasogastric tube is preferable to total parental nutrition in these patients.

Physical Therapy

The department of physical therapy should be included in the initiation of any transplant program. Specialized protocols for the transplant patient with graded exercise programs designed to return the patient to full activity and rehabilitation are developed. The extended goals of cardiac rehabilitation are to decrease the total recovery time, provide a progressive structured exercise program, develop and maintain cardiovascular and pulmonary fitness, and initiate a regimen that will prepare patients to return to their normal or previous activity level. This program is generally begun within the first week after the transplant procedure and extends to the next 6 to 8 weeks. The role of physical therapy in the hospitalized preoperative patient can also be beneficial.

Discharge teaching is an important aspect of the postoperative care of the transplant patient. Patients are required to be familiar with their medications and side effects. In addition to the responsibility of learning and taking medications, the patient becomes familiar with the exercise program and important signs that should be monitored. These include testing urine for sugar, testing stool for occult blood, daily heart rate, excessive increase in weight, and elevation of temperature.

Cardiomyoplasty

More than 2 million Americans have congestive heart failure (CHF) and more than 400,000 new cases of CHF are diagnosed every year. Present medical therapy certainly improves symptoms and perhaps exercise tolerance, but improvement in survival has been minimal. Heart transplantation has been proven to improve survival, but fewer than 1% of patients with CHF undergo transplantation, because of donor inavailability and medical contraindications to heart transplantation. Another therapeutic alternative that is now being investigated is the use of a patient's own skeletal muscle to assist the failing heart.

Skeletal muscle has the ability to alter its physiologic, mechanical, and biochemical properties in response to long-term electrical stimulation to become capable of cardiac-like work. This property of muscle plasticity has been exploited in the development of a new operation for the treatment of end-stage CHF called cardiomyoplasty. In this operation the patient's own latissimus dorsi muscle is mobilized on its neurovascular pedicle, placed into the chest, and then wrapped around the patient's heart. This muscle is stimulated to contract in synchrony with cardiac systole by a specially designed cardiomyostimulator. During a period of 8 to 12 weeks the muscle is gradually conditioned to provide increasing cardiac assistance. Cardiomyoplasty seems best suited for patients with New York Heart Association class III CHF, and 85% of survivors report a dramatic increase (to classes I or II) in their exercise tolerance. This operation has been performed in more than 100 patients worldwide, and clinical trials are presently under way in this country to assess the safety and effectiveness of this new operation. If proved effective, this operation would avoid the

problems of donor availability, chronic rejection, and immunosuppression associated with heart transplantation.

References

1. Augustine SM et al: Gastrointestinal complications in heart and in
   heart-lung transplant patient, *J Heart Transplant* 10:547, 1991.
2. Baumgartner WA: Operative techniques utilized in heart transplantation. In Baumgartner WA, Reitz BA, Achuff SC, eds: *Heart and
   heart-lung transplantation,* Philadelphia, 1990, WB Saunders.
3. Fowles RE, Reitz BA, Ream AK: Drug actions in a transplanted or
   artificial heart. In Kaplan JA, ed: *Cardiac anesthesia II: cardiovascular pharmacology,* New York, 1983, Grune & Stratton.
4. Gamberg P, Miller J, Lough ME: Impact of protective isolation on
   the incidence of infection after heart transplantation, *J Heart Transplant* 6:147, 1987.
5. Griepp RB et al: Hemodynamic performance of the transplanted human
   heart, *Surgery* 70:88, 1971.
6. Heck CF, Shumway SJ, Kaye MP: The Registry of the International
   Society for Heart Transplantation: sixth official report—1989, *J Heart
   Transplant* 8:271, 1989.
7. Hess N et al: Complete isolation: Is it necessary? *J Heart Transplant*
   4:458, 1985.
8. Horn JE, Bartlett JG: Infectious complications following heart transplantation. In Baumgartner WA, Reitz BA, Achuff SC, eds: *Heart
   and heart-lung transplantation,* Philadelphia, 1990, WB Saunders.
9. Hosenpud JD et al: Successful intermediate-term outcome for patients
   with cardiac amyloidosis undergoing heart transplantation: results of
   a multicenter survey, *J Heart Transplant* 9:364, 1990.
10. Icenogle T et al: DHPG effectively treats CMV infection in heart and
    heart-lung transplant patients: a preliminary report, *J Heart Transplant*
    6:199, 1987.
11. Kaye MP: The Registry of the International Society for Heart Trans-
    plantation: seventh official report—1990, *J Heart Transplant,* 9:323,
    1990.
12. Lower RR, Shumway NE: Studies on the orthotopic homotransplan-
    tation of the canine heart, *Surg Forum* 11:18, 1960.
13. McKelvey SA: Effects of denervation in the cardiac transplant recip-
    ient. In Douglas MK, Shinn JA, eds: *Advances in cardiovascular
    nursing,* Rockville, Md, 1985, Aspen Systems.
14. Pope SE et al: Exercise response of the denervated heart in long-term
    cardiac transplant recipients, *Am J Cardiol* 46:213, 1980.
15. Reitz BA: Heart and lung transplantation. In Baumgartner WA, Reitz
    BA, Achuff SC eds: Heart and heart-lung transplantation, Philadel-
    phia, 1990, WB Saunders.

16. Savin WM, Schoeder JS, Haskell WL: Response of cardiac transplant recipients to static and dynamic exercise: a review, *J Heart Transplant* 1:72, 1986.
17. Shaver JA et al: Hemodynamic observations after cardiac transplantation, *N Engl J Med* 281:822, 1969.
18. Sinnott J, Collison J, Rogers K: Treatment of cytomegalovirus gastrointestinal ulceration in a heart transplant patient, *J Heart Transplant* 6:186, 1987.
19. Stinson EB et al: Hemodynamic observations one and two years after cardiac transplantation in man, *Circulation* 14:1183, 1972.
20. Watson F et al: Treatment of cytomegalovirus pneumonia in heart transplant recipients with 9(1,3-dehydroxy-2-propoxymethyl)-quanine (DHPG), *J Heart Transplant* 7:102, 1988.

Artificial Devices for Mechanical Support

21

Peter W. Cho, David Johnson, Janice Wallop,
Dennis Rivard, and Duke E. Cameron

A thorough understanding of cardiovascular physiology and recent advances in biomedical engineering now permit surgeons confronted with cardiac failure to intervene directly with mechanical devices to support the patient's circulation. Where surgeons were previously limited to relying on the natural course of recovery after injury, aided only by inotropic drugs, they can now optimize available cardiac function, partially take over pump function, or replace the malfunctioning heart altogether. Problems with cost and blood-surface incompatibility, leading to blood element trauma and the activation of inflammation-coagulation cascades, prevent the techniques described here from providing long-term solutions to cardiac failure, but they have proven themselves to be effective, life-saving measures for the patient awaiting natural recovery (e.g., stunned myocardium after cardiac surgery) or a definitive procedure (e.g., coronary artery bypass graft or transplantation).

This discussion of mechanical circulatory support considers the broad classes of devices rather than the wide variety of proprietary systems available and focuses on the most frequently used devices, the intraaortic balloon pump (IABP) and the ventricular assist device (VAD). Device-specific indications for use are presented, but for particulars of hemodynamic management in the clinical setting the reader is referred to Chapter 7.

General Considerations

Currently no device has been approved for permanent assistance or replacement of the heart. Consequently, mechanical circulatory support is indicated only for resuscitation to allow recovery of heart function or as a bridge to heart transplantation. Because mechanical assistance often requires invasive procedures and itself causes significant physiologic derangements, all other less invasive measures must first be exhausted. When cardiac failure after a technically adequate repair has been judged reversible, the accepted sequence of interventions is (1) inotropes, (2) IABP, and finally (3) VAD.

Accurate assessment of cardiac function is essential when mechanical assistance is contemplated and during the time of assistance and weaning. Doppler-flow echocardiography, particularly transesophageal echocardiography (TEE), is indispensible in this role. Similarly useful is a left atrial pressure monitoring line; the surgeon should have a low threshold for placing such a line in the operating room. Information yielded by pulmonary artery catheters has been only moderately helpful. Whatever the circumstances, the surgeon will ultimately do best by relying on clinical judgment rather than slavishly adhering to "the numbers."

Intraaortic Balloon Counterpulsation

The inflation and deflation of the intraaortic balloon in synchrony with the cardiac cycle can optimize myocardial oxygen consumption. Inflation during diastole augments coronary perfusion and hence oxygen delivery, whereas deflation during systole reduces the afterload against which the heart must work, thereby decreasing myocardial oxygen demand. The indications and contraindications for this relatively noninvasive device are listed in Tables 21-1 and 21-2, respectively. Generally speaking, the cardiac surgical patient who would benefit from a balloon pump is the one who weans poorly from cardiopulmonary bypass (CPB) or decompensates in the intensive care unit (ICU) as a result of cardiogenic shock unresponsive to volume loading, afterload reduction, inotropic drugs, and epicardial pacing.

The balloon catheter is customarily placed through the femoral artery either by an open or precutaneous Seldinger technique (see Chapter 4). The transthoracic route is seldom used, because most surgeons elect to place a VAD if the aorta is accessible only through

***Table* 21-1**   Indications for IABP Placement

Postcardiotomy cardiogenic shock (inability to wean from CPB)
Cardiogenic shock after acute MI, unresponsive to medical
   treatment
   Primary myocardial dysfunction
   Ventricular septal defect
   Mitral regurgitation, papillary muscle rupture
Unstable angina
   Pre-MI and post-MI
   Failed angioplasty (during preparation for operation)
Ventricular tachyarrhythmias caused by ischemia
Bridge to transplantation
High-risk cardiac patients undergoing general surgical proce-
   dures
Adjunct to mechanical ventricular assistance

MI, Myocardial infarction.

***Table* 21-2**   Contraindications to IABP Placement

Aortic regurgitation
Aortic dissection
Thoracic aneurysm
Severe peripheral vascular disease
Severe blood dyscrasias
Irreversible brain injury
Irreversible, end-stage ventricular failure

the thorax. Balloon catheters are available in a wide variety of sizes, from 4.5 to 12.0F, with balloon volumes between 2.5 and 40.0 cc. (The typical adult requires an 8.5 to 9.0F catheter with a 40 cc balloon.) The correctly placed balloon lies just distal to the left subclavian artery takeoff and lies well above the renal arteries (Fig. 21-1); a chest film verifies this position. If the surgeon chooses, patients undergo anticoagulation with 10% low-molec-ular-weight dextran (40 kd) or low-dose heparin infusions.

Three parameters can be adjusted during operation of the bal-loon pump, according to the changing requirements of the patient's condition. Synchronization of balloon inflation or deflation with the cardiac cycle can be achieved in a variety of *trigger modes,*

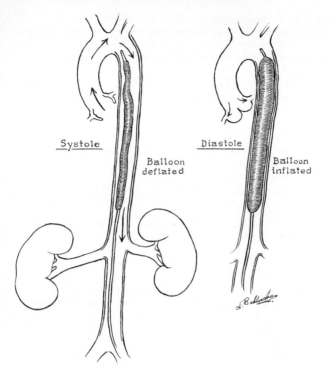

Fig. 21-1 Correct positioning of IABP.

each of which has its advantages (Table 21-3); most frequently the balloon is triggered from the electrocardiogram (ECG). Once the trigger mode has been selected, the *timing* of balloon inflation and deflation within the cardiac cycle must be carefully set, for the efficacy of the device depends principally on this. Inflation must occur just after aortic valve closure for proper diastolic augmentation, and deflation must be complete just as the aortic valve opens for proper afterload reduction. Optimal timing can be determined simply by reference to the aortic pressure waveform (Fig. 21-2) as appropriate adjustments are made with the inflation and deflation timing dials. The same waveform and the patient's hemodynamic status reveal timing errors (Fig. 21-3). Finally, the *amount of augmentation* can be varied by the ratio of heart rate

Text continued on p. 492.

***Table* 21-3** IABP Trigger Modes

ECG
    Most frequently used mode
    HR >150 beats/min decreases IABP efficiency
    Can be used during arrests
    Can be used in atrial fibrillation
Pressure
    Used in case of inconsistent ECG trigger
    Used during electrocautery use
    Requires systolic BP >50 mm Hg
    Not recommended for irregular rhythm
Pacer
    For atrioventricular, ventricular-pacing
    Requires 100% pacing
Internal
    Used when patient cannot generate cardiac output
    Set rate
    May be used when systolic BP <50 mm Hg
    Augmentation should be <½

BP, Blood pressure.

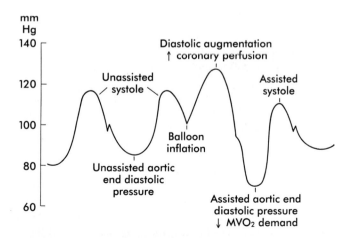

Fig. 21-2 Arterial waveform during IABP use.

Early Deflation

Premature deflation of the IAB during the diastolic phase

Waveform Characteristics:
- Deflation of IAB is seen as a sharp drop following diastolic augmentation
- Suboptimal diastolic augmentation
- Assisted aortic end diastolic pressure may be equal to or greater than the unassisted aortic end diastolic pressure
- Assisted systolic pressure may rise

Physiologic Effects:
A
- Sub-optimal coronary perfusion
- Potential for retrograde coronary and carotid blood flow
- Angina may occur as a result of retrograde coronary blood flow
- Sub-optimal afterload reduction
- Increased MVO_2 demand

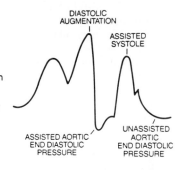

Early Inflation

Inflation of the IAB prior to aortic valve closure

Waveform Characteristics:
- Inflation of IAB prior to dicrotic notch.
- Diastolic augmentation encroaches onto systole (may be unable to distinguish)

Physiologic Effects:
B
- Potential premature closure of aortic valve
- Potential increased in LVEDV and LVEDP or PCWP
- Increased left ventricular wall stress or afterload
- Aortic Regurgitation
- Increased MVO_2 demand

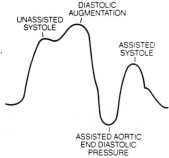

Fig. 21-3 IABP timing errors. **A,** Early deflation. **B,** Early inflation. **C,** Late deflation. **D,** Late inflation.

Late Deflation

C

Deflation of the IAB late in diastolic phase as aortic valve is beginning to open

Waveform Characteristics:
- Assisted aortic end-diastolic pressure may be equal to the unassisted aortic end diastolic pressure
- Rate of rise of assisted systole is prolonged
- Diastolic augmentation may appear widened

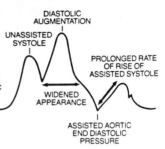

Physiologic Effects:
- Afterload reduction is essentially absent
- Increased MVO$_2$ consumption due to the left ventricle ejecting against a greater resistance and a prolonged isovolumetric contraction phase
- IAB may impede left ventricular ejection and increase the afterload

Late Inflation

D

Inflation of the IAB markedly after closure of the aortic valve

Waveform Characteristics:
- Inflation of the IAB after the dicrotic notch.
- Absence of sharp V
- Sub-optimal diastolic augmentation

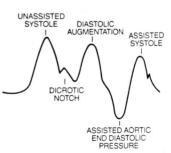

Physiologic Effects:
- Sub-optimal coronary artery perfusion

Fig. 21-3 *cont'd.* For legend see opposite page.

to inflation frequency (1:1, 2:1, etc.) and by the degree to which the balloon is inflated each time (percent augmentation).

Weaning from the IABP is accomplished in various ways, but the guiding principle is to withdraw support incrementally and to assess the hemodynamic consequences at each step. The patient must be hemodynamically stable before weaning can be considered; while receiving minimal inotropes the patient should demonstrate the following:

Cardiac index greater than 2.0 L/min/m^2

Systolic blood pressure greater than 90 mm Hg

Left atrial and right atrial pressure less than 20 mm Hg

Heart rate less than 100 beats/min

Urine output greater than 0.5 ml/kg/hr

In our cardiac surgical ICU inflation frequency is decreased (1:1, to 2:1 to 3:1) at 1 to 2-hour intervals and then the amount of augmentation is decreased to a minimum of 50% (to minimize thrombosis). If minimal balloon support is tolerated for several hours, the catheter is withdrawn, with care taken to purge the proximal and distal femoral artery to allow the egress of intravascular thrombi. Direct pressure is manually applied to the insertion site for 20 minutes, followed by a sandbag for 4 to 6 hours; the patient is confined to bed for at least 12 hours.

Serious complications can arise at any time during the use of the balloon catheter (Table 21-4). At insertion the femoral artery or aorta can be injured, leading to leg ischemia, retroperitoneal hemorrhage, or aortic dissection; those patients with severe peripheral vascular disease are naturally at greater risk for these injuries. While the balloon remains in the patient, the clinician must routinely reconfirm balloon position and monitor perfusion to vascular distributions at risk (extremities, viscera, spinal cord). The balloon that has migrated can cause hemodynamic embarrassment by encroaching on the aortic valve or by becoming kinked and can obstruct blood flow to major branch vessels. Minimal patient movement, daily chest films, routine monitoring of visceral function (e.g., blood chemistry, urine output), and frequent extremity neurovascular checks are appropriate. Of all balloon catheter–associated complications leg ischemia is the most frequent, occurring in 5% to 19% of patients, and obliges the surgeon to remove the catheter and perform thrombectomy and arterioplasty. Less frequently pseudoaneurysm formation, wound infection, and catheter failure can occur. Of these, the first two can largely be

***Table* 21-4**   Complications of IABP

Vessel perforation
    More common in shock, peripheral vascular disease
    Superficial femoral artery → thrombosis, leg ischemia
    High perforation → retroperitoneal hemorrhage
Incorrect position
    Visceral ischemia
    Aortic insufficiency
Limb ischemia
    Most common complication: 5%-19%
    Related to cardiac output, vessel and catheter diameter, intimal injury, thromboembolic phenomena
    Requires removal, thrombectomy, patch angioplasty
Aortic dissection
    Incidence <5%
    Dissection is retrograde; often seals on own
Wound problems
    Infection (1%-3%) → antibiotic prophylaxis
    Pseudoaneurysm
    Lymphatics injury
Gas escape and catheter failure
    Exceedingly rare

---

avoided by applying adequate pressure after catheter removal and by the use of prophylactic antibiotics and strict aseptic technique, respectively; the latter rarely occurs.

Ventricular Assist Devices

When insufficient native function remains in the heart even with the assistance of inotropes and the balloon pump, use of a VAD may be considered. In contrast to the balloon pump, which at best can only optimize existing cardiac function, the VAD takes over the pump function of a ventricle. One or both ventricles may be assisted in this manner. For short-term purposes centrifugal pump systems are clearly favored for their ease of use, cost, and ability to adapt to changing hemodynamic conditions; roller pumps are now rarely used to drive VADs. Longer-term devices typically used as bridges to transplantation include the various sac-type pumps driven electrically (e.g., Novacor LVAS, Baxter Healthcare Corp., Oakland, Calif.) or pneumatically (e.g., Thermedics Heart-

Table **21-5**   Contraindications to VAD Placement

Technically imperfect procedure
Severe preoperative organ dysfunction
Severe infection (bacterial endocarditis)
Advanced age (few survivors >70 yr)
Prolonged CPB
Metastatic cancer
Irreversible cardiac dysfunction in patient not a candidate for
  transplantation

mate, Thermo Cardiosystems, Inc., Woburn, Mass., Thoratec
Pierce-Donachy, Thoratec Laboratories Corp., Berkeley, Calif.,
Abiomed BVS-5000 Abiomed Cardiovascular, Inc., Danvers,
Mass.). Less common devices are based on the Archimedes screw
principle (Interventional Systems Hemopump, Johnson and Johnson, New Brunswick, NJ) or on direct mechanical ventricular
actuation.

Because implantation of a VAD entails significant risks, certain
criteria must be met by candidate patients: (1) the surgical repair
must be technically satisfactory; (2) potential metabolic (acid-base,
electrolyte, temperature) and electrophysiologic causes of cardiac
failure must be ruled out; (3) manipulation of preload and afterload,
and inotropic support, have failed; and (4) IABP assistance is
inadequate. Contraindications for use are listed in Table 21-5. Once
an appropriate indication has been established, the failing ventricle
or ventricles must be identified. Isolated left ventricular failure is
distinguished by the usual criteria (Table 21-6). Care must be taken
in diagnosing independent right ventricular failure in the presence
of left ventricular failure, because right-sided failure may be purely
the result of left-sided failure; accordingly, an IABP or left VAD
should be placed first and right ventricular function reassessed. If
true biventricular function exists, a right VAD may be added, or
extracorporeal membrane oxygenation (ECMO) may be initiated
(particularly in children). Finally, the surgeon must verify that
independent right ventricular failure is not caused by pulmonary
hypertension, because a right VAD in that setting could cause fatal
endobronchial hemorrhage.

When the centrifugal pump system is used, device insertion is
similar to cannulation for standard CPB. To assist the left ventricle,
VAD inflow is from a 24 to 32F cannula placed in the left atrium

***Table* 21-6**   Criteria for Ventricular Failure

Left ventricular failure
    Cardiac index <1.8 L/min/m²
    Aortic pressure (systolic) <90 mm Hg
    Left atrial or pulmonary capillary wedge pressure >20 mm
       Hg
    Right atrial pressure <15 mm Hg
Right ventricular failure
    Cardiac index <1.8 L/min/m²
    Aortic pressure (systolic) <90 mm Hg
    Left atrial or pulmonary capillary wedge pressure <10 mm
       Hg
    Right atrial pressure >20 mm Hg

(through the right superior pulmonary vein or atrial appendage) and outflow is to the ascending aorta through a 20 to 22F cannula. In the case of the right ventricular assistance, inflow is taken from the right atrium and directed into the pulmonary artery. A left atrial pressure line should routinely accompany VAD placement; it is invaluable for distinguishing between hypovolemia and cannula malposition in case of poor left VAD flow. With a right VAD, pressure readings from a pulmonary artery catheter are unreliable. Cannulas exit the mediastinum through separate sites near the inferior portion of the incision, similar to thoracostomy tube placement. Whenever practicable the chest is closed to minimize bleeding. IABPs are typically retained as an adjunct for later weaning.

During ventricular assistance patients are sedated and generally remain intubated. Heparinization is recommended for roller and centrifugal pumps (activated clotting times, 180 to 200 seconds) but is unnecessary for some sac-type pumps. In the adult blood flow is maintained at 2 to 4 L/m²/min, with adequacy of systemic perfusion monitored by physical examination and by arterial blood gas and mixed venous oxygen saturation determinations, blood chemistry analysis, and urine output. TEEs are intermittently obtained to evaluate ventricular distention and to assess quality of ventricular ejection with decreased VAD flow, especially during weaning (occasional ejection every few hours is also encouraged to prevent intraventricular stasis).

Weaning should not be attempted within the first 24 hours after institution of assistance. The usual sequence of weaning begins with tapering of inotropes, followed by removal first of the VAD and then finally the IABP. Here again TEE is helpful for assessing ventricular function as assistance is withdrawn. The protocol followed in our ICU requires that the heart maintain a cardiac index greater than 2.0 L/m^2/min with filling pressures less than 20 mm Hg as VAD flow is decreased by 25% every 4 to 6 hours to a minimum flow of 0.5 L/min. In the event of failure at any step, VAD flow is increased to the level where the hemodynamic criteria were last fulfilled and the wean trial resumed after 12 to 24 hours. As a rule, if no significant ventricular recovery is seen within 72 hours, successful weaning is unlikely.

The most common complications attending VAD use are excessive bleeding, infection, renal failure, and central nervous system events. Risk factors predisposing to bleeding are prolonged CPB and preexisting coagulopathy. Rates of blood loss and coagulation indexes should be carefully monitored and appropriate replacements made. In addition to strict observance of aseptic technique, prophylactic antibiotics are administered and the centrifugal pump head changed every 72 hours. Because of the great risk of cannula dislodgement, closed chest cardiac massage is absolutely contraindicated; sternal wire-cutters must be kept at hand for open chest massage in case of cardiac arrest.

Cardiopulmonary Bypass

Total CPB is seldom used outside the operating room except for combined cardiopulmonary failure and occasionally for biventricular failure. Pump systems incorporating an oxygenator and a heat exchanger, such as the CardioPulmonary Support System (C.R. Bard, Inc., Tewksbury, Mass.), provide total CPB but only up to about 6 hours. For continued total bypass the patient must undergo ECMO. Although ECMO has been successfully used in children for up to 28 to 30 days, adults tolerate it poorly beyond 5 to 7 days.

Total Artificial Heart

The total artificial heart has had a disappointing record in its intended role as an indefinite replacement for the heart. Consequently, its use is strictly investigational and limited to a few institutions around the country. Bridging to transplantation has been accomplished with the total artificial heart.

Appendix A
Cardiovascular Drugs

Kirk J. Fleischer and R. *Scott Stuart*

Adrenergic receptors
Antiarrhythmic agents
   Atropine
   Bretylium (Bretylol)
   Lidocaine (Xylocaine)
   Procainamide (Procan)
Amrinone (Inocor)
β-Receptor antagonists
   Atenolol (Tenormin)
   Esmolol (Brevibloc)
   Propranolol (Inderal)
Calcium chloride
Clonidine (Catapres)
Dobutamine (Dobutrex)
Dopamine (Intropin)
Epinephrine

Hydralazine (Apresoline)
Isoproterenol (Isuprel)
Labetolol (Normodyne)
Loop diuretics
   Furosemide (Lasix)
   Bumetadine (Bumex)
Nifedipine (Procardia)
Nitroglycerin
Norepinephrine (Levophed)
Phenylephrine (Neo-Synephrine)
Prazosin (Minipress)
Prostaglandin E_1
Sodium nitroprusside (Nipride)
Thiazide diuretics
   Chlorothiazide (Diuril)
   Metolazone (Zaroxolyn)

Table A-1 Adrenergic Receptors

Receptor	Location	Physiologic response
α_1	Blood vessels	Vasoconstriction
α_2	Central nervous system	Vasodilation
β_1	Heart	Positive inotrope
		Positive chronotrope
		Increased automaticity
		Increased rate of conduction
β_2	Blood vessels	Vasodilation (primarily muscle vascular beds)
DA	Central nervous system	Splanchnic (renal and mesenteric) vasodilation

Antiarrhythmic Agents (see Chapter 10)

Atropine

Indications
1. Bradycardia
2. Atrioventricular (AV) block

Dosage: 0.5-1.0 mg intravenous (IV) push, may repeat q 5 min to maximum total of 2.0 mg

Bretylium (Bretylol)

Indication: Refractory ventricular arrhythmias

Dosage: 5-10 mg/kg IV over 10 to 20 min, followed by continuous infusion at 1-5 mg/min

Lidocaine (Xylocaine)

Indications
1. Ventricular arrhytmias (first-line agent)
2. Acute myocardial infarction (prophylaxis against ventricular arrhythmias)

Dosage: 1 mg/kg IV push (may repeat), followed by continuous infusion at 1-4 mg/min

Procainamide (Procan)

Indications
1. Ventricular arrhythmias
2. Supraventricular arrhythmias

Dosage: 20-25 mg/min IV to total loading dose of 1000 mg, followed by continuous infusion of 2-6 mg/min

Amrinone (Inocor)

Class: Phosphodiesterase inhibitor

Pharmacologic effects
1. Vasodilator (arterial and venous)
2. Weak positive inotrope (in some patients)
3. Increased AV nodal conduction

Indications
1. Low cardiac output syndrome (LCOS) refractory to standard therapy
2. Right ventricular failure and/or pulmonary hypertension
3. Severe congestive heart failure (CHF)

Dosage

> Loading dose: 0.75-1.5 mg/kg IV over 3-5 min (may repeat after 15-30 min)
>
> Continuous infusion: Start at 5-10 μg/kg/min, may titrate up to 15-20 μg/kg/min

Untoward effects

1. Arrhythmias (supraventricular and ventricular)
2. Hypotension
3. Thrombocytopenia, gastrointestinal distress, and hepatotoxicity

Note:

1. Hemodynamic effects analogous to those of dobutamine; synergistic in combined therapy with β agonists
2. May increase ventricular rate in setting of atrial fibrillation or flutter
3. Difficult to titrate because of long half-life (3.5-6 hr)
4. Contraindications
   a. Acute myocardial infarction (risk of arrhythmia)
   b. Thrombocytopenia

β-receptor Antagonists

Agents:

1. β₁ (Cardioselective) agents
   a. *Atenolol (Tenormin)*
   b. *Esmolol (Brevibloc)*
2. β₁/β₂ (Nonselective) agents: *Propranolol (Inderal)*

Pharmacologic effects

1. Negative inotrope
2. Negative chronotrope
3. Prolongation of AV conduction
4. Reduction of atrial and ventricular automaticity

Indications

1. Hypertension
2. Arrhythmias (supraventricular and ventricular)
3. Hypercatecholamine states (including hyperdynamic myocardium syndrome)
4. Acute myocardial ischemia or infarction

Dosage

> *Atenolol:* 50-100 mg orally (PO) qd

Esmolol

Loading dose: 0.5-1.0 mg/kg over 1 min

Continuous infusion: Start at 50 μg/kg/min, titrate to effect by increasing infusion by increments of 50 μg/kg/min; repeat bolus with 0.5 mg/kg before *each* increase

Propranolol

0.5-1.0 mg IV q 5 min to effect (maximum 0.1 mg/kg), then 1-5 mg IV q 6 hr

10-80 mg PO q 6 hr

Untoward effects

1. Exacerbation of CHF
2. Bronchospasm (less with cardioselective agents)
3. Hypotension
4. Bradycardia
5. Exacerbation of preexisting cardiac conduction abnormalities
6. Rebound hypertension
7. Reduced clearance of some drugs
   a. Digoxin (Esmolol)
   b. Theophylline and lidocaine (propranolol)

Note

1. Consult attending surgeon or fellow before initiation of β-blocker therapy
2. Use extreme caution when administering β blockers concomitantly with calcium channel blockers. May cause asystole, heart block, or systolic ventricular failure.
3. β blockers mask signs of the following:
   a. Hypoglycemia (diaphoresis, tachycardia)
   b. Hypovolemia or anemia (tachycardia)
4. Abrupt withdrawal of β blocker may precipitate the following:
   a. Sudden death
   b. Rebound hypertension
5. Treatment of β blocker–induced bradycardia: Atropine, glucagon (2.5-7.5 mg/hr), or pacer
6. Treatment of β blocker–induced hypotension: β agonist (dobutamine or dopamine, 15 μg/kg/min)
7. Absolute contraindications
   a. Significant chronic obstructive pulmonary disease or asthma
   b. Significant CHF

c. Severe bradycardia (heart rate [HR] <45 beats/min)
d. AV block
e. Hypotension

Calcium Chloride

Pharmacologic effects
1. Positive inotrope
2. Vasoconstrictor

Indications
1. Acute hypotension
2. Reversal or blunting of vasodilating effects of calcium channel blockers

Dosage: 250-500 mg IV bolus. May repeat q 5-10 min prn up to 3 times until patient is stabilized. No continuous infusion.

Note:
1. For emergency use only. Beneficial effects can be dramatic but are short lived. Provides time to assess situation and initiate acute therapeutic interventions.
2. Cardiopulmonary bypass can cause hypocalcemia. Although agent is effective even if ionized calcium level is normal, the lower the ionized calcium level, the more dramatic improvement noted with calcium chloride.

Clonidine (Catapres)

Class: α_2-Adrenergic receptor agonist
Pharmacologic effect: Vasodilator
Indication: Hypertension
Dosage:
Acute management: 0.2 mg PO, then 0.1 mg PO q 1 hr; maximum total: 0.8 mg
Maintenance therapy: Start with 0.1 mg PO bid; may increase by 0.1-0.2 mg/day until desired blood pressure (BP) achieved; maximum total daily dose: 2.4 mg

Untoward effects:
1. Bradycardia
2. Rebound hypertension and tachycardia
3. Drowsiness, fatigue

Note:
1. Do not discontinue suddenly because rebound hypersympathetic state can occur

2. Concurrent use with β blockers may result in paradoxic hypertension

Dobutamine (Dobutrex)

Class: β_1/β_2-Adrenergic agonist
Pharmacologic effects
1. Positive inotrope
2. Positive chronotrope
3. Increased AV conduction
4. Vasodilator
Indications:
1. LCOS
2. Right-sided ventricular failure associated with pulmonary hypertension
3. Acute mitral regurgitation with or without right-sided ventricular failure
4. Acute ventricular septal defect
Dosage: Continuous infusion: 2-20 μg/kg/min IV; titrate to effect
Untoward effects
1. Tachycardia
2. Arrhythmias (ventricular)
3. Hypotension (at high doses)
Note:
1. Inotrope of choice in LCOS under following conditions:
   a. If patient is normotensive
   b. Associated with myocardial ischemia (coronary artery autoregulation undisturbed by dobutamine)
   c. Accompanied by evidence of left ventricular failure (elevated pulmonary capillary wedge pressure [PCWP], pulmonary edema)
2. Although dobutamine causes vasodilation, BP usually remains unchanged because of the augmented CO
3. At doses <15 μg/kg/min, incidence of tachycardia or arrhythmia less than with dopamine; thus dobutamine is an alternative, equally effective drug if these contraindications for dopamine are present
4. Tachyphylaxis (gradually increasing drug tolerance) to dobutamine can develop within 24 hr
5. Contraindication: Hypertrophic cardiomyopathy

Dopamine (Intropin, DA)

Class: $\alpha_1/\beta_1/DA$-Adrenergic receptor agonist
Pharmacologic effects: Dose-dependent

Dosage	Predominant receptor stimulated	Hemodynamic effect
0-3 μg/kg/min	DA	Splanchnic vasodilator
5-8 μg/kg/min	β_1	Positive inotrope/ chronotrope
>10 μg/kg/min	α	Vasoconstrictor

Note: Doses are only general trends. Some β and α effects can be seen at lower doses.

Indications
1. LCOS
2. Acute oliguria
3. Acute hypotension (as temporizing measure)

Dosage: Continuous infusion: 1-15 μg/kg/min IV, titrate to desired effect

Untoward effects
1. Tachycardia
2. Arrhythmias (ventricular)
3. Elevation of PCWP (via pulmonary venoconstriction)

Note:
1. First-line inotrope in LCOS if patient hypotensive (including cardiogenic shock)
2. Tachycardia is often limiting factor in use of DA
3. Risk of arrhythmia significantly increased and splanchnic vasodilation reduced with doses >10 μg/kg/min
4. If dose requirement exceeds 15 μg/kg/min do the following:
   a. Add dobutamine or vasodilator (i.e., nitroprusside), *or*
   b. Select another agent (epinephrine). Continue DA at "renal dose" (2-3 μg/kg/min) to preserve renal blood flow.
5. Use renal dose DA (if patient does not have tachycardia) to assist in maintaining adequate urine output during early postoperative period (first 12-24 hr); later, can be used as adjunct to standard diuretic therapy for resistant fluid retention

6. Local extravasation causes soft tissue necrosis (due to vasoconstriction). Treat with local infiltration of phentolamine (α antagonist).
7. Tachyphylaxis (gradually increasing drug tolerance) to the inotropic effect of DA can develop within 24 hr
8. Contraindication: Tachycardia or arrhythmias

Epinephrine

Class: $\alpha_1/\beta_1/\beta_2$-Adrenergic receptor agonist
Pharmacologic effects: Dose-dependent
1. Positive inotrope
2. Positive chronotrope
3. Increased automaticity
4. Vasodilator (at low doses β_2 predominates)
5. Vasoconstrictor (at higher doses α_1 predominates)

Indications:
1. Hypotension refractory to first-line agents
2. Severe LCOS

Dosage: Continuous infusion: 0.01-0.2 μg/kg/min IV, titrate to effect (β_1 and some α_1 [kidney and skin]: at all doses. β_2, 0.01-0.05 μg/kg/min; α_1: >0.05 μg/kg/min)

Untoward effects
1. Tachycardia
2. Arrhythmias (ventricular)
3. Renal failure (caused by reduction in renal blood flow)
4. Myocardial ischemia (caused by tachycardia)
5. Hypertension and associated cerebrovascular hemorrhage

Note:
1. Second-line inotrope after dopamine and dobutamine. May be combined with these first-line agents to provide more inotropic support.
2. Tachycardia and arrhythmia limit its use to refractory or severe cases.
3. Extreme care must be taken in patients with marginal renal function because renal vasoconstriction occurs at all doses. Concurrent administration of vasodilator or low-dose dopamine may attenuate splanchnic vasoconstriction.
4. Contraindications
   a. Myocardial ischemia
   b. Arrhythmias
   c. Renal insufficiency

d. Glaucoma
e. However, often no alternative is available once resort to epinephrine

Hydralazine (Apresoline)

Pharmacologic effects: Vasodilator (arterial)
Indications: Hypertension
Dosage: Maintenance therapy: 25-75 mg PO q 6-8 hr (unfortunately, at time of publication, parenteral form of hydralazine is no longer available)
Untoward effects
1. Reflex tachycardia
2. Myocardial ischemia (caused by tachycardia and reduced diastolic pressure)
3. Lupus-like syndrome
4. Headache, nausea and vomiting, dizziness
Note:
1. Reflex tachycardia limits use of hydralazine if not given concurrently with β blocker
2. Difficult to titrate because of long half-life (3-7 hr)
3. Contraindications
   a. Myocardial ischemia
   b. Mitral valve stenosis

Isoproterenol (Isuprel)

Class: β_1/β_2-Adrenergic receptor agonist
Pharmacologic effects (β_1 effect > β_2 effect)
1. Positive inotrope
2. Positive chronotrope
3. Increased myocardial automaticity
4. Vasodilator
Indications
1. Pulmonary hypertension
2. Right ventricular failure
3. Bradycardia in heart transplantation (denervated heart)
4. Bradycardia or AV conduction block unresponsive to atropine
5. β blocker or calcium channel blocker overdose
Dosage: Continuous infusion: 0.01-0.1 μg/kg/min, titrate to effect

Untoward effects
  1. Tachycardia
  2. Arrhythmias (ventricular)
  3. Myocardial ischemia

Note:
  1. Risks of tachycardia and arrhythmias significantly limit use of isoproterenol in coronary bypass patients
  2. Furthermore, ischemia may result from increase in myocardial oxygen demand from tachycardia and reduction in oxygen supply from reduced coronary perfusion associated with reduced diastolic pressures seen with isoproterenol
  3. Can be used as temporizing adjunct in the acute management of pericardial tamponade (maintain cardiac output by increasing HR as stroke volume fixed or diminishing)
  4. Contraindications
     a. Arrhythmias
     b. Myocardial ischemia

Labetolol (Normodyne)

Class: Mixed α- and β-adrenergic antagonist (α effect < β effect)
Pharmacologic effects
  1. Vasodilator (α_1)
  2. Negative inotrope and chronotrope (β)
Indication: Hypertension
Dosage
  1. Bolus therapy for acute control of BP: 5-20 mg IV slowly. Repeat q 5-10 min until effect achieved. Maximum total: 200 mg.
  2. Continuous infusion: Start at 1-2 mg/min, titrate to effect
  3. Oral dose: Start with 100-200 mg PO bid, may increase up to 400 mg bid
Untoward effects
  1. Exacerbation of CHF and bronchospasm (see β-receptor antagonists section for complete list of β receptor–mediated sequelae)
  2. Orthostatic hypotension (>50%)
  3. Nausea and vomiting

Note:
  1. Much faster acting than pure β blocker for treatment of acute hypertension
  2. Reduction in BP without reflex tachycardia

3. Difficult to titrate because of long half-life (4 hr)
4. Contraindications are same as for other β-blocking agents (e.g., CHF, chronic obstructive pulmonary disease)

Loop Diuretics

Agents
   1. *Furosemide (Lasix)*
   2. *Bumetanide (Bumex)*
Pharmacologic effects
   1. Diuresis
   2. Venodilator (furosemide)
Indications
   1. Acute oliguria
   2. CHF
   3. Hypertension (chronic)
Dosage:
   Furosemide
      10-40 mg IV slow push (20 mg/min in patient with normal renal function, 4 mg/min if impaired); if no effect in 20-30 min, double dose and may continue doubling dose until approximately 300-350 mg is reached (at which time trial with another agent is indicated)
      20-80 mg PO QD-q 6 hr
   Bumetanide: 0.5-1.0 mg IV q 2-4 hr as needed (to maximum 10 mg/24 hr)
      0.5-2.0 mg PO QD-q 6 hr
   Potency: 1 mg bumetanide = 40 mg furosemide
Untoward effects
   1. Hypokalemia, hypomagnesemia
   2. Impaired glucose tolerance
Note:
   1. Furosemide is first-line diuretic agent in cardiac surgery
   2. Closely follow serum electrolytes. Hypokalemia is associated with increased digoxin toxicity and arrhythmogenicity.
   3. Increased risk of ototoxicity (and nephrotoxicity) when administered concurrently with aminoglycosides or as rapid IV push
   4. High doses often required in following conditions:
      a. Severe CHF
      b. Renal failure

   c. Elderly patients
   d. History of preoperative diuretic use
5. Acute reduction of CO may occur with furosemide because of venodilation and associated preload reduction
6. Furosemide (like metolazone) is effective even in patients with significantly reduced renal function (to glomerular filtration rate of 10 ml/min).
7. Bumetanide usually given concurrently with thiazide diuretic chlorothiazide (Diuril) at our institution
8. Contraindicated in patients with sulfa allergy

Nifedipine (Procardia)

Class: Calcium channel antagonist
Pharmacologic effects
   1. Vasodilator (arterial)
   2. Coronary vasodilator
   3. Negative inotrope
   4. Reduction of myocardial conduction and automaticity
Indications
   1. Hypertension (systemic and pulmonary)
   2. Coronary vasospasm, internal mammary vasospasm
Dosage
   Acute management: 10-20 mg sublingually (SL) or PO (bite-and-swallow) every 30 min prn. *Note:* In elderly start with 5 mg to avoid cerebral underperfusion associated with acute hypotensive episode.
   Maintenance therapy: 10-20 mg PO q 6 hr
Untoward effects
   1. Tachycardia (sympathetic reflex)
   2. Myocardial ischemia (caused by tachycardia)
   3. Rebound vasospasm (if abruptly discontinue)
   4. High degree AV block (rare)
Note:
   1. Nifedipine is first-line oral antihypertensive used in the postoperative cardiac surgery patient. It is a potent and rapidly acting vasodilator.
   2. Although bite-and-swallow route consistently provides fastest absorption, SL route permits discontinuation (rinse out mouth) if patient becomes hypotensive
   3. Risk of administering nifedipine concurrently with β blockers is less than with verapamil. The negative chronotropic

effect of β blockers can protect against tachycardia-induced myocardial ischemia.
4. Causes elevated digoxin levels (increased by 45%). Monitor levels when initiate, adjust, and discontinue nifedipine.

Nitroglycerin (TNG)

Pharmacologic effects
1. Vasodilator (venous); at high doses also arterial vasodilator
2. Coronary vasodilator
3. Increased blood flow via coronary collaterals to ischemic myocardium

Indications
1. Myocardial ischemia or infarction
2. Coronary vasospasm
3. Hypertension (systemic and pulmonary)
4. Right ventricular failure

Dosage

Sublingual (for acute chest pain): 0.3-0.6 mg SL q 5 min up to 3 times

Continuous infusion: 10-200 μg/min IV; start at 10 μg/min, increase by 10 μg/kg/min every 5-10 min; titrate to desired effect (in setting of acute ischemia, 100 μg/min)

Topical (Nitropaste): ½-2 inches q 6-8 hr

Oral: Isosorbide dinitrate 30, 60, or 120 mg PO qid

Untoward effects
1. Headache, facial flushing
2. Mild hypoxia (caused by mild ventilation-perfusion mismatching)
3. Methemoglobinemia

Note:
1. Tolerance or tachyphylaxis develops with continuous treatment periods >24-48 hr
2. High doses of TNG can achieve adequate BP control in most (up to 85%) patients after coronary bypass. Unlike nitroprusside, TNG demonstrates no coronary steal phenomenon, no rebound hypertension, and only mild intrapulmonary shunting. However, high doses are costly and require large volume of fluid.
3. TNG metabolized to nitrites, which mediate oxidation of hemoglobin to methemoglobin. Cyanosis, low O_2 saturation,

and impaired O_2 delivery appear despite adequate Pao_2 as levels of methemoglobin increase. Treatment: methylene blue, 1 mg/kg IV.

4. Contraindications
   a. Pericardial tamponade (elevated preload crucial for survival)
   b. Elevated intracranial pressure

Norepinephrine (Levophed, NE)

Class: α_1/β_1-Adrenergic receptor agonist

Pharmacologic effects
1. Vasoconstrictor (arterial and venous)
2. Positive inotrope (but no positive chronotropic effect)

Indications
1. Severe cardiogenic shock
2. Severe septic shock

Dosage: Continuous infusion: 0.01-0.2 µg/kg/min IV, titrate to effect

Untoward effects
1. Tissue ischemia resulting from intense vasoconstriction (e.g., renal failure)
2. Myocardial ischemia
3. Hypertension and associated cerebrovascular hemorrhage
4. Reflex bradycardia

Note:
1. Infrequently used in cardiac surgery. Primary indication is septic shock (high CO, low SVR) refractory to phenylephrine
2. Extreme caution must be taken in patients with marginal renal function. Concurrent administration of dopamine may attenuate splanchnic vasoconstriction.
3. Local extravasation causes soft tissue necrosis (caused by vasoconstriction). Treat with local infiltration of 5-10 mg of phentolamine (α antagonist) as soon as possible.
4. Contraindications
   a. Myocardial ischemia
   b. Renal failure
   c. However, often no alternative once resort to norepinephrine

Phenylephrine (Neo-Synephrine)

Class: α_1-Adrenergic receptor agonist
Pharmacologic effect: Vasoconstrictor (arterial and venous)
Indications
  1. Inflammatory-mediated vasodilation associated with cardio-pulmonary bypass
  2. Sepsis
Dosage: Continuous infusion: start at 0.15-0.5 μg/kg/min, titrate to desired effect
Untoward effects
  1. Myocardial ischemia
  2. Reduced visceral perfusion
  3. Reflex bradycardia
Note: May cause arrhythmias when used concurrently with digoxin or β blockers

Prostaglandin E_1 (PGE_1)

Pharmacologic effect: Vasodilator
Indication: Refractory right-sided ventricular failure from pulmonary hypertension
Dosage: Continuous infusion: 0.01-0.15 μg/kg/min IV, titrate to effect
Untoward effect: Profound systemic hypotension
Note: Administer concurrent norepinephrine therapy to counteract systemic hypotension. Infuse PGE_1 through central venous pressure port/line (pulmonary circulation), norepinephrine through left atrial line (systemic circulation).

Prazosin (Minipress)

Class: α_1-Adrenergic receptor antagonist
Pharmacologic effect: Vasodilator (arterial and venous)
Indication: Hypertension
Dosage: 0.5-1.0 mg PO bid initially; may gradually increase to 5-10 mg PO bid
Untoward effects
  1. Syncope (because of orthostatic hypotension)
  2. Dizziness, headache, weakness
Note: Syncope may occur with first dose. Incidence can be dramatically reduced by starting with low dose and administering to patient in supine position (usually given at bedtime).

Sodium Nitroprusside (Nipride, SNP)

Pharmacologic effects
1. Vasodilator (arterial and venous)
2. Coronary vasodilator

Indications
1. Hypertension
2. LCOS

Dosage: Continuous infusion: 0.1-10.0 μg/kg/min, titrate to desired afterload and blood pressure

Untoward effects
1. Cyanide or thiocyanate toxicity
2. Hypoxia (caused by ventilation perfusion mismatch resulting from attenuation of hypoxia-induced pulmonary vasoconstriction)
3. Coronary steal phenomenon (caused by reduction of coronary perfusion pressure without augmentation of collateral blood flow to ischemic myocardium)
4. Rebound hypertension

Note:
1. Parenteral drug of choice for afterload reduction and BP control in cardiac surgery
2. Invasive arterial pressure monitoring essential
3. Do not discontinue acutely because significant rebound hypertension may develop
4. Hypoxia more pronounced in elderly and in patients with preexisting lung disease
5. Easily titratable because onset and cessation of action are virtually immediate
6. Toxicity
   a. SNP metabolized to cyanide then thiocyanate (in liver), which is excreted by kidneys. Thus use cautiously in patients with renal or hepatic insufficiency.
   b. Risk of toxicity increased with elevated doses and prolonged infusions (>48 hr); however, it also occurs at low doses in early postoperative period (mechanism uncertain, but apparently associated with hypothermia)
   c. Signs and symptoms: Mental status changes, dilated pupils, headache, absent reflexes, nausea, coma, dyspnea
   d. Laboratory reveals metabolic acidosis and elevated mixed venous O_2 saturation

e. Tachyphylaxis (gradually increasing tolerance to anti-hypertensive effects of SNP) is perhaps most reliable sign of toxicity
f. Treatment
   i. Discontinue SNP, begin alternative antihypertensive therapy, determine thiocyanate levels
   ii. Sodium thiosulfate, 150 mg/kg IV; amyl nitrate in-halation (10 min); sodium nitrite (3%), 10 ml IV; methylene blue, 1 mg/kg IV over 5 min; hydroxo-cobalamin infusion, 25 mg/hr IV
7. Contraindications
   a. Myocardial ischemia
   b. Increased intracranial pressure

Thiazide Diuretics

Agents*
1. *Chlorothiazide (Diuril)*
2. *Metolazone (Zaroxolyn)*
Pharmacologic effect: Diuresis
Indications
1. Acute oliguria
2. CHF
3. Hypertension (chronic)
Dosage
Chlorothiazide: 250-500 mg IV q 6 hr; 250-1000 mg PO qd-q12 hr
Metolazone: 2.5-10 mg PO qd
Untoward effects
1. Hypokalemia, hypomagnesemia
2. Impaired glucose tolerance
Note:
1. Closely follow serum electrolytes. Hypokalemia is associ-ated with increased digoxin toxicity and arrhythmogenicity.
2. Increased risk of arrhythmia (torsade de pointes) if thiazide diuretics are used in combination with class IA or III an-tiarrhythmics

---

*A multitude of thiazide diuretics are available, but few differences exist between them. Chlorothiazide and metolazone are the agents most frequently used at our institution.

3. Metolazone (like furosemide) is effective even in patients with significantly reduced renal function
4. Chlorothiazide is usually given concurrently with loop diuretic bumetanide (Bumex) at our institution
5. Contraindicated in patients with sulfa allergy

Table A-2   Inotropic and Vasopressor Agents

	Dosage (μg/kg/min)	Predominant sympathomimetic effect			
		α	β₁	β₂	DA
Dopamine	0-3.0				DA
	5.0-8.0		β1		
	>10.0	α			
Dobutamine	2.0-20.0		β1	β2	
Epinephrine	0.01-0.05		β1	β2	
	>0.05	α	β1		
Norepinephrine	0.01-0.2	α	β1		
Isoproterenol	0.01-0.10		β1	β2	
Amrinone	5.0-20.0*	Inhibits phosphodiesterase			
Phenylephrine	0.15-0.50	α			

*After loading dose of 0.75-1.5 μg/kg.

Table A-3 Antihypertensive and Afterload Reducing Agents

Agent	Dose IV	Dose PO*
Amrinone	Loading dose: 0.75-1.5 mg/kg; infusion: 5-20 μg/kg/min	NA
β-blockers	(See specific agent for doses)	
Clonidine	NA	0.2 mg, then 0.1 mg q 1 hr (maximum: 0.8 mg)
Hydralazine	NA	25-50 mg q 6-8 hr
Labetolol	Bolus therapy: 5-20 mg (slowly); infusion, 1-2 mg/min	100-200 mg bid
Nifedipine	NA	5-20 mg q 30 min as needed acutely, then q 6 hr
Nitroglycerin	Infusion: 10-200 μg/min	0.3-0.6 mg (SL, acutely for ischemia)
Prazosin	NA	30-60 mg PO qid (isosorbide)
Sodium nitroprusside	Infusion: 0.1-10.0 μg/kg/min	0.5-1.0 mg bid
		NA

NA, Not available.
*Starting oral doses.

Appendix B: Management Summaries

Kirk J. Fleischer and R. Scott Stuart

Management of Postoperative Low Cardiac Output Syndrome

I. Key principles
   A. Constantly reevaluate hemodynamic status (particularly after intervention)
   B. Follow trends in hemodynamics (not absolute numbers)
   C. Seek assistance *early* whenever one is uncertain about management
   D. Use systematic and physiologic approach to optimization of determinants of cardiac output (CO). One should address these hemodynamic parameters in the following sequence: Heart rate/arrhythmia→preload→afterload→ contractility.

II. Listed here are possible therapeutic interventions (or goals) for the most common causes of low cardiac output syndrome (LCOS). It is meant only as a brief review for those who already have a thorough understanding of the principles governing CO.
   A. Dysrhythmias
      1. Bradycardia: Atropine, isoproterenol, pacer
      2. Tachycardia: Fluids, O_2, morphine, anxiolytic, esmolol
      3. Other arrhythmias: See Chapter 10
   B. Inadequate preload: Administer fluids, control mediastinal bleeding, rule out cardiac tamponade
   C. Elevated afterload: Warming light or blanket, fluids, vasodilator therapy
   D. Reduced contractility: Rule out myocardial ischemia (see

following section); administer O_2; correct acidosis and optimize ventilation; use warming light or blanket; administer inotropic therapy, mechanical assist device

Management of Postoperative Myocardial Ischemia

I. ABC's of resuscitation (*a*irway, *b*reathing, *c*irculation)

II. Admit patient to monitored bed

III. Immediate therapy
   A. O_2 (100% face mask or intubation)
   B. Nitroglycerin sublingually: 0.4 mg STAT and q 5 min and nitropaste 1-2 inches)
   C. Establish intravenous (IV) access (large-gauge if hypotension present)
   D. Morphine, 1-2 mg IV STAT

IV. *Notify attending surgeon or fellow!*

V. Acute therapy
   A. Follow-up 12-lead electrocardiogram q 5-10 min until ischemic changes resolve
   B. If blood pressure (BP) adequate, consider nifedipine, 10 mg SL, and/or nitroglycerin infusion, 10-100 µg/min
   C. If hemodynamically unstable, initiate invasive monitoring (intraarterial and Swan-Ganz catheters)
   D. If hematocrit $< 30\%$ and no evidence of congestive heart failure, transfuse packed red blood cells. If pulmonary edema is present, diurese (furosemide) *before* transfusions.

VI. Determine cardiac hemodynamics and optimize determinants of CO (see section on LCOS). In brief, usual goals are treatment of tachyarrhythmias and bradyarrhythmias, reduction of preload and afterload, and judicious use of inotropes to maintain adequate contractility (while also minimizing myocardial O_2 consumption).

VII. Consider mechanical assist device (intraaortic balloon pump) early in setting of myocardial ischemia!

VIII. Ventricular arrhythmia prophylaxis
   A. Correct K^+ and Mg^{++}
   B. Lidocaine, 1 mg/kg IV bolus (procainamide, bretylium, or amiodarone for refractory arrhythmias)

IX. Consider heparinization

X. Emergent coronary catheterization and/or surgical intervention

Management of Postoperative Hypertension

I. Warming lights or blankets
II. Sedation and analgesia; verbal reassurance
III. Optimize oxygenation and ventilation
IV. Determine cardiac hemodynamics (cardiac index [CI] and systemic vascular resistance [SVR])
    A. If CI <2.0 L/min/m², follow algorithm for treatment of LCOS
    B. If SVR elevated, initiate vasodilator therapy
    C. If CI >3.0 L/min/m², consider β-blocker therapy for hyperdynamic syndrome (consult attending surgeon or fellow)
V. Other
    A. Foley catheter or nasogastric tube if visceral distention is suspected
    B. Antipyretic agent if patient is febrile
    C. Paralytic agent (Pavulon) if intubated patient is shivering

Management of Postoperative Hypotension

I. Immediate management: Address ABC's of resuscitation (*a*irway, *b*reathing, *c*irculation)
    A. Place patient in Trendelenberg position
    B. O₂ (100% face mask or intubation if indicated)
    C. IV fluid bolus (through cordis port or large peripheral IV)
    D. Calcium chloride 1 amp IV bolus (may repeat)
    E. If in early postoperative period, dopamine is often already infusing at renal dose. Increase dopamine rate to achieve pressor effect (15-20 μg/kg/min).
    F. *Notify fellow or attending surgeon.*
II. Definitive therapy
    A. Assessment (physical examination, 12-lead electrocardiogram and telemetry, arterial blood gases, chest x-ray, Swan-Ganz catheterization)
    B. Evaluate and optimize hemodynamic parameters (preload, afterload, and contractility)
    C. Etiologies of acute postoperative hypotension
        1. Hypovolemia*
        2. Decreased contractility*
            a. Myocardial ischemia or infarction

---

*Most common causes.

Frequently Used Formulae in the Cardiac Surgery ICU

Parameter	Formula	Normal values
Mean arterial pressure (MAP)	$MAP = DBP + 1/3(SBP - DBP)$	65-100 mm Hg
Cardiac output (CO)	$CO = SV \times HR$	4-8 L/min
Cardiac index (CI)	$CI = CO \div BSA$	2.5-4 L/min/m^2
Systemic vascular resistance (SVR)	$SVR = \dfrac{MAP - CVP}{CO} \times 80$	900-1400 dynes/sec/cm^{-5}
Pulmonary vascular resistance (PVR)	$PVR = \dfrac{MPAP - PCWP}{CO} \times 80$	150-250 dynes/sec/cm^{-5}
Alveolar-arterial (A-a) gradient	A-a Gradient $= [713(Fio_2) - (Paco_2 \div 0.8)] - Pao_2$	Age dependent: 20 yr, ≈ 10; 70 yr, $\approx 20\text{-}25$

BSA, Body surface area; CVP, central venous pressure; DBP, diastolic blood pressure; Fio_2, fraction of inspired oxygen; HR, heart rate; $MPAP$, mean pulmonary artery pressure; $Paco_2$, arterial carbon dioxide pressure; Pao_2, arterial oxygen pressure; $PCWP$, pulmonary capillary wedge pressure; SBP, systolic blood pressure; SV, stroke volume.

b. Other causes (e.g., hypothermia, acidosis) (see section on LCOS)
3. Cardiac tamponade
4. Arrhythmias
5. Decreased SVR (sepsis, inflammatory-mediated vasodilation, transfusion or drug reaction)
6. Pneumothorax
7. Pulmonary embolus
D. Treat primary cause of hypotension

Index